The Evidence Base of Clinical Diagnosis

Theory and methods of diagnostic research

The Evidence Base of Clinical Diagnosis

Theory and methods of diagnostic research

Second Edition

EDITED BY

J. André Knottnerus, MD, PhD

Professor of General Practice
Netherlands School of Primary Care Research
Maastricht University
President of the Health Council of The Netherlands
The Hague, The Netherlands

Frank Buntinx, MD, PhD

Professor
Department of General Practice
Catholic University Leuven, Belgium
Netherlands School of Primary Care Research
Maastricht University
Maastricht, The Netherlands

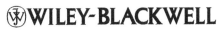
A John Wiley & Sons, Ltd., Publication

BMJ | Books

This edition first published 2009, © 2002, 2009 by Blackwell Publishing Ltd.

BMJ Books is an imprint of BMJ Publishing Group Limited, used under licence by Blackwell Publishing which was acquired by John Wiley & Sons in February 2007. Blackwell's publishing programme has been merged with Wiley's global Scientific, Technical and Medical business to form Wiley-Blackwell.

Registered office: John Wiley & Sons Ltd, The Atrium, Southern Gate, Chichester, West Sussex, PO19 8SQ, UK

Editorial offices: 9600 Garsington Road, Oxford, OX4 2DQ, UK
   The Atrium, Southern Gate, Chichester, West Sussex, PO19 8SQ, UK
   111 River Street, Hoboken, NJ 07030-5774, USA

For details of our global editorial offices, for customer services and for information about how to apply for permission to reuse the copyright material in this book please see our website at www.wiley.com/wiley-blackwell

The right of the author to be identified as the author of this work has been asserted in accordance with the Copyright, Designs and Patents Act 1988.

A catalogue record for this book is available from the British Library.

Library of Congress Cataloging-in-Publication Data
The evidence base of clinical diagnosis : theory and methods of diagnostic research / edited by J. André Knottnerus, Frank Buntinx. – 2nd ed.
   p. ; cm.
   Includes bibliographical references.
   ISBN 978-1-4051-5787-2
   1. Diagnosis–Research–Methodology.   2. Evidence-based medicine.   I. Knottnerus, J. André.
II. Buntinx, Frank.
   [DNLM: 1. Biomedical Research–methods.   2. Biomedical Research–standards.   3. Diagnostic Techniques and Procedures–standards.   4. Evidence-Based Medicine. WB 141 E931 2008]
RC71.3.E95 2008
616.07′5–dc22
                            2008015530

ISBN: 978-1-4051-5787-2

Set in 9.5/12 pt Meridien by Aptara® Inc., New Delhi, India

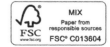

Contents

List of Contributors

Marc Aerts, PhD
Professor in Biostatistics
Center for Statistics
Hasselt University
Diepenbeek, Belgium

Bert Aertgeerts, MD, PhD
Professor of General Practice K.U. Leuven
Director of the Belgian Centre of
  Evidence-Based Medicine
Kapucijnenvoer
Leuven, Belgium

Patrick M. M. Bossuyt
Professor of Clinical Epidemiology
Department Clinical Epidemiology and
  Biostatistics, Academic Medical Center
University of Amsterdam
Amsterdam, The Netherlands

Rudi Bruyninckx, MD, MSc
Department of General Practice
KU Leuven
Leuven, Belgium

Frank Buntinx, MD, PhD
Professor, Department of General Practice
Catholic University Leuven, Belgium
Department of General Practice
Maastricht University
Maastricht, The Netherlands

Geert-Jan Dinant, MD, PhD
Professor of Clinical Research in
  General Practice
Maastricht University
School for Public Health and Primary Care
  (Caphri), Maastricht University
Maastricht, The Netherlands

René Eijkemans
Department of Public Health
Erasmus MC
University Medical Center Rotterdam
Rotterdam, The Netherlands

Arthur S. Elstein, PhD
Department of Medical Education
University of Illinois at Chicago
Chicago, Illinois, USA

Tom Fahey, MSc, MD, MFPH, FRCGP
Department of General Practice
Royal College of Surgeons in Ireland
  Medical School
Dublin, Ireland

Constantine Gatsonis, PhD
Professor of Medical Science (Biostatistics)
Director, Center for Statistical Sciences
Brown University
Providence
Rhode Island, USA

Paul P. Glasziou, FRACGP, PhD
Director, Centre for Evidence-Based
  Medicine
Department of Primary Health Care
University of Oxford
Oxford, UK

J. Dik F. Habbema, PhD
Professor, Department of Public Health
Erasmus MC—Erasmus University Medical
  Centre
Rotterdam, The Netherlands

R. Brian Haynes, MD, PhD, FRCPC, FRSC
Michael Gent Chair
Department of Clinical Epidemiology and
  Biostatistics
Professor, Department of Medicine
DeGroote School of Medicine
McMaster University Faculty of Health
  Sciences
Hamilton,
Ontario, Canada

Les M. Irwig, MBBCh, PhD
Professor of Epidemiology
Screening and Test Evaluation Program
School of Public Health

University of Sydney
Sydney, Australia

J. André Knottnerus, MD, PhD
Professor of General Practice
Netherlands School of Primary Care
　Research
Maastricht University
President of the Health Council of
　The Netherlands
The Hague, The Netherlands

Pieta Krijnen
Integrated Cancer Centre West
Leiden, The Netherlands

Jeroen G. Lijmer, MD, PhD
Department of Psychiatry
Waterland Hospital
Purmerend, The Netherlands

Petra Macaskill, BA, MAppStat, PhD
Screening and Test Evaluation Program
School of Public Health
University of Sydney
Sydney, Australia

Jean W. Muris, MD, PhD
Research Institute Caphri
Department General Practice
Maastricht University
Maastricht, The Netherlands

Alan Schwartz, PhD
Associate Professor and Director of
　Research
Departments of Medical Education and
　Pediatrics
University of Illinois at Chicago
Chicago, Illinois, USA

Hans Severens
Professor of Medical Technology
　Assessment
Caphri
Maastricht University
Department of Health Organization
Policy and Economics Maastricht
University Hospital Maastricht

Department of Clinical Epidemiology MTA
Maastricht, The Netherlands

Nynke Smidt, PhD
Department of Clinical Epidemiology and
　Biostatistics
Academic Medical Center
University of Amsterdam
Amsterdam, The Netherlands

Ann van den Bruel, MD, PhD
Assistant Professor
Department of General Practice
Katholieke Universiteit Leuven
Leuven, Belgium

Jef van den Ende, MD, PhD
Professor in the Department of Clinical
　Sciences
Institute of Tropical Medicine
Antwerpen, Belgium

Johan van der Lei, MD, PhD
Professor of Medical Informatics
Department of Medical Informatics
Erasmus MC, University Medical Center
　Rotterdam
Rotterdam, The Netherlands

Trudy van der Weijden, PhD, MD
Associate Professor, Maastricht University
Department of General Practice
School for Public Health and Primary Care
　(Caphri)
Maastricht, The Netherlands

Onno P. van Schayck
Professor of Preventive Medicine
Scientific Co-director Research School
　Caphri
Maastricht University
Maastricht, The Netherlands

Chris van Weel, MD, FRCGP, FRACGP
Professor of General Practice
Hon. Fellow of the Royal College of General
　Practitioners and of the Royal Australian
　College of General Practitioners

Radboud University Medical Centre
Department of General Practice
Nijmegen, The Netherlands

Ron Winkens

General Practitioner and Associate
  Professor
Medical Co-ordinator of the Maastricht
  Diagnostic Centre
University Medical Centre Maastricht and
  School for Public Health and Primary
  Care (Caphri)

Maastricht University
Maastricht, The Netherlands

John J. You, MD, MSc, FRCP(C)
Assistant Professor
Departments of Medicine and Clinical
  Epidemiology and Biostatistics
McMaster University
Hamilton and
Adjunct Scientist, Institute for Clinical
  Evaluative Sciences
Toronto, Ontario
Canada

Preface

> *I consider much less thinking has gone into the theory underlying diagnosis, or possibly one should say less energy has gone into constructing the correct model of diagnostic procedures, than into therapy or prevention where the concept of "altering the natural history of the disease" has been generally accepted and a theory has been evolved for testing hypotheses concerning this.*[1]

Although seeking an evidence base for medicine is as old as medicine itself, in the past two decades the concept of evidence-based medicine (EBM) has strongly stimulated the application of the best available evidence from clinical research into medical practice.[2] At the same time, this process has revealed the need for a more extensive and more valid evidence base as input for EBM.[3] Accordingly, investigators have been encouraged to intensify the production and innovation of clinical knowledge, and clinical research has become more successful in seeing its results implemented in practice more completely in a shorter period.

In developing the evidence base of clinical management, more than 35 years after Archie Cochrane wrote the words cited above, the theory and methodology of diagnostic research still lags substantially behind that of research into the effectiveness of treatment. This is the more challenging because making an adequate diagnostic process is a prime requirement for appropriate clinical decision making, including prognostic assessment and the selection of the most effective treatment options. The reason for this lagging behind of diagnostic research methodology is not only less invested energy and resources. At least as importantly, diagnostic research is much more comprehensive and complex than treatment research as it encompasses not only accuracy, but the domains of prognosis and intervention as well.

In view of this apparent need for further methodological development of the evidence base of clinical diagnosis, this book, which is now published in its second edition, was initiated. The aim is to provide a comprehensive framework for (future) investigators who want to do diagnostic research, and for clinicians, practitioners, and students who are interested to learn more about its principles, relevant methodological options, and pitfalls. In preparing the work, the contributors were able to profit from the experience and insights collected and reported by many leading clinical researchers in the field. For those who wish to know more than could be described in this book, the references in the chapters can be a useful guide. This second edition is not only an update of the first version but is also enriched with some new chapters on important issues that, in the light of recent progress, needed to be more extensively covered.

First, a general outline of diagnostic research is presented. What are the key objectives, the challenges, and the corresponding options for study design? What should the architecture of diagnostic research look like to provide us with an appropriate research strategy, yielding the clinical information we are looking for, with a minimum burden for study patients and an efficient use of resources? Second, important design features for studying the accuracy and clinical impact of diagnostic tests and procedures are dealt with in more detail, addressing the cross-sectional study, the randomized controlled trial, and the before–after study. In addition, it is shown that the impact of diagnostic tests varies with different clinical settings and target populations, and indications are given as how to ensure that estimates of test accuracy will travel and be transferable to other settings. Also, overviews are presented of the analysis of data on the accuracy of diagnostic tests and of the principles of frequently used multivariable approaches.

A diagnostic study should be reported in such a way that readers can get a good impression of its research question, methodological quality, and added value. To improve the practice of reporting, the STARD statement (Standards for Reporting of Diagnostic accuracy studies) was initiated. Its development, uptake, and effects are described. These standards can be also helpful in prospectively planning a diagnostic accuracy study.

Nowadays, for both clinical investigators and readers of research articles, it is not enough to understand the methodology of original clinical studies. They must also know more about the techniques to summarize and synthesize results from various clinical studies on a certain topic. Guidelines for systematic reviews and meta-analysis of studies evaluating the accuracy of diagnostic tests are therefore presented.

To aid evidence-based clinical decision making, clinical prediction rules (CPRs) explicitly quantify the independent contribution from elements of the clinical examination and available diagnostic tests. Accordingly, methodological standards, construction, validation, implementation, and impact of CPRs, and their integration into computerized clinical decision support systems and decision aids for patients, are covered. Furthermore, as clinical research results can only be successfully incorporated into diagnostic decision making if the way clinicians tend to solve medical problems is taken into account, an overview of the domain of clinical problem solving is given. Eventually, we have to recognize that improving test use in daily care needs more than clinical research, and presenting insights, guidelines, and tools. Therefore, (cost) effective implementation of improved test ordering—which has become a field of study in itself—is also highlighted.

Finally, an overview of the diagnostic research strategy is given and related to challenges for future development. Innovation is especially expected from four fields: progress in (bio)medical knowledge, information and communication technology, the changing role of the patient, and continued methodological exploration.

This book includes contributions from a number of authors. To allow each chapter to keep a logical structure in itself, some key topics have been dealt with more than once, albeit to a varying extent and in different contexts. Instead of seeing this as a problem, we think this is an opportunity for readers to see important issues considered from different perspectives.

The field of diagnostic research is developing strongly and an increasing number of talented clinical investigators are working in (the methodology of) diagnostic research. In view of this dynamic field, we welcome comments from readers and suggestions for further improvement.

We wish to thank Richard Smith and Trish Groves from the *British Medical Journal*, who have so positively welcomed the initiative for this book, and Mary Banks and Simone Dudziak from Blackwell Publishing, who have encouraged and supported the preparation of this second edition until the work was done.

J. André Knottnerus and Frank Buntinx

References

1. Cochrane AL. *Effectiveness and efficiency: random reflections on health services*. The Nuffield Provincial Hospitals Trusts, 1972. Reprinted London: Royal Society of Medicine Press; 1999.
2. Sackett DL, Rosenberg WM, Gray JA, Haynes RB, Richardson WS. Evidence based medicine: what it is and what it isn't. *BMJ*. 1996;**312**:71–72.
3. Knottnerus JA, Dinant GJ. Medicine based evidence, a prerequisite for evidence based medicine. *BMJ*. 1997;**315**:1109–10.

CHAPTER 1

General introduction: evaluation of diagnostic procedures

J. André Knottnerus, Frank Buntinx, and Chris van Weel

Summary box

- Whereas the development of diagnostic technologies has greatly accelerated, the methodology of diagnostic research still lags behind that of evaluation of treatment.
- Diagnostic research appears to be more comprehensive and complex than treatment research as it evaluates the connection between diagnostic and prognostic assessment with choosing optimal interventions.
- Objectives of diagnostic testing are (1) detecting or excluding disorders, (2) contributing to further diagnostic and therapeutic management, (3) assessing prognosis, (4) monitoring clinical course, and (5) measuring general health or fitness.
- Methodological challenges include dealing with complex relations, the "gold standard" problem, spectrum and selection bias, "soft" outcome measures, observer variability and bias, optimizing clinical relevance, appropriate sample size, and rapid progress of applicable knowledge over time.
- Choosing the appropriate study design depends on the research question; the most important designs are the cross-sectional study (to determine the accuracy and added discriminatory value of diagnostic procedures) and the randomized controlled trial (to evaluate the clinical impact of [additional] testing).
- To synthesize the results of various studies on the same topic, diagnostic systematic reviews and meta-analyses are powerful tools.

(continued)

The Evidence Base of Clinical Diagnosis: Theory and Methods of Diagnostic Research. 2nd edition.
Edited by J. André Knottnerus and Frank Buntinx. © 2009 Blackwell Publishing,
ISBN: 978-1-4051-5787-2.

> *(continued)*
> - To make the step from research to practice, clinical decision analysis, cost-effectiveness studies, and quality-of-care research, including implementation studies, are important.

Introduction

The development and introduction of new diagnostic technologies have accelerated greatly over the past few decades. This is reflected in a substantial expansion of research on diagnostic tests and of publications on diagnostic research methodology. However, the evaluation of diagnostic techniques is far from being as established as the evaluation of therapies.

Apart from regulations for obvious safety aspects, at present—unlike the situation with regard to drugs—there are no widely accepted formal requirements for validity and effectiveness that diagnostic tests must meet to be accepted or retained as a routine part of health care. This is related to another point: in spite of important early initiatives[1,2] the methodology for evaluation of diagnostics is not yet as crystallized as the deeply rooted principles of the randomized controlled trial on therapeutic effectiveness[1,3] and of etiologic study designs.[4,5] It is not surprising, then, that serious methodological flaws are often found in published diagnostic studies.[6,7,8]

An additional challenge is the comprehensiveness of diagnostic research. Diagnostic evaluation is the first crucial medical intervention in an episode of illness, labeling symptoms and complaints as health problems, and indicating possible disease and its prognosis. Effective and efficient therapy—also including reassurance, "watchful waiting," and supporting patient self-efficacy—depends to a large extent on an accurate interpretation of (early) symptoms and the outcome of the diagnostic process. Accordingly, as diagnosis covers not only test accuracy but is also the basis for prognosis and appropriate treatment choice, diagnostic research is in fact much more complex than treatment research.

A special point of concern is that the funding of diagnostic evaluation studies is not well organized, especially if the research is not focused on particular body systems or disorders covered by strong research foundations. Rather than being limited to a particular body system, diagnostic evaluation studies frequently start from a complaint, a clinical problem, or certain tests.

Because the quality of diagnostic procedures is indicative for the quality of health care as a whole, it is vital to overcome the shortfall in standards, methodology, and funding. Accurate evaluation of diagnostic performance will contribute to the prevention of unjustified treatment, lack of treatment or mistreatment, and unnecessary costs. In this context, important steps forward toward the professionalizing of diagnostic studies have already been made with the work on the architecture of diagnostic studies[9] (see also Chapters 1, 2, and 14), the Standards for Reporting of Diagnostic Accuracy studies (STARD)[10] (see Chapter 9), and QUADAS, a tool for the Quality Assessment of Diagnostic Accuracy Studies included in systematic reviews.[11] As a general background, this introductory chapter presents an overview of the objectives of diagnostic testing and evaluation research, important methodological challenges, and research design options.

Objectives

Diagnostic testing can be seen as the collection of additional information intended to (further) clarify the character and prognosis of the patient's condition and can include patients' characteristics, symptoms and signs, history and physical examination items, or additional tests using laboratory or other technical facilities. A "test" not only must be considered but also the specific question the test is supposed to answer. Therefore, the performance of tests must be evaluated in accordance with their intended objectives. Objectives may include:

- *Detecting or excluding disorders, by increasing diagnostic certainty as to their presence or absence.* This can only be achieved if the test has sufficient discrimination. Table 1.1 shows the most common measures of discrimination. Most of these can be simply derived from a 2 × 2 table comparing the test result with the diagnostic reference standard, as demonstrated by the example of ankle trauma. A more elaborate and comprehensive explanation of how to calculate these and other measures from collected data is presented in Chapter 7. Examples of tests for which such measures have been assessed are given in Table 1.2. Such a representation allows various tests for the same purpose to be compared. This can show, for example, that less invasive tests (such as ultrasonography) may be as good as or even better diagnostically than more invasive or hazardous ones (e.g., angiography). Also, it can be shown that history data (e.g., change in bowel habit) may be at least as valuable as laboratory data. What is important is not just the discrimination per se, but rather what a test may add to what cheaper and less invasive diagnostics already provided to the diagnostic process. This is relevant, for instance, in assessing the added value of liver function tests to history taking and physical examination in ill-defined, nonspecific complaints. Finally, using the measures defined in Table 1.1 allows the comparison of the value of a test in different settings, for example, general practice versus the hospital emergency department.[12]
- *Contributing to the decision-making process with regard to further diagnostic and therapeutic management,* including the indications for therapy (e.g., by determining the localization and shape of a lesion) and choosing the preferred therapeutic approach.
- *Assessing prognosis* on the basis of the nature and severity of diagnostic findings. This is a starting point for planning the clinical follow-up and for informing and—if justified—reassuring the patient

Table 1.1 Commonly used measures of the discrimination of a diagnostic test T for disease D, illustrated with physical examination for detecting a fracture in ankle trauma, using x-ray film as the reference standard

T: (conclusion of) physical examination	D: (result of) x-ray		Total
	Fracture	No fracture	
Fracture	190	80	270
No fracture	10	720	730
Total	200	800	1,000

The SENSITIVITY of test T is the probability of a positive (abnormal) test result in people with disease D: $P(T+|D+) = 190/200 = 0.95$.

The SPECIFICITY of T is the probability of a negative (normal) test result in people without D: $P(T-|D-) = 720/800 = 0.90$.

Note: Sensitivity and specificity together determine the discrimination of a test in a given situation.

The LIKELIHOOD RATIO (LR) of test result T_X is the ratio of probability of test result T_X in people with D, and by the probability of T_X in people without D.

The general formula for LR_X is $\dfrac{P(T_X|D+)}{P(T_X|D-)}$

For a positive result, LR+ is $\dfrac{P(T+|D+)}{P(T+|D-)}$

which is equivalent to $\dfrac{\text{Sensitivity}}{1-\text{specificity}} = \dfrac{190/200}{1-720/800} = 9.5$

For a negative result, LR- is $\dfrac{P(T-|D+)}{P(T-|D-)}$

which is equivalent to $\dfrac{1-\text{Sensitivity}}{\text{specificity}} = \dfrac{1-190/200}{720/800} = 0.06$

Note: LR is an overall measure of the discrimination of test result T_X. The test is useless if LR = 1. The test is better the more LR differs from 1, that is, greater than 1 for LR+ and lower than 1 for LR−.

For tests with multiple outcome categories, LR_X can be calculated for every separate category x, as the ratio of the probability of outcome category x among diseased and the probability of outcome category x among nondiseased.

The PREDICTIVE VALUE of a test result T_X is:

for a positive result, the probability of D in persons with a positive test result: $P(D+|T+) = 190/270 = 0.70$.

for a negative result, the probability of absence of D in persons with a negative result: $P(D-|T-) = 720/730 = 0.99$.

Note: The predictive value of a positive test result (posterior or post-test probability) must be compared with the estimated probability of D before T is carried out (the prior or pretest probability). For a good discrimination, the difference between the posttest and the pretest probability should be large.

The (diagnostic) ODDS RATIO (OR), or the cross-product ratio, represents the overall discrimination of a dichotomous test T, and is equivalent to the ratio of LR+ and LR−. $OR = (190 \times 720)/(80 \times 10) = 171$.

Note: If OR=1, T is useless. T is better the more OR differs from 1.

The receiver operating characteristic (ROC) curve graphically represents the relation between sensitivity and specificity for tests with a variable cutoff point, on an ordinal scale (e.g., in case of 5 degrees of suspicion of ankle fracture; or cervical smear) or interval scale (e.g., if degree of suspicion of ankle fracture is expressed in a percentage; or ST changes in exercise ECG testing). If the AUC (area under the curve) = 0.5, the test is useless. For a perfect test, the AUC=1.0 (see Chapter 7).

Table 1.2 Discrimination of some diagnostic tests for various target disorders, expressed in sensitivity, specificity, likelihood ratios, and odds ratio (examples based on several sources)

Test	Target Disorder	Sensitivity (%)	Specificity (%)	Likelihood ratio Positive result	Likelihood ratio Negative result	Odds ratio
Exercise ECG*[13]	Coronary stenosis	65	89	5.9	0.39	15.0
Absence of chest wall tenderness in chest pain[14]	Myocardial infarction	92	34	1.4	0.23	5.9
Stress thallium scintigraphy[13]	Coronary stenosis	85	85	5.7	0.18	32.1
Ultrasonography[13]	Pancreatic cancer	70	85	4.7	0.35	13.2
CT scan[13]	Pancreatic cancer	85	90	8.5	0.17	51.0
Angiography[13]	Pancreatic cancer	75	80	3.8	0.31	12.0
Gross hematuria in men[15]	Urological cancer	64	99	99	0.51	195
Gross hematuria in women[15]	Urological cancer	47	99	83	0.66	126
ESR ≥28 mm/1 h**[16]	Malignancy	78	94	13.0	0.23	56.0
ESR ≥28 mm/1 h**[16]	Inflammatory disease	46	95	9.2	0.57	16.2
Intermittent claudication**[17]	Peripheral arterial occlusive disease	31	93	4.4	0.74	5.6
Posterior tibial/dorsalis pedis artery pulse**[17]	Peripheral arterial occlusive disease	73	92	9.1	0.29	30.4
Change in bowel habit**[18]	Colorectal cancer	88	72	3.1	0.17	18.4
Weight loss**[18]	Colorectal cancer	44	85	2.9	0.66	4.6
Rectal bleeding[19]	Colorectal cancer	29	99	68	0.70	97
ESR ≥30 mm/1 h**[18]	Colorectal cancer	40	96	10.0	0.42	14.0
White blood cell count .10⁹**[18]	Colorectal cancer	75	90	7.5	0.28	26.3
Occult blood test ≥1 positive out of 3**[18]	Colorectal cancer	50	82	2.7	0.61	4.6

*Cut-off point: ST depression ≥1 mm.
**In a general-practice setting.

- *Monitoring the clinical course* of a disorder, or a state of health such as pregnancy, or the clinical course of an illness during or after treatment.
- *Measuring physical fitness* in relation to specific requirements, for example, for sports or employment.

The evaluation of a diagnostic test concentrates on its added value for the intended application, taking into consideration the burden for the patient (such as pain, cost, or waiting time) and any possible complications resulting from the test (such as intestinal perforation in endoscopy). This requires a comparison between the situations with and without the use of the test or a comparison with the use of other tests.

Prior to the evaluation, one must decide whether to focus on maximizing the health perspectives of the individual patient (which is usually the physician's aim) or on the best possible cost-effectiveness (as economists are likely to do). The latter can be expressed in the amount of money to be invested per number of life years gained, whether or not adjusted for quality of life. Between these two approaches, which do not necessarily yield the same outcome, there is the tension between strictly individual and collective interests. This becomes especially obvious when policy makers have to decide which options would be accepted as the most efficient in a macroeconomic perspective.

Another prior decision is whether one would be satisfied with a qualitative understanding of the diagnostic decision-making process or would need a detailed quantitative analysis.[20] In the first case, one would chart the stages and structure of the decision-making process in relation to the test to be evaluated. This may already provide sufficient insight, for instance, if it becomes clear beforehand that the result will not influence the decision to be taken. Examples of useless testing are (1) the value of the routine electrocardiogram in acute chest pain for exploring the likelihood of a suspected myocardial infarction, with the consequent decision whether to admit the patient to hospital; and (2) the value of "routine blood tests" in general practice for deciding whether to refer a patient with acute abdominal pain to a surgeon. In addition to qualitatively mapping the structure of the decision-making process, quantitative analysis attempts to assess test discrimination and the (probability of the) ultimate clinical outcome, taking the risks (and the costs) of the test procedure into account. The choice of a qualitative or a quantitative approach depends on the question to be answered and the data available.

If a test has not yet been introduced in clinical practice, the prospects for a good evaluation are better than if it is already in general use. It is then still possible to define an appropriate control group the test is not applied to, so that its influence on the prognosis can be investigated. In addition, at such an early stage, the conclusion of the analysis can still be used in the decision regarding the introduction. Furthermore, it is possible to prospectively plan a monitoring procedure and an evaluation after the introduction. All of this emphasizes the importance of developing an evaluation program before a test is introduced.

A common misunderstanding is that only expensive, advanced diagnostic technology cause unacceptable increases in health care costs. Cheap but frequently used (routine) tests not only account for a major part of direct costs but also greatly influence other costs, as they often preselect patients for more expensive procedures. Yet the performance of such low-threshold diagnostics has often not been adequately evaluated. Examples include many applications of hematological, clinicochemical, and urine tests.[21,22,23]

Methodological challenges

In the evaluation of diagnostic procedures, a number of methodological challenges have to be considered.

Complex relations

Most diagnostics have more than one indication or are relevant for more than one nosological outcome. In addition, tests are often not applied in isolation but in combination, for instance, in the context of clinical protocols. Ideally, clinical research should reflect the health care context,[24] but it is generally impossible to investigate all aspects in one study. One limitation is that the inclusion of a large number of interacting variables calls for large sample sizes that are not easy to obtain. Generally, choices must be made about which issues are the most important. Multivariable statistical techniques are available to allow for the (added) value of various diagnostic data, both separately and in combination, also in the form of diagnostic prediction rules.[25,26,27] In epidemiologic research, such techniques were earlier used for the purpose of analyzing etiologic data, generally focusing on the overall etiologic impact of a factor adjusted for covariables. Diagnostic analysis aims to specify test performance in clinical subgroups or to identify the set of variables that yield the best individual diagnostic prediction, which is a completely different perspective. Much work remains to be done to improve the methodology of diagnostic data analysis.

Diagnostic data analysis will be discussed further in Chapter 7 and multivariable analysis in Chapter 8.

The "gold" standard problem

To evaluate the discriminatory power of a test, its results must be compared with an independently established standard diagnosis. However, a "gold" standard, providing full certainty on the health status, rarely exists. Even x-rays, CT scans, and pathological preparations may produce false positive and false negative results. The aim must then be to define an adequate reference standard that approximates the gold standard as closely as possible.

Sometimes one is faced with whether any appropriate reference standard procedure exists at all. For example, in determining the discrimination of liver tests for diagnosing liver pathology, neither imaging techniques nor biopsies can detect all abnormalities. In addition, as a liver biopsy is an invasive procedure, it is unsuitable for use as a standard in an evaluation study. A useful independent standard diagnosis may not even exist conceptually, for example, when determining the predictive value of symptoms that are themselves part of the disease definition, as in migraine, or when the symptoms and functionality are more important for management decisions than the anatomical status, as in prostatism. Also, in studying the diagnostic value of clinical examination to detect severe pathology in nonacute abdominal complaints, a comprehensive invasive standard screening, if at all possible or ethically allowed, would yield many irrelevant findings while not all relevant pathology would be immediately found. An option, then, is diagnostic assessment after a follow-up period by an independent panel of experts, representing a "delayed type" cross-sectional study.[28] This may not be perfect but can be the most acceptable solution.[1]

A further issue is the dominance of prevailing reference standards. For example, as long as classic angiography is considered the standard when validating noninvasive vascular imaging techniques, the latter will always seem inferior because perfect agreement is never attainable. However, as soon as a new method comes to be regarded as sufficiently valid to be accepted as the standard, the difference will, from then on, be explained in favor of this new method. In addition, one must accept that two methods may actually measure different concepts. For example, when comparing advanced ultrasound measurements in blood vessels with angiography, the first measures blood flow, relevant to fully explain the symptoms, whereas the second reflects the anatomical situation, which is important for the surgeon. Furthermore, the progress of clinicopathological insights is of great importance. For instance, although clinical pattern X may first be the standard to evaluate the significance of microbiological findings, it will become of secondary diagnostic importance once the infectious agent-causing X has been identified. The agent will then be the diagnostic standard, as illustrated by the history of the diagnosis of tuberculosis.

In Chapters 3 and 6, more will be said about reference standard problems.

Spectrum and selection bias

The evaluation of diagnostics may be flawed by many types of bias.[1,29,30] The most important of these are spectrum bias and selection bias.

Spectrum bias may occur when the discrimination of the diagnostic is assessed in a study population with a different clinical spectrum (for instance, in more advanced cases) than among those in whom the test is to be applied in practice. This may, for example, happen with tests calibrated in a hospital setting but applied in general practice. Also, sensitivity may be determined in seriously diseased subjects, whereas specificity is tested in clearly healthy subjects. Both will then be grossly overestimated relative to the practical situation, where testing is necessary because it is impossible to clinically distinguish in advance who is healthy and who is diseased.

Selection bias is to be expected if there is a relation between the test result and the probability of being included in the study population in which the test is calibrated. For example, subjects with an abnormal exercise electrocardiogram are relatively likely to be preselected for coronary angiography. Consequently, if this exercise test is calibrated among preselected subjects, a higher sensitivity and a lower specificity will be found than if this preselection had not occurred.[31] Similarly, on the basis of referral patterns alone, it is to be expected that the sensitivity of many tests is higher in the hospital than in general practice and the specificity lower. Considering selection is especially relevant given the nature of medical practice. If a patient enters the consultation room, the physician immediately has information about the patient's gender, age, and general health. The patient can look tired or energetic, visit the physician in his or her office or ask for a house call, or be rushed into the emergency department by ambulance. Such characteristics are in fact results of previous "tests," providing prior information before the physician asks the first question or performs physical examination. This may influence not only the prior probability of disease but also the discrimination of subsequent diagnostic tests.[12]

Although spectrum and selection biases are often related, the clinical picture is the primary point of concern with spectrum bias, whereas the mechanism of selection is the principal issue with selection bias. These types of bias may affect not only sensitivity and specificity but also all other measures of discrimination listed in Table 1.1.[32]

Chapters 2 and 6 will further address the issue of dealing with spectrum and selection phenomena.

"Soft" measures

Subjective factors such as pain, feeling unwell, and reassurance are important in diagnostic management. Most decisions for a watchful waiting strategy in the early phase of an episode of illness are based on the appraisal of such "soft" measures. These often determine the indication for diagnostic examinations and may themselves be part of the diagnostics (e.g., a symptom or complaint) to be evaluated. Also, weighing such factors is generally indispensable in the assessment of the overall clinical outcome and the related impact on quality of life.[33] Evaluation studies should, on the one hand, aim as much as possible to objectify these subjective factors in a reproducible way. On the other hand, interindividual and even intraindividual differences will always play a part[34] and should be acknowledged in the clinical decision-making process.

Observer variability and observer bias

Variability between different observers, as well as for the same observer in reading and interpreting diagnostic data, should not only be acknowledged for "soft" diagnostics such as history taking and physical examination but also for "harder" ones like x-rays, CT and MRI scans, and pathological slides. Even tests not involving any human assessment show inter- and intra-instrument variability. Such variability should be limited if the diagnostic is to produce useful information.

At the same time, researchers should beware of systematic observer bias because of prior knowledge about the subjects examined, especially if subjective factors play a role in determining test results or the reference standard.[35] Clearly, if one wishes to evaluate whether a doctor can accurately diagnose an ankle fracture based on history and clinical examination, it must be certain that the doctor is unaware of an available x-ray result; and a pathologist making an independent final diagnosis should not have previous knowledge about the most likely clinical diagnosis.[36] In such situations, "blinding" is required. A different form of observer bias could occur if the diagnosticians are prejudiced in favor of one of the methods to be compared, as they may unconsciously put greater effort into that technique. A further challenge is that the experience and skill required should be equal for the methods compared, if these are to have a fair chance in the assessment. In this respect, new methods are at risk of being disadvantaged, especially shortly after being introduced.

Discrimination does not mean usefulness

For various reasons, a test with good discrimination does not necessarily influence management.

To begin with, a test may add too little to what is already known clinically to alter management. Furthermore, the physician may take insufficient account of the information provided by the test. This is a complex issue. For instance, studies of the consequences of routine blood testing have shown that in some cases an unaltered diagnosis still led to changes in the considered policy.[16] In a classic study on the clinical impact of upper gastrointestinal endoscopy, a number of changes (23%) in management were made in the absence of a change in diagnosis, whereas in many patients (30%) in which the diagnosis was changed, management was not altered.[37] A test may detect a disorder for which no effective treatment is available. For example, the MRI scan provides refined diagnostic information with regard to various brain conditions for which no therapy is yet in prospect. Finally, as already discussed, supplementary test results are not always relevant for treatment decisions.

For this reason, it is important that studies evaluating diagnostic tests increasingly also investigate the tests' influence on management.[38,39,40]

Indication area and prior probability

Whether a test can effectively detect or exclude a particular disorder is influenced by the prior probability of that disorder. A test is generally not useful if the prior probability is either very low or very high: not only will the result rarely influence patient management, but the risk of, respectively, a false positive or a false negative result is relatively high. In other words, there is an "indication area" for the test between these extremes of prior probability.[2,20] Evaluation of diagnostics should therefore address the issue of whether the test could be particularly useful for certain categories of prior probability. For example, tests with a moderate specificity are not useful for screening in an asymptomatic population (with a low prior probability) because of the high risk of false positive results.

Small steps and large numbers

Compared with therapeutic effectiveness studies, evaluation studies of diagnostic procedures have often neglected the question of whether the sample size is adequate to provide the desired information with a sufficient degree of certainty. A problem is that progress in diagnostic decision making often takes the form of a series of small steps to gain in certainty, rather than one big breakthrough. Evaluating the importance of a small step, however, requires a relatively large study population.

Changes over time and the mosaic of evidence

Innovations in diagnostic technology may proceed at such a speed that a thorough evaluation may take longer than the development of even more advanced techniques. For example, the results of evaluation studies on the clinical impact and cost-effectiveness of the CT scan had not yet fully crystallized when the MRI and PET scans appeared on the scene. So, the results of evaluation studies may already be lagging behind when they appear. Therefore, there is a need for general models (scenarios) for the evaluation of particular (types of) tests and test procedures, whose overall framework is relatively stable and into which information on new tests can be entered by substituting the relevant pieces in the whole mosaic. It may be possible to insert new test opportunities for specific clinical pathways or certain subgroups.[41] The mosaic approach allows for a quick evaluation of the impact of new imaging or DNA techniques with better discrimination on the cost-effectiveness of breast cancer screening, if other pieces of the mosaic (such as treatment efficacy) have not changed. Discrimination can often be relatively rapidly assessed by means of a cross-sectional study, which may avoid new prospective studies. The same can be said for the influence of changes in relevant costs, such as fees for medical treatment or the price of drugs.

Research designs

Various methodological approaches are available to evaluate diagnostic technologies, including original clinical research, on the one hand, and systematically synthesizing the findings of already performed empirical studies and clinical expertise, on the other.

For empirical clinical studies, there is a range of design options. The appropriate study design depends on the research question to be answered (Table 1.3). In diagnostic accuracy studies, the relationship between test result and reference standard has to be assessed cross-sectionally. This can be achieved by a cross-sectional survey (which may also include the delayed type cross-sectional design), but especially in early validation studies other approaches (case–referent or test result–based sampling) can be most efficient. Design options for studying the impact of diagnostic testing on clinical decision making and patient prognosis are the "diagnostic randomized controlled trial" (RCT), which is methodologically the strongest approach, and the before–after study. Also, cohort and case–control designs have been shown to

Table 1.3 Methodological options in diagnostic research in relation to study objectives

Study objective	Methodological options
Clinical studies	
Diagnostic accuracy	Cross-sectional study
	—survey
	—case–referent sampling
	—test result–based sampling
Impact of diagnostic testing on prognosis or management	Randomized controlled trial
	Cohort study
	Case–control study
	Before–after study
Synthesizing findings and expertise	
Synthesizing results of multiple studies	Systematic review
	Meta-analysis
Evaluation of most effective or cost-effective diagnostic strategy	Clinical decision analysis
	Cost-effectiveness analysis
Translating findings for practice	Integrating results of the above mentioned approaches
	Developing clinical prediction rules
	Expert consensus methods
	Developing guidelines
Integrating information in clinical practice	ICT support studies
	Studying diagnostic problem solving
	Evaluation of implementation in practice

ICT, information and communication technology.

have a place in this context. In Chapter 2, the most important strategic considerations in choosing the appropriate design in diagnostic research will be specifically addressed.

Current knowledge can be synthesized by systematic reviews, meta-analyses, clinical decision analysis, cost-effectiveness studies, and consensus methods, with the ultimate aim of integrating and translating research findings for implementation in practice.

In the following sections, issues of special relevance to diagnostic evaluation studies will be briefly outlined.

Clinical studies

A common type of research is the cross-sectional study, assessing the relationship between diagnostic test results and the presence of particular disorders.[42] This relationship is usually expressed in the measures of discrimination included in Table 1.1. Design options are (1) a survey in an "indicated population," representing subjects in whom the studied test would be considered in practice; (2) sampling groups with (cases) and without disease (referents) to compare their test distributions; or (3) sampling groups with different test results, between which the occurrence of a disease is compared. It is advisable to include in the evaluation already adopted tests, as this is a direct way to obtain an estimate of the added value of the new test. The cross-sectional study will be dealt with in more detail in Chapter 3.

In an RCT, the experimental group undergoes the diagnostic procedure to be evaluated, while a control group undergoes a different (for example, the usual) or no test. This allows the assessment of not only differences in the percentage of correct diagnoses but also the influence of the evaluated test on management and prognosis. A variant is to apply the diagnostic test to all patients but to disclose its results to the caregivers for a random half of the patients, if ethically justified. This constitutes an ideal placebo procedure for the patient. Not only the (added) value of single tests can be evaluated but also different test strategies and even test-treatment protocols can be compared. Although diagnostic RCTs are not easy to carry out and not always necessary or feasible,[43] several important ones have been carried out already some time ago.[44,45,46,47,48,49] Among the best known are the early trials on the effectiveness of breast cancer screening, which have often linked a standardized management protocol to the screening result.[50,51] The randomized controlled trial in diagnostic research is further discussed in Chapter 4.

If the prognostic value of a test is to be assessed and an RCT is not feasible, its principles can serve as the paradigm in applying other methods, such as the cohort study. The difference from the RCT is that the diagnostic information is not randomly assigned, but a comparison is made between two otherwise composed groups.[52] It has the methodological problem that one can never be sure, especially regarding unknown or unmeasurable covariables, whether the compared groups have similar disease or prognostic spectra to begin with. A method providing relatively rapid results regarding the clinical impact of a test is the case–control study. This is often (although not necessarily) carried out retrospectively, that is, after the course and the final status of the patients are known, in subjects who have been eligible for the diagnostic test to be evaluated. It can be studied whether "indicated subjects" showing an adverse outcome (cases) underwent the diagnostic test more or less frequently than indicated subjects without such outcome (controls). A basic requirement is that the diagnostic must have been available to all involved at the time. Well-known examples are case–control studies on the relationship between mortality from breast cancer and participation in breast cancer screening programs.[53,54] This approach is efficient, although potential bias because of lack of prior comparability of tested and nontested subjects must be considered.

The influence of a diagnostic examination on the physician's management can also be investigated by comparing the intended management policies before and after test results are available. Such before–after comparisons (management impact studies) have their own applications, limitations, and precautionary measures, as reviewed by Guyatt *et al.*[55] The method has, for example, been applied early in determining the added value of the CT scan and in studying the diagnostic impact of hematological tests in general practice.[56, 57] The before–after study design will be outlined in Chapter 5.

Although appropriate inclusion and exclusion criteria for study subjects are as important as in therapeutic research, in diagnostic research using and defining such criteria is less well developed. Appropriate criteria are indispensable in order to focus on the clinical question at issue, the relevant spectrum of clinical severity, the disorders to be evaluated, and the desired degree of selection of the study population (e.g., primary care or referred population).[58]

Another issue that deserves attention is the external (clinical) validity of results of diagnostic studies, as prediction models tend to perform better on data from which they were derived than on data in other, comparable populations.[59, 60] In addition, differences in settings often play an important role.[32, 61] Deciding whether estimates of test accuracy are generalizable and transferable to other settings depends on an understanding of the possible reasons for variability in test discrimination and calibration across settings, as will be highlighted in Chapter 6.

Synthesizing research findings and clinical expertise

Often the problem is not so much a lack of research findings but the lack of a good summary and systematic processing of those findings. A diagnostic systematic review and meta-analysis of the pooled data of a number of diagnostic studies can synthesize the results of those studies, which provides an overall assessment of the value of diagnostic procedures[62, 63] and can also help to identify differences in test accuracy between clinical subgroups. In this way, an overview of the current state of knowledge is obtained within a relatively short time. While until recently making diagnostic systematic reviews faced a methodological backlog compared with systematic reviews of treatment, the decision of the Cochrane Collaboration to include the meta-analysis of studies on diagnostic and screening tests has boosted methods development in this field. As differences in spectrum, setting, and subgroups are quite usual in the application and evaluation of diagnostics, between-study heterogeneity is a frequent phenomenon. This largely complicates the quantitative approach to diagnostic reviews and asks for hierarchical (sometimes also called "multilevel") methods. The methodology of systematically reviewing studies on the accuracy of diagnostic tests is elaborated in Chapter 10.

Another important approach is clinical decision analysis, systematically comparing various diagnostic strategies based on their clinical outcome or cost-effectiveness, supported by probability and decision trees. If good estimates of the discrimination and risks of testing, the occurrence and prognosis of suspected disorders, and the "value" of various clinical outcomes are available, a decision tree can be evaluated quantitatively to identify the clinically optimal or most cost-effective strategy. An important element in the decision analytic approach is the combined analysis of diagnostic and therapeutic effectiveness. In this context, a qualitative analysis can already be very useful. For example, nowadays, noninvasive techniques show a high level of discrimination in diagnosing carotid stenoses, even in asymptomatic patients. These techniques allow improved patient selection (triage) for the invasive and more hazardous carotid angiography, which is needed to make final decisions regarding surgical intervention. But if surgery has not been proven to influence the prognosis of asymptomatic patients clearly favorably compared with nonsurgical management,[64,65] the decision tree is greatly simplified because it no longer would include either angiography or surgery and maybe not even noninvasive testing.

Decision analysis does not always provide an answer. The problem may be too complex to be summarized in a tree, essential data may be missing, and often a lack of agreement on key assumptions regarding the value of outcomes may occur. Therefore, consensus procedures are often an indispensable step in the translational process from clinical research to guidelines for practice. In these procedures, clinical experts integrate the most recent state of knowledge with their experience to agree on clinical guidelines regarding the preferred approach of a particular medical problem, differentiated for relevant subgroups.[66]

In the context of developing guidelines, clinical prediction rules (CPRs) can be important to aid evidence-based clinical descision making.[67] Chapter 11 will discuss CPRs in relation to the clinical context in which they are used and will review methodological challenges in developing and validating them and in assessing their impact.

Integrating information in clinical practice

To help clinical investigators harvest essential diagnostic research data from clinical databases and to support clinicians in making and in improving diagnostic decisions, medical informatics, and ICT (information and communication technology) innovations are indispensable. Therefore, the issue of implementation of CPRs in relation to ICT will be addressed in Chapter 11, including future developments.

The information processing approaches outlined in the previous section constitute links between research findings and clinical practice and can be applied in combination to support evidence-based medicine. How such input can have optimal impact on the diagnostic decision making of individual doctors is, however, far from simple or straightforward. Therefore, given the growing cognitive requirements of diagnostic techniques, studies to increase our insight in diagnostic problem solving by clinicians is an important part of diagnostic research. This topic is discussed in Chapter 12.

Information from good clinical studies, systematic reviews, and guideline construction is necessary but in many cases not sufficient for improving routine practice. In view of this, during the past decade, implementation research has been strongly developed to face this challenge and to facilitate the steps from clinical science to patient care. Accordingly, Chapter 13 deals with improving test ordering and its cost-effectiveness in clinical practice.

Concluding remarks

Diagnostic technology assessment would be greatly stimulated if formal standards for the evaluation of diagnostics were to be adopted as a requirement for admittance to the market. Health authorities could initiate assembling panels of experts to promote and monitor the evaluation of both new and traditional diagnostic facilities as to effectiveness, efficiency, and safety, as a basis for acceptance and retention of diagnostics in clinical practice. Furthermore, professional organizations have a great responsibility to set, to implement, to maintain, and to improve clinical standards. More effective international cooperation would be useful, as it has proved to be in the approval and quality control of drugs. In this way, the availability of resources for industrial, private, and governmental funding for diagnostic research and technology assessment would also be stimulated.

Regarding the feasibility of diagnostic evaluation studies, the required size and duration must be considered in relation to the speed of technological progress. This speed can be very great, for instance, in areas where molecular genetic knowledge and information and communication technology play an important part. Especially in such areas, updating of decision analyses, expert assessments, and scenarios by inserting new pieces of the "mosaic" of evidence may be more useful than fully comprehensive, lengthy trials. This may be, for example, relevant for the evaluation of diagnostic areas where current tests will be replaced by new DNA diagnostics in the years to come.

References

1. Feinstein AR. *Clinical epidemiology: The architecture of clinical research*. Philadelphia: W. B. Saunders; 1985.
2. Sackett DL, Haynes RB, Tugwell P. *Clinical epidemiology: A basic science for clinical medicine*. Boston: Little, Brown; 1985.
3. Pocock SJ. *Clinical trials, a practical approach*. New York: John Wiley & Sons; 1983.
4. Kleinbaum DG, Kupper LL, Morgenstern H. *Epidemiologic research, principles, and quantitative methods*. Belmont (CA): Wadsworth; 1982.
5. Miettinen OS. *Theoretical epidemiology, principles of occurrence research in medicine*. New York: John Wiley & Sons; 1985.
6. Sheps SB, Schechter MT. The assessment of diagnostic tests: A survey of current medical research. *JAMA*. 1984;**252**:2418–22.
7. Reid ML, Lachs MS, Feinstein AR. Use of methodological standards in diagnostic research: Getting better but still not good. *JAMA*. 1995;**274**:645–51.
8. Lijmer JG, Mol BW, Heisterkamp S, et al. Empirical evidence of design-related bias in studies of diagnostic tests. *JAMA*. 1999;**282**:1061–66.
9. Sackett DL, Haynes RB. The architecture of diagnostic research. *BMJ*. 2002; **324**:539–41.

10. Bossuyt PM, Reitsma JB, Bruns DE, et al. The Standards for Reporting of Diagnostic Accuracy group: Towards complete and accurate reporting of studies of diagnostic accuracy: The STARD initiative. *Clin Radiol.* 2003;**58**:575–80.
11. Whiting PF, Weswood ME, Rutjes AW, et al. Evaluation of QUADAS, a tool for the quality assessment of diagnostic accuracy studies. *BMC Med Res Methodol.* 2006;**6**:9.
12. Buntinx F, Knockaert D, de Blaey N, et al. Chest pain in general practice or in the hospital emergency department: Is it the same? *Fam Pract.* 2001;**18**:591–94.
13. Panzer RJ, Black ER, Griner PF, eds. *Diagnostic strategies for common medical problems.* Philadelphia: American College of Physicians; 1991. 2nd ed. Black ER, Bordley DR, Tape TG, Panzer RJ, eds.; 1999.
14. Bruyninckx R, Aertgeerts B, Buntinx F. Signs and symptoms in diagnosing acute myocardial infarction and acute coronary syndrome: A diagnostic meta-analysis. Report. 2007: University of Leuven, 2007.
15. Bruyninckx R, Buntinx F, Aertgeerts B, et al. The diagnostic value of macroscopic haematuria for the diagnosis of urological cancer in general practice. *Br J Gen Pract.* 2003;**53**:31–35.
16. Dinant GJ, Knottnerus JA, Van Wersch JW. Discriminating ability of the erythrocyte sedimentation rate: A prospective study in general practice. *Br J Gen Pract.* 1991;**41**:365–70.
17. Stoffers HEJH, Kester ADM, Kaiser V, et al. Diagnostic value of signs and symptoms associated with peripheral arterial obstructive disease seen in general practice: A multivariable approach. *Med Decis Making.* 1997;**17**:61–70.
18. Fijten GHF. *Rectal bleeding, a danger signal?* Amsterdam: Thesis Publishers; 1993.
19. Wouters H, Van Casteren V, Buntinx F. Rectal bleeding and colorectal cancer in general practice: diagnostic study. *BMJ.* 2000;**321**:998–99.
20. Knottnerus JA, Winkens R. Screening and diagnostic tests. In: Silagy C, Haines A, eds. *Evidence based practice in primary care.* London: BMJ Books; 1998.
21. Dinant GJ. *Diagnostic value of the erythrocyte sedimentation rate in general practice.* PhD thesis, University of Maastricht; 1991.
22. Hobbs FD, Delaney BC, Fitzmaurice DA, et al. A review of near patient testing in primary care. *Health Technol Assess.* 1997;**1**:i–iv, 1–229.
23. Campens D, Buntinx F. Selecting the best renal function tests: A meta-analysis of diagnostic studies. *Int J Technol Assess Health Care.* 1997;**13**:343–56.
24. van Weel C, Knottnerus JA. Evidence-based interventions and comprehensive treatment. *Lancet.* 1999;**353**:916–8.
25. Spiegelhalter DJ, Crean GP, Holden R, et al. Taking a calculated risk: predictive scoring systems in dyspepsia. *Scand J Gastroenterol.* 1987;**22** Suppl 128:152–60.
26. Knottnerus JA. Diagnostic prediction rules: Principles, requirements, and pitfalls. *Prim Care.* 1995;**22**:341–63.
27. Knottnerus JA. Application of logistic regression to the analysis of diagnostic data. *Med Decis Making.* 1992;**12**:93–108.
28. Knottnerus JA, Dinant GJ. Medicine based evidence, a prerequisite for evidence based medicine. *BMJ.* 1997;**315**:1109–10.
29. Ransohoff DF, Feinstein AR. Problems of spectrum and bias in evaluating the efficacy of diagnostic tests. *N Engl J Med.* 1978;**299**:926–30.
30. Begg CB. Biases in the assessment of diagnostic tests. *Stat Med.* 1987;**6**:411–23.
31. Green MS. The effect of validation group bias on screening tests for coronary artery disease. *Stat Med.* 1985;**4**:53–61.

32. Knottnerus JA, Leffers P. The influence of referral patterns on the characteristics of diagnostic tests. *J Clin Epidemiol.* 1992;**45**:1143–54.
33. Feinstein, AR. *Clinimetrics.* New Haven (CT): Yale University Press; 1987.
34. Zarin OA, Pauker SG. Decision analysis as a basis for medical decision making: The tree of Hippokrates. *J Med Philos.* 1984;**9**:181–213.
35. Moons KG, Grobbee DE. When should we remain blind and when should our eyes remain open in diagnostic studies? *J Clin Epidemiol.* 2002;**55**:633–36.
36. Schwartz WB, Wolfe HJ, Pauker SG. Pathology and probabilities, a new approach to interpreting and reporting biopsies. *N Engl J Med.* 1981;**305**:917–23.
37. Liechtenstein JI, Feinstein AR, Suzio KD, et al. The effectiveness of pandendoscopy on diagnostic and therapeutic decisions about chronic abdominal pain. *J Clin Gastroenterol.* 1980;**2**:31–36.
38. Sachs S, Bilfinger TV. The impact of positron emission tomography on clinical decision making in a university-based multidisciplinary lung cancer practice. *Chest.* 2005;**128**(2):698–703.
39. Milas M, Stephen A, Berber E, et al. Ultrasonography for the endocrine surgeon: a valuable clinical tool that enhances diagnostic and therapeutic outcomes. *Surgery.* 2005;**138**:1193–200.
40. Kymes SM, Lee K, Fletcher JW, et al. Assessing diagnostic accuracy and the clinical value of positron emission tomography imaging in patients with solitary pulmonary nodules (SNAP). *Clin Trials.* 2006;**3**:31–42.
41. Bossuyt PM, Irwig L, Craig J, et al. Comparative accuracy: assessing new tests against existing diagnostic pathways. *BMJ.* 2006;**332**:1089–92.
42. Knottnerus JA, Muris JW. Assessment of the accuracy of diagnostic tests: the cross-sectional study. *J Clin Epidemiol.* 2003;**56**:1118–28.
43. Guyatt GH, Sackett DL, Haynes RB. Evaluating diagnostic tests. In: Haynes RB, Sackett DL, Guyatt GH, Tugwell P, eds. *Clinical epidemiology: How to do clinical practice research.* Philadelphia: Lippincott, Williams & Wilkins; 2006.
44. Dronfield MW, Langman MJ, Atkinson M, et al. Outcome of endoscopy and barium radiography for acute upper gastrointestinal bleeding: controlled trial in 1037 patients. *BMJ.* 1982;**284**:545–48.
45. Brett GZ. The value of lung cancer detection by six-monthly chest radiographs. *Thorax.* 1968;**23**:414–20.
46. Brown VA, Sawers RS, Parsons RJ, et al. The value of antenatal cardiotocography in the management of high risk pregnancy: a randomised controlled trial. *Br J Obstet Gynaecol.* 1982;**89**:716–22.
47. Flynn AM, Kelly J, Mansfield H, et al. A randomised controlled trial of non-stress antepartum cardiotocography. *Br J Obstet Gynaecol.* 1982;**89**:427–33.
48. Durbridge TC, Edwards F, Edwards RG, et al. An evaluation of multiphasic screening on admission to hospital. *Med J Aust.* 1976;**1**:703–5.
49. Hull RD, Hirsch J, Carter CJ, et al. Diagnostic efficacy of impedance phletysmography for clinically suspected deep-vein thrombosis: A randomized trial. *Ann Intern Med.* 1985;**102**:21–28.
50. Shapiro S, Venet W, Strax Ph, et al. Ten- to fourteen-year effect of screening on breast cancer mortality. *J Natl Cancer Inst.* 1982;**69**:349–55.
51. Tabár L, Fagerberg CJG, Gad A, et al. Reduction in mortality from breast cancer after mass screening with mammography. *Lancet.* 1985;**1**:829–31.
52. Harms LM, Schellevis FG, van Eijk JT, et al. Cardiovascular morbidity and mortality among hypertensive patients in general practice: the evaluation of long-term systematic management. *J Clin Epidemiol.* 1997;**50**:779–86.

53. Collette HJA, Day NE, Rombach JJ, et al. Evaluation of screening for breast cancer in a non-randomised study (the DOM project) by means of a case control study. *Lancet.* 1984;**1**:1224–6.
54. Verbeek ALM, Hendriks JHCL, Holland R, et al. Reduction of breast cancer mortality through mass-screening with modern mammography. *Lancet.* 1984;**1**:1222–4.
55. Guyatt GH, Tugwell P, Feeny DH, et al. The role of before–after studies of therapeutic impact in the evaluation of diagnostic technologies. *J Chronic Dis.* 1986;**39**:295–304.
56. Fineberg HV, Bauman R. Computerized cranial tomography: effect on diagnostic and therapeutic planns. *JAMA.* 1977;**238**:224–7.
57. Dinant GJ, Knottnerus JA, van Wersch JW. Diagnostic impact of the erythrocyte sedimentation rate in general practice: A before–after analysis. *Fam Pract.* 1991;**9**:28–31.
58. Knottnerus JA. Medical decision making by general practitioners and specialists. *Fam Pract.* 1991;**8**:305–7.
59. Starmans R, Muris J, Schouten HJA, et al. The diagnostic value of scoring models for organic and non-organic gastrointestinal disease in non-acute abdominal pain. *Med Decis Making.* 1994;**14**:208–15.
60. Bleeker SE, Moll HA, Steyerberg EW, et al. External validation is necessary in prediction research: a clinical example. *J Clin Epidemiol.* 2003;**56**:441–7.
61. Irwig L, Bossuyt P, Glasziou P, et al. Designing studies to ensure that estimates of test accuracy are transferable. *BMJ.* 2002;**324**:669–71.
62. Irwig L, Macaskill P, Glasziou P, et al. Meta-analytic methods for diagnostic test accuracy. *J Clin Epidemiol.* 1995;**48**:119–30.
63. Buntinx F, Brouwers M. Relation between sampling device and detection of abnormality in cervical smears: A meta-analysis of randomised and quasi-randomised studies. *BMJ.* 1996;**313**:1285–90.
64. Chambers BR, Donnan GA. Carotid endarterectomy for asymptomatic carotid stenosis. *Cochrane Database Syst Rev.* 2005;Oct 19(4):CD001923.
65. Ederle J, Brown MM.The evidence for medicine versus surgery for carotid stenosis. *Eur J Radiol.* 2006;**60**:3–7.
66. Woolf SH, Grol R, Hutchinson A, et al. Clinical guidelines: Potential benefits, limitations, and harms of clinical guidelines. *BMJ.* 1999;**318**:527–30.
67. McGinn T, Guyatt G, Wyer P, et al. Diagnosis: Clinical prediction rules: Users' guides to the medical literature. Chicago: AMA Press, 2004. pp. 471–83.

CHAPTER 2

The architecture of diagnostic research*

R. Brian Haynes and John J. You

Summary box

- Because diagnostic testing aims to discriminate between clinically "normal" and "abnormal," the definition of "normal" is a basic issue in diagnostic research. Although "the normal range" has been typically been defined according to the distribution of test results (the "bell curve" or "Gaussian" distribution), the "therapeutic definition" of normal (test result beyond which intervention does more good than harm) is the most clinically relevant.
- The diagnostic research question to be answered has to be carefully formulated and determines the appropriate research approach. The five most relevant types of question are:
  - **Phase I questions: Do patients with the target disorder have different test results from normal individuals?** The answer requires a comparison of the distribution of test results among patients known to have the disease and people known not to have the disease.
  - **Phase II questions: Are patients with certain test results more likely to have the target disorder than patients with other test results?** This can be studied in the same dataset that generated the Phase I answer, but now test characteristics such as sensitivity and specificity and predictive values are estimated.

---

* David L. Sackett was the lead author of the first edition of this chapter. While he has retired from matters related to evidence-based medicine, his outstanding contributions to the concepts and contents of this chapter are gratefully acknowledged.

The Evidence Base of Clinical Diagnosis: Theory and Methods of Diagnostic Research. 2nd edition.
Edited by J. André Knottnerus and Frank Buntinx. © 2009 Blackwell Publishing.
ISBN: 978-1-4051-5787-2.

- Only if Phase I and Phase II studies, performed in "ideal circumstances," are sufficiently promising as to allow dependable discrimination between diseased and nondiseased subjects, is it worth evaluating the test under "usual" circumstances. Phase III and IV questions must then be answered.
- **Phase III questions: Among patients in whom it is clinically sensible to suspect the target disorder, does the test result distinguish those with and without the target disorder?** To get the appropriate answer, a consecutive series of such patients should be studied. The validity of Phase III studies is threatened if the reference standard or diagnostic test is lost, not performed, or indeterminate.
- **Phase IV questions: Do patients who undergo the diagnostic test fare better (in their ultimate health outcomes) than similar patients who do not?** These questions have to be answered by randomizing patients to undergo the test of interest or some other (or no) test.
- **Phase V questions: Does use of the diagnostic test lead to better health outcomes at an acceptable cost?** Answers to these questions can also be obtained from randomized clinical trials. The external validity, or generalizability, of the findings is threatened if patients enrolled in the trials or the management strategies used are importantly different from those in real practice.
• Because of a varying patient mix, test characteristics, such as sensitivity, specificity, and likelihood ratios may vary between different health-care settings.

Introduction

When making a diagnosis, clinicians may not have access to reference or "gold" standard tests for the target disorders they suspect. Even if they do have access, they may often wish to avoid the risks, or costs, of these reference standards, especially when they are invasive, painful, or dangerous. No wonder, then, that clinical researchers examine relationships between a wide range of more easily measured phenomena and final diagnoses. These phenomena include elements of the patient's history, physical examination, images from all sorts of penetrating waves, and the levels of myriad constituents of body fluids and tissues.

Alas, even the most promising phenomena, when nominated as diagnostic tests, almost never exhibit a one-to-one relation with their respective target disorders, and several different diagnostic tests may compete for primacy in diagnosing the same target disorder. As a result, considerable effort has been expended at the interface between clinical medicine and scientific methods in an effort to maximize the validity and usefulness of diagnostic tests. This book describes the result of those efforts, and this chapter focuses on the specific sorts of questions posed in diagnostic research and the study architectures used to answer them.

As this book is being written, considerable interest is being directed to questions about the usefulness of the plasma concentration of B-type natriuretic peptide in diagnosing left ventricular dysfunction.[1] This interest is justified on two grounds: first, left ventricular dysfunction is difficult to diagnose on clinical examination; and second, randomized trials have shown that treating it reduces its morbidity and mortality. Because real examples are far better than hypothetical ones in illustrating not just the overall strategies but also the down-to-earth tactics of clinical research, we will employ this one in the following paragraphs. To save space and tongue twisting, we will refer to the diagnostic test, B-type natriuretic peptide, as BNP and the target disorder it is intended to diagnose, left ventricular dysfunction, as LVD. The starting point in evaluating this or any other promising diagnostic test is to decide how we will define its normal range.

What do you mean by "normal" and "the normal range"?

This chapter deals with the strategies (a lot) and tactics (a little) of research that attempt to distinguish patients who are "normal" from those who have a specific target disorder. Before we begin, however, we need to acknowledge that several different definitions of normal are used in clinical medicine, and we confuse them at our (and patients') peril. We know six of them[2] and credit Tony Murphy for pointing out five.[3] A common "Gaussian" definition (fortunately falling into disuse) assumes that the diagnostic test results for BNP (or some arithmetic manipulation of them) for everyone, or for a group of presumably normal people, or for a carefully characterized "reference" population, will fit a specific theoretical distribution known as the *normal* or *Gaussian* distribution. Because the mean of a Gaussian distribution plus or minus 2 standard deviations encloses 95% of its contents, it became a tempting way to define the normal many years ago, and came into general use. It is unfortunate that it did, for three logical consequences of its use have led to enormous confusion and the creation of a new field of medicine: the diagnosis of nondisease. First, diagnostic test results usually do not fit the Gaussian distribution. (Actually, we should be grateful that they do not; the Gaussian distribution extends to infinity in both directions, necessitating occasional patients with impossibly high BNP results and others on the minus side of zero.) Second, if the highest and lowest 2.5% of diagnostic test results are called abnormal, then all the diseases they represent have exactly the same estimated frequency, a clinically nonsensical conclusion.

The third harmful consequence of the use of the Gaussian definition of normal is shared by its more recent replacement, the *percentile*. Recognizing the failure of diagnostic test results to fit a theoretical distribution such as the Gaussian, some laboratory specialists suggested that we ignore the shape of the distribution and simply refer (for example) to the lower (or upper) 95% of BNP or other test results as normal. Although this percentile definition does avoid the problems of infinite and negative test values, it still suggests that the underlying prevalence of all diseases is exactly the same, 5%, which is silly and still contributes to the "upper-limit syndrome" of nondisease because its use means that the only "normal" patients are the ones who are not yet sufficiently worked up. This inevitable consequence arises as follows: if the normal range for a given diagnostic test is defined as including the lower 95% of its results, then the probability that a given patient will be called "normal" when subjected to this test is 95%, or 0.95. If this same patient undergoes two independent diagnostic tests (independent in the sense that they are probing totally different organs or functions), the likelihood of this patient being called normal is now $(0.95) \times (0.95) = 0.90$. So, the likelihood of any patient being called normal is 0.95 raised to the power of the number of independent diagnostic tests performed on them. Thus, a patient who undergoes 20 tests has only 0.95 to the 20th power, or about 1 chance in 3, of being called normal; a patient undergoing 100 such tests has only about 6 chances in 1,000 of being called normal at the end of the workup.

Other definitions of normal, in avoiding the foregoing pitfalls, present other problems. The *risk factor* definition is based on studies of precursors or statistical predictors of subsequent clinical events. By this definition, the normal range for BNP or serum cholesterol or blood pressure consists of those levels that carry no additional risk of morbidity or mortality. Unfortunately, however, many of these risk factors exhibit steady increases in risk throughout their range of values; indeed, some hold that the "normal" total serum cholesterol (defined by cardiovascular risk) might lie well below 3.9 mmol/L (150 mg%), whereas our local laboratories employ an upper limit of normal of 5.2 mmol/L (200 mg%), and other institutions employ still other definitions.

Another shortcoming of this risk factor definition becomes apparent when we examine the health consequences of acting upon a test result that lies beyond the normal range: will altering BNP or any other risk factor really change risk? For example, although obesity is a risk factor for hypertension, controversy continues over whether weight reduction improves mild hypertension. One of us led a randomized trial in which we peeled 4.1 kg (on average) from obese, mildly hypertensive women with a behaviorally oriented weight reduction program (the control women lost less than 1 kg).[4] Despite both their and our efforts (the cost of the experimental group's behaviorally oriented weight reduction program came to US$60 per kilo), there was no accompanying decline in blood pressure.

A related approach defines the normal as that which is *culturally desirable*, providing an opportunity for what H. L. Mencken called "the corruption of medicine by morality" through the "confusion of the theory of the healthy with the theory of the virtuous,"[5] Although this definition does not fit our

BNP example, one sees such definitions in their mostly benign form at the fringes of the current lifestyle movement (e.g., "It is better to be slim than fat,"[†] and "Exercise and fitness are better than sedentary living and lack of fitness") and in its malignant form in the health care system of the Third Reich. Such a definition has the potential for considerable harm and may also serve to subvert the role of medicine in society.

Two final definitions are highly relevant and useful to the clinician because they focus directly on the clinical acts of diagnosis and therapy. The *diagnostic* definition identifies a range of BNP (or other diagnostic test) results beyond which LVD (or another specific target disorder) is (with known probability) present. This is the definition we focus on. The "known probability" with which a target disorder is present is known formally as the positive predictive value and depends on where we set the limits for the normal range of diagnostic test results. This definition has real clinical value and is a distinct improvement over the definitions described earlier. It does, however, require that clinicians keep track of diagnostic ranges and cutoffs.

The final definition of normal sets its limits at the level of BNP beyond which specific treatments for LVD (such as ACE inhibitors) have been shown conclusively to do more good than harm. This *therapeutic* definition is attractive because of its link with action. The therapeutic definition of the normal range of blood pressure, for example, avoids the hazards of labeling patients as diseased unless they could benefit from treatment. Thus, in the early 1960s, the only levels of blood pressure conclusively shown to benefit from antihypertensive drugs were diastolic pressures in excess of 130 mmHg (Phase V). Then, in 1967, the first of a series of randomized trials demonstrated the clear advantages of initiating drugs at 115 mmHg, and the upper limit of normal blood pressure, under the therapeutic definition, fell to that level. In 1970, it was lowered further to 105 mmHg with a second convincing trial, and current guidelines about which patients have abnormal blood pressures that require treatment add an element of the risk factor definition and recommend treatment based on the combination of blood pressure with age, sex, cholesterol level, blood sugar, and smoking habit. These days one can even obtain evidence for blood pressure treatment levels based on the presence of a second disease: for example, in diabetes the "tight control" of blood pressure reduces the risk of major complications in a cost-effective way, with the current recommendation being to intervene if the blood pressure exceeds 130/85 mmHg. Obviously, the use of this therapeutic definition requires that clinicians (and guideline developers) keep abreast of advances in therapeutics, and that is as it should be.

In summary, then, before you start any diagnostic study you need to define what you mean by normal, and be confident that you have done so in a sensible and clinically useful fashion.

[†] But the tragic consequences of anorexia nervosa teach us that even this definition can do harm.

The question is everything

As in other forms of clinical research, there are several different ways in which one could carry out a study into the potential or real diagnostic usefulness of a physical sign or laboratory test, and each of them is appropriate to one sort of question and inappropriate for others. Among the questions one might pose about the relation between a putative diagnostic test (say, BNP) and a target disorder (say, LVD), five are most relevant:

- **Phase I questions:** Do patients with the target disorder have different test results from normal individuals? (Do patients with LVD have higher BNP than normal individuals?)
- **Phase II questions:** Are patients with certain test results more likely to have the target disorder than patients with other test results? (Are patients with higher BNP more likely to have LVD than patients with lower BNP?)
- **Phase III questions:** Among patients in whom it is clinically sensible to suspect the target disorder, does the level of the test result distinguish those with and without the target disorder? (Among patients in whom it is clinically sensible to suspect LVD, does the level of BNP distinguish those with and without LVD?)
- **Phase IV questions:** Do patients who undergo this diagnostic test fare better (in their ultimate health outcomes) than similar patients who do not? (Of greatest interest in evaluating early diagnosis through screening tests, this might be phrased: Do patients screened with BNP [in the hope of achieving the early diagnosis of LVD] have better health outcomes [mortality, function, quality of life] than those who do not undergo screening?).
- **Phase V questions:** Does use of the diagnostic test lead to better health outcomes at an acceptable cost? (Are the health outcomes associated with BNP testing worth the associated costs when compared to a conventional diagnostic strategy? Or, does BNP testing represent good "value-for-money"?)

At first glance, the first three questions may appear indistinguishable. They are not, because the strategies and tactics employed in answering them are crucially different and so are the conclusions that can be drawn from their answers. The first two differ in the "direction" in which their results are analyzed and interpreted, and the third differs from the first two in the fashion in which study patients are assembled. The fourth question gets at what we and our patients would most like to know: are they better off for having undergone it? The conclusions that can (and, more importantly, cannot) be drawn from the answers to these questions are crucially different, and there are plenty of examples of the price paid by patients and providers when the answers to Phase I or II questions are interpreted as if they were answering a Phase III (or even a Phase IV) question. Finally, Phase V studies address the question of most importance to managers and policy makers: is the test worth the cost, compared with other uses of the available funds?

Table 2.1 Answering a Phase I question: Do patients with LVD have higher BNP than normal individuals?

	Patients known to have the target disorder (LVD)	Normal controls
Average diagnostic test (BNP precursor) result (and its range)	493.5, range from 248.9 to 909	129.4, range from 53.6 to 159.7

BNP, B-type natriuretic peptide; LVD, left ventricular dysfunction.

These questions also nicely describe an orderly and efficient progression of research into the potential usefulness of a clinical sign, symptom, or laboratory result, and we will use the BNP story to show this sequence.

Phase I questions: Do patients with the target disorder have different test results from normal individuals?

Question 1 often can be answered with a minimum of effort, time, and expense, and its architecture is displayed in Table 2.1.

For example, a group of investigators at a British university hospital measured BNP precursor in convenience samples of "normal controls" and in patients who had various combinations of hypertension, ventricular hypertrophy, and LVD.[6] They found statistically significant differences in median BNP precursors between patients with and normal individuals without LVD and no overlap in their range of BNP precursor results. It was not surprising, therefore, that they concluded that BNP was "a useful diagnostic aid for LVD."

Note, however, that the direction of interpretation here is from known diagnosis back to diagnostic test. Answers to Phase I questions cannot be applied directly to patients because they are presented as overall (usually average) test results. They are not analyzed in terms of the diagnostic test's sensitivity, specificity, or likelihood ratios. Moreover, Phase I studies are typically conducted among patients known to have the disease and people known not to have the disease (rather than among patients who are suspected of having, but not known to have, the disease). As a result, this phase of diagnostic test evaluation cannot be translated into diagnostic action.

Why, then, ask Phase I questions at all? There are two reasons. First, such studies add to our biologic insights about the mechanisms of disease, and may serve later research into therapy as well as diagnosis. Second, such studies are quick and relatively cheap, and a negative answer to their question removes the need to ask the tougher, more time-consuming, and costlier questions of Phases II–IV. Thus, if a convenience (or "grab") sample of patients with LVD already known to the investigators displays the same average levels and distribution of BNP as apparently healthy laboratory technicians or captive medical students, it is time to abandon it as a diagnostic test and devote scarce resources to some other lead.

Table 2.2 Answering a Phase II question: Are patients with higher BNP more likely to have LVD than patients with lower BNP?

	Patients known to have the target disorder (LVD)	Normal controls
High BNP	39	2
Normal BNP	1	25

Tests characteristics and their 95% intervals

	Lower	Upper
Sensitivity = 98%	87%	100%
Specificity = 92%	77%	98%
Positive predictive value = 95%	84%	99%
Negative predictive value = 96%	81%	100%
Likelihood ratio for an abnormal test result = 13	3.5	50
Likelihood ratio for a normal test result = 0.03	0.0003	0.19

BNP, B-type natriuretic peptide; LVD, left ventricular dysfunction.

Phase II questions: Are patients with certain test results more likely to have the target disorder than patients with other test results?

Following a positive answer to a Phase I question, it is logical to ask a Phase II question, this time changing the direction of interpretation so that it runs from diagnostic test result forward to diagnosis. Although the Phase II questions often can be asked in the same dataset that generated the Phase I answer, the architecture of asking and answering them differs. For example, a second group of investigators at a Belgian university hospital measured BNP in "normal subjects" and three groups of patients with coronary artery disease and varying degrees of LVD.[7] Among the analyses they performed (including the creation of ROC curves; see Chapter 7) was a simple plot of individual BNP results, generating the results shown in Table 2.2 by picking the cutoff that best distinguished their patients with severe LVD from their normal controls.

As you can see, the results in Table 2.2 are extremely encouraging. Whether it is used to "rule out" LVD on the basis of its high sensitivity (SnNout – a *Sen*sitive test that is *N*egative helps to rule *out* the diagnosis)[2p83] or to "rule-in" LVD with its high specificity (SpPin – a *Sp*ecific test that is *P*ositive serves to rule *in* the diagnosis),[2p77] BNP looks useful, so it is no wonder that the authors concluded: "BNP concentrations are good indicators of the severity and prognosis of congestive heart failure."

But is Table 2.2 overly encouraging? It compares test results between groups of patients who already have established diagnoses (rather than those who are merely suspected of the target disorder) and contrasts extreme groups of normals and those with severe disease. Thus, it tells us whether the test shows diagnostic promise under ideal conditions for the test, not for usual practice. A useful way to think about this difference between Phase II and Phase III studies is by analogy with randomized clinical trials, which range from addressing explanatory (efficacy) issues of therapy (Can the new treatment work under ideal circumstances?) to management (pragmatic, effectiveness) issues (Does the new treatment work under usual circumstances?). We have summarized this analogy in Table 2.3.

As shown in Table 2.3, the Phase II study summarized in Table 2.2 is explanatory in nature: preselected groups of normal individuals ("ducks") and those who clearly have the target disorder ("yaks") undergo testing under the most rigorous circumstances possible, with the presence or absence of the target disorder being determined by the same reference standard. No attempt is made to validate these initial ("training set") results (especially the cutoff used to set the upper limit of normal BNP) in a second, independent "test" set of ducks and yaks. However, and as with the Phase I study, this relatively easy Phase II investigation tells us whether the promising diagnostic test is worth further, costlier evaluation; as we have said elsewhere,[2p57] if the test cannot tell the difference between a duck and a yak it is worthless in diagnosing either one. As long as the writers and readers of a Phase II explanatory study report make no pragmatic claims about its usefulness in routine clinical practice, no harm is done. Furthermore, criticisms of Phase II explanatory studies for their failure to satisfy the methodological standards employed in Phase III pragmatic studies do not make sense.

Phase III questions: Among patients in whom it is clinically sensible to suspect the target disorder, does the level of the test result distinguish those with and without the target disorder?

Given its promise in Phase I and II studies, it is understandable that BNP would be tested in the much costlier and more time-consuming Phase III study, to determine whether it was useful among patients in whom it is clinically sensible to suspect LVD. An Oxfordshire group of clinical investigators reported that they did just that by inviting area general practitioners "to refer patients with suspected heart failure to our clinic."[8] Once there, these 126 patients underwent independent, blind BNP measurements and echocardiography. Their results are summarized in Table 2.4.

About one-third of the patients referred by their general practitioners had LVD on echocardiography. These investigators documented that BNP measurements did not look nearly as promising when tested in a Phase III study in the pragmatic real-world setting of routine clinical practice and concluded that "introducing routine measurement [of BNP] would be unlikely to improve the

Table 2.3 Explanatory and pragmatic studies of diagnostic tests and treatments

Feature	Promising diagnostic test		Promising treatment	
	Explanatory (Phase II study)	Pragmatic (Phase III study)	Explanatory	Pragmatic
Question	Can this test discriminate under ideal circumstances?	Does this test discriminate in routine practice?	Efficacy: Can this treatment work under ideal circumstances?	Effectiveness: Does this treatment work in routine practice?
Selection of patients	Preselected groups of normal individuals and of those who clearly have the target disorder	Consecutive patients in whom it is clinically sensible to suspect the target disorder	Highly compliant, high-risk, high-response patients	All comers, regardless of compliance, risk of responsiveness
Application of maneuver	Carried out by expert clinician or operator on best equipment	Carried out by usual clinical or operator on usual equipment	Administered by experts with great attention to compliance	Administered by usual clinicians under usual circumstances
Definition of outcomes	Same reference standard for those with and without the target disorder	Often different standards for patients with and without the target disorder; may invoke good treatment-free prognosis as proof of absence of target disorder	May focus on pathophysiology, surrogate outcomes, or cause-specific mortality	"Hard" clinical events or death (often all-cause mortality)
Exclusions of patients or events	Often exclude patients with lost results and indeterminate diagnoses	Include all patients, regardless of lost results or indeterminate diagnoses	May exclude events before or after treatment is applied	Includes all events after randomization
Results confirmed in a second, independent ("test") sample of patients	Usually not	Ideally yes		
Incorporation into systematic review	Usually not	Ideally yes	Sometimes	Ideal

Table 2.4 Answering a Phase III question: Among patients in whom it is clinically sensible to suspect LVD, does the level of BNP distinguish patients with and without LVD?

	Patients with LVD on echocardiography	Patients with normal echos
High BNP (>17.9 pg/mL)	35	57
Normal BNP (<18 pg/mL)	5	29
Prevalence or pretest probability of LVD	40/126 = 32%	

Test characteristics and their 95% confidence intervals

	Lower	Upper
Sensitivity = 88%	74%	94%
Specificity = 34%	25%	44%
Positive predictive value = 38%	29%	48%
Negative predictive value = 85%	70%	94%
Likelihood ratio for an abnormal test result = 1.3	1.1	1.6
Likelihood ratio for a normal test result = 0.4	0.2	0.9

BNP, B-type natriuretic peptide; LVD, left ventricular dysfunction.

diagnosis of symptomatic [LVD] in the community." However, their report of the study also documented the effect of two other cut-points for BNP.

This led both to a counterclaim on the usefulness of BNP in the subsequent e-mail letters to the editor, and to an opportunity for us to describe an alternative way of presenting information about the accuracy of a diagnostic test: the multilevel likelihood ratio (LR). The original report makes it possible for us to construct Table 2.5.

By using multilevel likelihood ratios to take advantage of the full range of BNP results, we can be slightly more optimistic about the diagnostic usefulness of higher levels: the LR for BNP results >76 pg/mL was 5.1. These levels were found in 29% of the patients in this study, and their presence raised the pretest probability of LVD in the average patient from 32% to a posttest probability of 70%. This can be determined directly from Table 2.5 for this "average" patient

Table 2.5 Answering a Phase III question with likelihood ratios

	Patients with LVD on echocardiography	Patients with normal echoes	Likelihood ratio and 95% CI
High BNP (>76 pg/mL)	26 (0.650)	11 (0.128)	5.1 (2.8–9.2)
Mid BNP (10–75 pg/mL)	11 (0.275)	60 (0.698)	0.4 (0.2–0.7)
Low BNP (<10 pg/mL)	3 (0.075)	15 (0.174)	0.4 (0.1–1)
Total	40 (1.000)	86 (1.000)	

BNP, B-type natriuretic peptide; CI, confidence interval; LVD, left ventricular dysfunction.

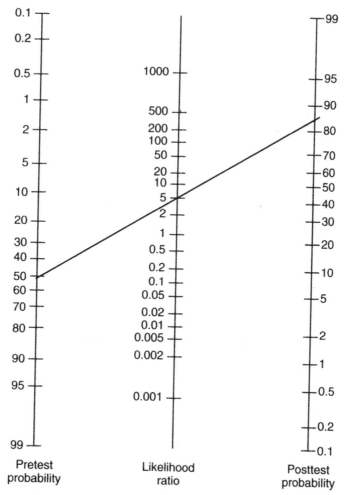

Figure 2.1 Nomogram for converting pretest likelihoods (left column) to posttest likelihoods (right column) by drawing a straight line from the pretest likelihood through the likelihood ratio for the test result.

with a pretest probability of 32% and a high BNP: reading horizontally across the top row, the result is $26/(26 + 11) = 70\%$.

However, if the patient has a different pretest likelihood, say 50%, then either the table must be reconstructed for this higher figure, or the pretest likelihood needs to be converted to a pretest odds (50% is a pretest odds of $(1 - 0.5)/0.5 = 1$), and then multiplied by the likelihood ratio for the test result (5.1 in this case), giving a post test odds of 5.1, which then can be converted back into a posttest percentage of $5.1/(1 + 5.1) = 84\%$. These calculations are rendered unnecessary by using a nomogram, as in Figure 2.1.

Table 2.6 The ideal Phase III study meets the real world

The ideal study	Reference standard		
	Target disorder present		Target disorder absent
Diagnostic test result			
Positive	*a*		*b*
Negative	*c*		*d*

The real study	Reference standard		
	Target disorder present	Lost, not performed, or indeterminate	Target disorder absent
Diagnostic test result			
Positive	*a*	*v*	*b*
Lost, not perfomed, or indeterminate	*w*	*x*	*y*
Negative	*c*	*z*	*d*

Threats to the validity of Phase III studies

Several threats to the validity of Phase III studies can distort their estimates of the accuracy of the diagnostic test. The first batch is violations of the old critical appraisal guide: "Has there been an independent, blind comparison with a gold standard of diagnosis?"[2p52] By *independence* we mean that *all* study patients have undergone *both* the diagnostic test *and* the reference ("gold") standard evaluation and, more specifically, that the reference standard is applied *regardless of the diagnostic test result*. By blind, we mean that the reference standard is applied and interpreted in total ignorance of the diagnostic test result and vice versa. By anticipating these threats at the initial question-forming phase of a study, they can be avoided or minimized.

Although we prefer to conceptualize diagnostic test evaluations in terms of 2 × 2 tables such as the upper panel of Table 2.6 (and this is the way that most Phase II studies are performed), in reality Phase III studies generate the 3 × 3 tables shown in the lower panel of Table 2.6. Reports get lost, their results are sometimes incapable of interpretation, and sometimes we are unwilling to apply the reference standard to all the study patients.

The magnitude of the cells *v*–*z* and the method of handling patients who fall into these three cells will affect the validity of the study. In the perfect study, these cells are kept empty or so small that they cannot exert any important effect on the study conclusion.

However, there are six situations in which they become large enough to bias the measures of test accuracy. First, when the reference standard is expensive, painful, or risky, investigators will not wish to apply it to patients with negative diagnostic test results. Consequently, such patients risk winding up in cell z. Furthermore, there is an understandable temptation to shift them to cell d in the analysis. Because no diagnostic test is perfect, some of them surely belong in cell c. Shifting all of them to cell d falsely inflates both sensitivity and specificity. If this potential problem is recognized before the study begins, investigators can design their reference standard to prevent such patients from falling into cell z. This is accomplished by moving to a more pragmatic study and adding another, prognostic dimension to the reference standard, namely, the clinical course of patients with negative test results who receive no intervention for the target disorder. If patients who otherwise would end up in cell z develop the target disorder during this treatment-free follow-up, they belong in cell c. If they remain free of disease, they join cell d. The result is an unbiased and pragmatic estimate of sensitivity and specificity.

Second, the reference standard may be lost; and third, it may generate an uninterpretable or indeterminate result. As before, arbitrarily analyzing such patients as if they really did or did not have the target disorder will distort measures of diagnostic test accuracy. If these potential biases are identified in the planning stages, they can be minimized, a pragmatic solution such as that proposed previously for cell z considered, and clinically sensible rules established for shifting them to the definitive columns in a manner that confers the greatest benefit (in terms of treatment) and the least harm (in terms of labeling) to later patients.

Fourth, fifth, and sixth, the diagnostic test result may be lost, never performed, or indeterminate, so that the patient winds up in cells w, x, or y. Here the only unforgivable action is to exclude such patients from the analysis of accuracy. As before, anticipation of these problems before the study begins should minimize tests that are lost or never performed to the point where they would not affect the study conclusion regardless of how they were classified. If indeterminate results are likely to be frequent, a decision can be made before the study begins about whether they will be classified as positive or negative. Alternatively, if multilevel likelihood ratios are to be used, these patients can form their own stratum.

In addition to the six threats to validity related to cells v–z, there are two more. The seventh threat to validity noted in the previous critical appraisal guide arises when a patient's reference standard is applied or interpreted by someone who already knows that patient's diagnostic test result (and vice versa). This is a risk whenever there is any degree of interpretation (even in reading off a scale) involved in generating the result of the diagnostic test or reference standard. We know that these situations lead to biased inflations of sensitivity and specificity.

The eighth and final threat to the validity of accuracy estimates generated in Phase III studies arises whenever the selection of the "upper limit of normal" or cut-point for the diagnostic test is under the control of the investigator. When they can place the cut-point wherever they want, it is natural for them to select the point where it maximizes sensitivity (for use as a SnNout), specificity (for use as a SpPin), or the total number of patients correctly classified in that particular "training" set. If the study were repeated in a second, independent "test" set of patients, employing that same cut-point, the diagnostic test would be found to function a little or a lot worse. Thus, the true accuracy of a promising diagnostic test is not known until it has been evaluated in one or more independent studies.

The foregoing threats apply whether the diagnostic test comprises a single measurement of a single phenomenon or a multivariate combination of several phenomena. For example, Philip Wells and his colleagues determined the diagnostic accuracy of the combination of several items from the medical history, physical examination, and noninvasive testing in the diagnosis of deep vein thrombosis.[9] Although, their study generated similar results in three different centers (two in Canada and one in Italy), even they recommended further prospective testing before widespread use.

Limits to the applicability of Phase III studies

Introductory courses in epidemiology introduce the concept that predictive values change as we move back and forth between screening or primary care settings (with their low prevalence or pretest probability of the target disorder) to secondary and tertiary care (with their higher probability of the target disorder). This point is usually made by assuming that sensitivity and specificity remain constant across all settings. However, the mix (or spectrum) of patients also varies among these locations; for example, screening is applied to asymptomatic individuals with early disease, whereas tertiary care settings deal with patients with advanced or florid disease. No wonder, then, that sensitivity and specificity often vary between these settings. Moreover, because primary care patients with positive diagnostic test results (which comprise false positive as well as true positive results) are referred forward to secondary and tertiary care, we might expect specificity to fall as we move along the referral pathway.

Very little empirical evidence addresses this issue, and we acknowledge our debt to Dr. James Wagner of the University of Texas at Dallas for tracking down and systematically reviewing diagnostic data from over 2000 patients with clinically suspected appendicitis seen in primary care and on inpatient surgical wards (J. Wagner, personal communication, 2000). The diagnostic tests comprised the clinical signs that are sought when clinicians suspect appendicitis, and the reference standard is a combination of pathology reports on appendices when operations were performed, and a benign clinical course when they were not. The results for the diagnostic test of right lower quadrant tenderness are shown in Table 2.7.

A comparison of the results in primary and tertiary care shows, as we might expect, an increase in the proportions of patients with appendicitis (from 14% to 63%). But, of course, this increase in prevalence occurred partly because patients with right lower quadrant tenderness (regardless of whether this was

Table 2.7 The accuracy of right lower quadrant tenderness in the diagnosis of appendicitis

	Primary care settings Appendicitis		Tertiary care settings Appendicitis	
	Yes (%)	No (%)	Yes (%)	No (%)
Right lower quadrant tenderness				
Present	84	11	81	84
Absent	16	89	19	16
Totals	100	100	100	100
Frequency of appendicitis	14%		63%	
Frequency of positive sign	21%		82%	
Sensitivity	84%		81%	
Specificity	89%		16%	
LR$^+$	7.6		1	
LR$^-$	0.2		1	

a true positive or false positive finding) tended to be referred to the next level of care, whereas patients without this sign tended not to be referred onward; this is confirmed by the rise in the frequency of this sign from 21% of patients in primary care to 82% of patients in tertiary care. Although this sort of increase in a positive diagnostic test result is widely recognized, its effect on the accuracy of the test is not. The forward referral of patients with false positive test results leads to a fall in specificity, in this case a dramatic one from 89% down to 16%. As a result, a diagnostic sign of real value in primary care (LR+ of 8, LR– of 0.2) is useless in tertiary care (LR+ and LR– both 1); in other words, its diagnostic value has been "used up" along the way.[‡]

This phenomenon can place major limitations on the applicability of Phase III studies carried out in one sort of setting to another setting where the mix of test results may differ. Overcoming this limitation is another bonus that attends the replication of a promising Phase III study in a second "test" setting attended by patients of the sort that the test is claimed to benefit.

Does specificity always fall between primary care and tertiary care settings? Might this be employed to generate a "standardized correction factor" for extrapolating test accuracy between settings? Have a look at the clinical sign of abdominal rigidity in Table 2.8.

[‡] Although not germane to this book on research methods, there are two major clinical ramifications of this phenomenon. First, because clinical signs and other diagnostic tests often lose their value along the referral pathway, tertiary care clinicians might be forgiven for proceeding immediately to applying invasive reference standards. Second, tertiary care teachers should be careful what they teach primary care trainees about the uselessness of clinical signs.

Table 2.8 The accuracy of abdominal rigidity in the diagnosis of appendicitis

	Primary care settings Appendicitis		Tertiary care settings Appendicitis	
	Yes (%)	No (%)	Yes (%)	No (%)
Rigid abdomen				
Present	40	26	23	6
Absent	60	74	77	94
Totals	100	100	100	100
Frequency of appendicitis	14%		47%	
Frequency of positive sign	28%		14%	
Sensitivity	40%		24%	
Specificity	74%		94%	
LR+	1.5		5	
LR−	0.8		0.8	

In this case, a clinical sign that is useless in primary care (LR+ barely above 1 and LR− close to 1) is highly useful in tertiary care (LR+ of 5), and in this case specificity has risen (from 74% to 95%), not fallen, along the referral pathway. The solution to this paradox is revealed in the frequency of the sign in these two settings; it has fallen (from 28% to 14%), not risen, along the pathway from primary to tertiary care. We think that the explanation is that primary care clinicians, who do not want to miss any patient's appendicitis, are "overreading" abdominal rigidity compared with their colleagues in tertiary care. At this stage in our knowledge of this phenomenon, we do not think the "standard correction factors" noted in the previous paragraph are advisable, and this paradox once again points to the need to replicate promising Phase III study results in "test" settings attended by patients (and clinicians) of the sort that the test is claimed to benefit. In this regard, we welcome the creation of the CARE consortium of over 500 clinicians from over 25 countries[10] for their performance of web-based, large, simple, fast studies of the clinical examination.[11] It is hoped that this group, which can be contacted at www.carestudy.com, can make a large contribution to determining the wide applicability of the diagnostic test information obtained from the medical history and physical examination.

For clinicians who wish to apply the Bayesian properties of diagnostic tests, accurate estimates of the pretest probability of target disorders in their locale and setting are required. These can come from five sources: (1) personal experience, (2) population prevalence statistics, (3) practice databases, (4) the publication that described the test, or (5) one of a growing number of primary studies of pretest probability in different settings.[12]

Table 2.9 Answering a Phase IV question: Do patients undergoing BNP testing fare better than those who do not? (using improvement in the percentage of correct diagnoses as a surrogate for improved health outcomes)

	GP diagnosis at initial visit	GP diagnosis at next visit
BNP group, % correct diagnoses	49%	70%
Control group, % correct diagnoses	52%	60%

BNP, B-type natriuretic peptide; GP, general practitioners.

Phase IV questions: Do patients who undergo this diagnostic test fare better (in their ultimate health outcomes) than similar patients who do not?

The ultimate value of a diagnostic test is measured in the health outcomes produced by the further therapeutic interventions it precipitates. Sometimes, this benefit can be hinted at in Phase III studies if the reference standard for the absence of the target disorder is a benign clinical course despite the withholding of treatment. At other times, this benefit is self-evident, as in the correct diagnosis of patients with life-threatening target disorders who thereby receive life-saving treatments, and in these situations, demonstration of an increased number of correct diagnoses using the diagnostic test may be a suitable surrogate for "hard" clinical outcomes. Such a study of BNP testing was performed by investigators in New Zealand, who enrolled 307 patients presenting to their general practitioner (GP) with dyspnea and/or edema into a randomized trial.[13] The study results are summarized in Table 2.9.

Patients randomized to the BNP group had an initial diagnosis made by their GP followed by measurement of BNP precursor levels. The GP's initial diagnosis was correct in 49% of patients at the initial visit. At the subsequent visit, after receiving the BNP results, the proportion of correct diagnoses improved to 70%. In the control group, 52% of diagnoses were correct at the initial visit and only improved to 60% at the next visit. Upon further examination of their data, the investigators found that improved diagnostic accuracy in the BNP group was mainly due to the GPs improved ability to correctly rule out heart failure. Such studies of comparative accuracy, though rarely performed, may provide very useful information. If the new diagnostic test is not more accurate than existing diagnostic strategies, it would be difficult to envision how the test would lead to an improvement in health outcomes, and further investment in Phase IV studies that examine "hard" outcomes would not be worth pursuing.

Most often, Phase IV questions about health outcomes are posed for diagnostic tests that achieve the early detection of asymptomatic disease and can only be answered by the follow-up of patients randomized to undergo the diagnostic test of interest or some other (or no) test. In a systematic review of

Table 2.10 A systematic review of randomized trials of screening for colorectal cancer

Outcome	Unscreened group	Screened group	Relative risk reduction	Absolute risk reduction	Number needed to screen to prevent one more colorectal cancer death
Colorectal cancer mortality	0.58%	0.50%	16%	0.08%	1,237

several randomized trials of fecal occult blood testing,[14] over 400,000 patients were randomized to undergo annual or biennial screening or no screening, and then carefully followed for up to 13 years to determine their mortality from colorectal cancer. The results are summarized in Table 2.10.

In this example, patients were randomized to undergo or not undergo the diagnostic test. Because most of them remained cancer free, the sample size requirement was huge and the study architecture is relatively inefficient. It would have been far more efficient (but unacceptable in this case) to randomize the disclosure of positive test results, and this latter strategy was employed in a randomized trial of a developmental screening test in childhood.[15] In this study, the experimental children whose positive test results were revealed and who subsequently received the best available counseling and interventions fared no better in their subsequent academic, cognitive, or developmental performance than control children whose positive test results were concealed. However, parents of the "labeled" experimental children were more likely to worry about their school performance, and their teachers tended to report more behavioral problems among them. Indeed, the important warning that diagnostic tests can harm as well as help those undergoing them is not often stated in the literature. Potential harms include the anxiety caused by false positive diagnosis; the downstream costs of the often invasive work-ups that result from the discovery of "incidentalomas" (findings of uncertain significance that are unrelated to the original reason the test was performed);[16] and the detection of pseudodisease (disease that never would become apparent to patients during their lifetime had they not undergone the diagnostic test, but once detected, may lead to treatment in situations where the risks outweigh the benefits).[17]

Phase V questions: Does use of the diagnostic test lead to better health outcomes at an acceptable cost?

Expenditures for diagnostic testing are spiraling upward,[18] and accordingly, assessing the cost-effectiveness of these technologies is becoming increasingly important. While the architecture of cost-effectiveness studies can vary, their findings are reported using a common metric, the cost-effectiveness ratio: the additional cost (or cost savings) incurred for each additional unit of health

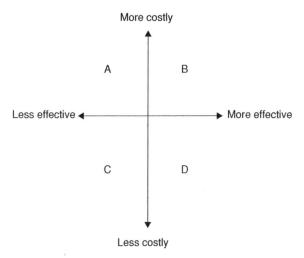

Figure 2.2 Four possible outcomes of a Phase V study: A, the test is more costly and less effective (undesirable); B, the test is more costly, but more effective; C, the test is less costly, but less effective; D, the test is less costly and more effective (most desirable).

benefit that is gained (or lost) by using the diagnostic test, compared with a conventional testing strategy. Figure 2.2 describes the four possible outcomes of a Phase V study (the cost-effectiveness "plane").

Given the encouraging findings of improved diagnostic accuracy in the Phase IV study of BNP testing described above (and given the large number of patients with suspected heart failure encountered in clinical practice), it would instructive to know whether BNP testing represents good "value-for-money." In a Phase V study of 452 patients presenting to the emergency department with acute dyspnea, Swiss investigators randomized patients to undergo either a diagnostic strategy that included rapid measurement of BNP or a conventional diagnostic strategy.[19] Their findings are summarized in Table 2.11.

Although all-cause mortality was not significantly different at 180 days, testing of BNP led to improvement in several health-related outcomes, including hospitalization and the use of intensive care (providing answers to Phase IV questions beyond improved accuracy). Total treatment cost was also significantly reduced in the BNP group. To address the "value-for-money" question, the investigators drew 5,000 random samples of their original data set (a technique known as bootstrapping) and plotted the outcome of each sample on the appropriate quadrants of Figure 2.2. In 80.6% of the replications, BNP testing was less costly and resulted in lower mortality; in 19.3% of the replications, BNP testing was less expensive and resulted in higher mortality; and in less than 0.1% of the replications, BNP guidance was more expensive, and resulted in either higher or lower mortality. Although the authors concluded

Table 2.11 Answering a Phase V question: Are the health outcomes associated with BNP testing worth the associated costs when compared to a conventional diagnostic strategy?

	BNP group	Control group	P value
Hospital admission rate	75%	85%	0.008
Intensive care unit admission rate	15%	24%	0.01
Days in hospital, median (interquartile range)	8 (1–16)	10 (5–18)	0.002
Mortality at 180 days	20%	23%	0.42
Total treatment cost at 180 days	$7,930	$10,503	0.006

that BNP testing was cost-effective, one might have been more confident in reaching this conclusion had 95% or more of the samples fallen into the lower mortality quadrants. Most often, promising diagnostic tests fall into quadrant B, that is, more costly but also more effective, and the difficult question to answer here is what one is willing to pay for a particular gain in health.

A limitation of Phase V studies that use a randomized design is that the external validity, or generalizability, of the findings is threatened if the patients enrolled in the trial and the management strategies used (which impact on costs) are not representative of real-world practice. Decision analytic models are often used as a substitute for, or to extrapolate the findings of, Phase V studies, allowing the investigator to explore cost-effectiveness under a wide range of assumptions. Because the findings from such exercises are only as good as the model inputs, the importance of basing such models on well-designed Phase I to V studies of diagnostic tests cannot be emphasized enough.

References

1. Hobbs R. Can heart failure be diagnosed in primary care? *BMJ.* 2000;**321**:188–89.
2. Sackett DL, Haynes RB, Guyatt GH, et al. *Clinical epidemiology: a basic science for clinical medicine.* 2nd ed. Boston: Little, Brown; 1991. pp. 58–61.
3. Murphy EA. The normal, and perils of the sylleptic argument. *Perspect Biol Med.* 1972;**15**:566.
4. Haynes RB, Harper AC, Costley SR, et al. Failure of weight reduction to reduce mildly elevated blood pressure: a randomized trial. *J Hypertens.* 1984;**2**:535.
5. Mencken HL. *A Mencken chrestomathy.* Westminster: Knopf; 1949. p. 12.
6. Talwar S, Siebenhofer A, Williams B, et al. Influence of hypertension, left ventricular hypertrophy, and left ventricular systolic dysfunction on plasma N terminal pre-BNP. *Heart.* 2000;**83**:278–82.
7. Selvais PL, Donickier JE, Robert A, et al. Cardiac natriuretic peptides for diagnosis and risk stratification in heart failure. *Eur J Clin Invest.* 1998;**28**:636–42.
8. Landray MJ, Lehman R, Arnold I. Measuring brain natriuretic peptide in suspected left ventricular systolic dysfunction in general practice: cross-sectional study. *BMJ.* 2000;**320**:985–86.

9. Wells PS, Hirsh J, Anderson DR, et al. A simple clinical model for the diagnosis of deep-vein thrombosis combined with impedance plethysmography: potential for an improvement in the diagnostic process. *J Intern Med.* 1998;**243**:15–23.

10. McAlister FA, Straus SE, Sackett DL (On behalf of the CARE-COAD group). Why we need large, simple studies of the clinical examination: the problem and a proposed solution. *Lancet.* 1999;**354**:1721–24.

11. Straus SE, McAlister FA, Sackett DL, et al. The accuracy of patient history, wheezing, and laryngeal measurements in diagnosing obstructive airway disease. *JAMA.* 2000;**283**:1853–57.

12. Sackett DL, Straus SE, Richardson WS, et al. *Evidence-based medicine: how to practice and teach EBM.* 2nd ed. Edinburgh: Churchill Livingstone; 2000. pp. 82–84.

13. Wright SP, Doughty RN, Pearl A, et al. Plasma amino-terminal pro-brain natriuretic peptide and accuracy of heart-failure diagnosis in primary care: A randomized, controlled trial. *J Am Coll Cardiol.* 2003;**42**:1793–800.

14. Hewitson P, Glasziou P, Irwig L, et al. Screening for colorectal cancer using the faecal occult blood test, Hemoccult. *Cochrane Database Syst Rev.* 1998(3):CD001216.

15. Cadman D, Chambers LW, Walter SD, et al. Evaluation of public health preschool child development screening: the process and outcomes of a community program. *Am J Public Health.* 1987;**77**:45–51.

16. Stone JH. Incidentalomas—clinical correlation and translational science required. *N Engl J Med.* 2006;**354**:2748–49.

17. Fisher ES, Welch HG. Avoiding the unintended consequences of growth in medical care: how might more be worse? *JAMA.* 1999;**281**:446–53.

18. Iglehart JK. The new era of medical imaging—progress and pitfalls. *N Engl J Med.* 2006;**354**:2822–28.

19. Mueller C, Laule-Kilian K, Schindler C, et al. Cost-effectiveness of B-type natriuretic peptide testing in patients with acute dyspnea. *Arch Intern Med.* 2006;**166**:1081–87.

CHAPTER 3

Assessment of the accuracy of diagnostic tests: the cross-sectional study

J. André Knottnerus and Jean W. Muris

Summary box

- In determining the accuracy of diagnostic testing, the first step is to specify the clinical diagnostic problem under study. Second, the contrast to be evaluated must be appropriately defined. Options are to evaluate one single test contrast; to compare two or more single tests; to evaluate further testing in addition to previous diagnostics; and to compare alternative diagnostic strategies. In addition, distinction should be made between evaluating testing in "extreme contrast" or "clinical practice" settings.
- For accuracy studies, general design types are (1) a survey of the total study population, (2) a case–referent approach, or (3) a test-based enrollment. The direction of the data collection should generally be prospective, but ambispective and retrospective approaches are sometimes appropriate.
- One should specify the determinants of primary interest (the test(s) under study) and other potentially important determinants (possible modifiers of test accuracy and confounding variables). As a matter of principle, the reference standard procedure to measure the target disorder should be applied on all included subjects, independently of the result of the test under study. Applying a reference standard procedure can be difficult because of classification errors, lack of a well-defined pathophysiological concept, incorporation bias, or too

---

The Evidence Base of Clinical Diagnosis: Theory and Methods of Diagnostic Research. 2nd edition. Edited by J. André Knottnerus and Frank Buntinx. © 2009 Blackwell Publishing, ISBN: 978-1-4051-5787-2.

invasive or too complex patient investigations. Possible solutions are an independent expert panel and the delayed-type cross-sectional study (clinical follow-up). Also, a prognostic criterion can be chosen to define clinical outcome.

- Inclusion criteria must be based on "the intention to diagnose" or "intention to screen" with respect to the studied clinical problem. Accordingly, the recruitment procedure is preferably a consecutive series of presenting patients or a target population screening, respectively. In the design phase, sample size estimation should be routine. Both bivariate and multivariable techniques can be used in the analysis, based on the evaluated contrast. Estimating test accuracy and prediction of outcome require different approaches.
- External (clinical) validation should preferably be based on repeated studies in other, similar populations. Also, systematic reviews and meta-analysis have a role.

Introduction

While the ultimate objective of the diagnostic phase is to optimize the patient's prognosis by enabling the clinician to choose an adequate therapeutic strategy, an accurate diagnostic assessment is a first and indispensable step in the process of clinical management.

Making a useful clinical diagnosis implies classifying the presented health problem of a patient in the context of accepted nosological knowledge. This diagnostic classification may result in confirmation or exclusion of the presence of a certain disease, in the choice for one disease from a set of possibly present diseases, or in the conclusion that a number of diseases are present simultaneously.[1] Also, it can be concluded that, given present knowledge, a further diagnostic classification than the observed symptomatology cannot be achieved. Sometimes a classification is not worthwhile, considering the balance between expected gain in certainty, the burden of making a definitive diagnosis, and the relevance of therapeutic consequences.

Apart from making a diagnostic classification, the diagnostic process may be aimed at assessing the clinical severity or monitoring the clinical course of a diagnosed condition. Another very important clinical application is documenting the precise localization or shape of a diagnosed lesion to support surgical, decision making.

A potential new diagnostic test must first go through a phase of pathophysiological and technical development, before its clinical effectiveness in terms of diagnostic accuracy or prognostic impact can be evaluated.[2, 3] The methodology discussed in this book, focused on clinical effectiveness, is applicable to the further evaluation of tests that have successfully passed this early development.

A basic question to be answered, then, is what is the probability that this particular patient with this particular symptomatology or these test results has a certain disorder or a combination of disorders? Obtaining an evidence-based answer, using clinical epidemiological research data, requires an analysis of the association between the presented symptomatology or test result and the appropriate diagnostic classification, that is, the presence or absence of certain diagnoses.

This chapter deals with principles, designs, and pitfalls of cross-sectional diagnostic accuracy research. In this context, cross-sectional research includes studies in which the measured test results and the health status to be diagnosed essentially represent one point in time for each study subject.[4]

Diagnostic research on test accuracy: the basic steps to take

All measures of diagnostic association[5] (Chapters 1 and 7) can be derived from appropriate research data on the relation between test results and a reference standard diagnosis. A valid data collection on this relation is the main point of concern,[6] while the various measures can be calculated by applying straightforward analytical methods. Research data for the purpose of diagnostic discrimination are generally collected in cross-sectional research, irrespective of the diagnostic parameters to be used.

As usual in research, a first requirement is to specify the research question. Second, the most appropriate study design to answer this question has to be outlined. A third step is to operationalize the determinants (test(s) to be evaluated, relevant modifiers of diagnostic accuracy, and possible confounding variables) and outcome (generally the presence or absence of the disorder to be diagnosed). Further, the study population, the corresponding inclusion and exclusion criteria, and the most appropriate recruitment procedure have to be further specified. Finally, an adequate sample size and data analysis must be planned and achieved.

The research question: contrast to be evaluated

In short, the diagnostic research question should define:
1 The clinical problem for which obtaining the diagnostic information is considered possibly relevant.
2 The test or test set to be evaluated.
3 Whether the planned study should evaluate (1) the potential of the test procedure to discriminate between subjects with and without a target disorder in an ideal situation of extreme contrast, or (2) to what extent it

could be useful in a daily practice clinical setting (where discrimination is, by definition, more difficult).

Box 3.1 The research question

Define the clinical problem
Contrast to be evaluated

- single test
- comparing single tests
- additional testing
- comparing diagnostic strategies

Extreme contrast or practice setting

Regarding the clinical problem studied (a), it is important not only to define the target disorder(s) to be diagnosed but also the clinical setting and clinical spectrum (e.g., early or later in the development of the disorder and degree of severity) at which one is primarily aiming. It is crucial whether the investigator wants to evaluate the validity of a test for diagnosing a possible disease in its early phase in a primary care setting or to diagnose more advanced disease in an outpatient clinic or hospital setting, with patients selected by referral based on suspect symptoms or previous tests.[7,8] This is dealt with in more detail in Chapters 2 and 6.

A key issue is the specific contrast to be evaluated (b). The question can be, for example, what is the discriminative power of one specific test or test procedure to be applied for a certain clinical diagnostic problem (single test)? However, the focus may also be on the discriminative power of a new test compared to the best test(s) already available for the clinical diagnostic problem under study (comparing single tests). For clinical practice, it is often important to determine the added value of further (e.g., more invasive) testing, given the tests already performed (additional testing),[9] or to evaluate the most accurate or efficient diagnostic test set or test sequence (diagnostic strategy) for a certain diagnostic problem. In general, we recommend that in studying a new, more invasive or more expensive test, already available, less invasive or less expensive tests with fewer adverse effects should be also included. This makes it possible to evaluate critically the new test's net contribution, if any. A new test can also be less invasive and therefore interesting to insert earlier in the process to preselect for more invasive tests (e.g., using blood testing as a criterion to carry out amniocentesis in prenatal screening). Such "triage" tests[10] may be less accurate than the existing more invasive ones, and it should then be evaluated whether the probability of more false negatives is outweighed by better preselection for more invasive testing, for example, in terms of less complications.

In general, it is informative to include the clinician's diagnostic assessment (without knowing the test result) as a separate test. The performance of new approaches can then be evaluated as to its added value compared with the doctor's usual diagnostic performance or "black box."

Regarding (c), critical appraisal of the state of current knowledge is important for defining an optimally efficient research strategy. For instance, if nothing at all is known yet about the discriminative power of a test, it is more efficient – in terms of reducing the burden for study patients, the sample size, the resources, and the time needed for the study – first to evaluate whether the test discriminates between clearly diseased and clearly nondiseased subjects. If the test does not discriminate in such a Phase I study (Feinstein,[4] Sackett and Haynes,[11] Chapter 2 of this book) any further, usually larger and longer, studies evaluating a more difficult contrast between clinically similar study subjects will be useless: the index test cannot be expected to add anything valuable to clinical practice anyhow.

The specification of these three aspects of the research question is decisive for designing the optimal study methodology. Aspect (c) was extensively addressed in Chapter 2.

Outline of the study design

Because study questions on diagnostic accuracy generally evaluate the association between (combinations of) test results and health status (mostly the presence or absence of a target disorder), a cross-sectional design is a natural basic design option. However, this basic design has various modifications, each with specific pros and cons in terms of scientific requirements, burden for the study subjects, and efficient use of resources.

Box 3.2 Study design

General approach

- – survey of total study population
- – case–referent approach
- – test-based enrolment

Direction of data collection

- – prospective
- – ambispective
- – retrospective

General approach

The most straightforward approach of the cross-sectional design is a survey of the study population to determine the test distribution and the presence of the target disorder simultaneously. Examples are a survey on the relationship between intermittent claudication and peripheral arterial occlusive disease in an elderly population[12] and a study in a consecutive series of sciatica patients to determine the accuracy of history and clinical examination.[13]

Another option is the case–referent approach, starting from an already known disease status (e.g., present or absent) as the criterion for enrollment, the test result being determined afterward in the study patients. This design type may be more efficient or more acceptable when the disease under study is infrequent or when the reference standard procedure is highly invasive to the patient, as with pancreatic cancer, or expensive.

A further approach is test-based enrollment, where the available test result (such as positive or negative) is the criterion for recruitment, with the disease status being determined afterward. This modification may be preferable when test results are easily available from routine health care. An example regarding the latter is a study on the diagnostic value of "fatigue" for detecting anemia in primary care, comparing patients presenting with fatigue and a control group without fatigue as to hematological parameters.[14]

In the context of the cross-sectional design, efficient sampling of the studied distributions may be artificially facilitated at the determinant (test) or the outcome (target disorder) side. For example, to achieve a balanced data collection over the relevant categories, a stratified sample can be drawn from the various test result levels or from various parts of the whole disease spectrum, from clearly no disease to most severe disease. Also, the contrast between the categories of the diseased and nondiseased subjects can be enhanced by limiting the sampling to those who have been proved to be clearly diseased and those proved to be completely healthy. The latter approach is applied in planning a Phase I study (Chapter 2), which is essentially a case–referent study. Because of a sharp contrast in disease spectrum between diseased and nondiseased, sensitivity and specificity will be optimal. In addition, as by sampling of cases and referents the "prevalence" in the study population can be artificially optimized (with, for example, a disease prevalence of 50%), Phase I studies generally need a relatively small number of subjects to be included. Moreover, for a Phase I study, the subjects in the "case group" (the diseased) and those in the reference group (the healthy or nondiseased subjects) can be specifically selected from populations consisting of subjects who have already undergone a "reference standard" procedure with maximum certainty.

Direction of data collection
Whereas Phase I and Phase II studies (according to Sackett and Haynes, Chapter 2) may be based on either retrospective or prospective identification of subjects with a certain diagnostic or test status, Phase III studies must usually be prospectively planned. The latter start from a study population of subjects comparable with those who will be tested in clinical practice. In such studies, it is not known in advance who is diseased and who is not, and the clinical

characteristics of the two are therefore similar (which in fact, is the reason that testing is clinically necessary at all). Because the clinical contrast is much less pronounced, and as the prevalence of diseased subjects is usually much lower than 50%, substantially larger sample sizes are generally needed than in Phase I studies.

Also, when the subject selection is prospective, the data collection can be partly retrospective (ambispective approach). For instance, if patient history is an important element of the diagnostic test to be evaluated (such as when studying the diagnostic value of rectal bleeding, palpitations, or psychiatric symptoms in the preceding 6 months), information about the past is included in the test result. Essential, however, is that the test result status, albeit based on historical information, is evaluated and interpreted as to its diagnostic accuracy when the patient "history" is taken.

The "direction" of the sampling and the data collection must be decided on in advance. In addition, secondary to scientific considerations, practical issues may play a role, such as the availability of data and the efficiency of its collection. Prospectively planned data collections often take more time but are generally more valid, as the procedure and the quality of the data collection can be optimized beforehand. But this is not always the case. Valid data may be already available in a well-documented database of an appropriate study population with an adequately described epidemiological (morbidity) numerator and (population) denominator and with all relevant covariables present. Especially when the clinical indication to perform the test is appropriately defined (e.g., coronary angiography in instable angina pectoris) and recorded, and when all eligible patients can be assumed to be included, this is an option. Also, a prospective data collection may sometimes imply a higher risk of bias than a retrospective approach. For example, if participating clinicians can know that they are being observed in a study of the accuracy of their usual diagnostic assessment compared with an independent standard or panel, their behavior could be easily influenced in the context of a prospective design (Hawthorne effect). However, in a retrospective design, the availability of complete and well-standardized data and the controlling of the subject selection process are often problematic.[15]

Operationalizing determinants and outcome

Determinants
As in any (clinical) epidemiological study, research questions on diagnostic accuracy can be operationalized in a central "occurrence relation"[16] between independent and dependent variables.

The independent variable or determinant of primary interest is the test result to be evaluated, and the primary dependent or outcome variable is (presence or absence of) the target disorder. When evaluating a single test, the test results in all study subjects are related to the reference standard. In fact, we are then comparing testing (yielding the posttest probabilities of the disorder D,

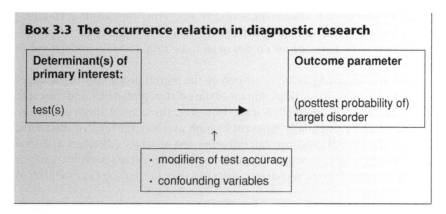

Box 3.3 The occurrence relation in diagnostic research

Determinant(s) of primary interest:		Outcome parameter
test(s)	⟶	(posttest probability of) target disorder

↑

- modifiers of test accuracy
- confounding variables

for example, for positive and negative test results) with not testing (expressed in the pretest probability of D). When two or more tests are compared, we have a number of separate determinants that are contrasted as to their discriminatory power. In studying the value of an additional (more invasive) test, given the tests already performed, the discrimination of applying all other tests is compared with that of applying all other tests plus the additional one. And to evaluate the most accurate or efficient diagnostic test set or strategy for a certain clinical problem, the performances of all the considered test combinations and sequences must be compared. To be able to make these comparisons, all separate tests have to be performed in all study subjects.

The accuracy of diagnostic tests may vary in relation to subject characteristics, such as gender, age, and comorbidity. For example, in studying the diagnostic accuracy of mammography in the detection of breast cancer, it is important to consider that this accuracy depends on age, gender, and the possible presence of fibroadenomatosis of the breasts. To evaluate the influence of such modifiers of test accuracy, these have to be measured and included in the analysis. In fact, we are dealing here with various subgroups in which the diagnostic accuracy may be different. Effect-modifying variables can be accounted for later in the analysis by stratified analysis (subgroup analysis) of the measures of diagnostic association or by introducing interaction terms in logistic regression analysis (Chapter 8).[17–18] Because diagnostic assessment can be seen as optimal discrimination between subgroups with a different probability of disease, effect-modifying variables can also be considered as additional diagnostic tests themselves.

Confounding variables are independent extraneous determinants of the outcome that may obscure or inflate an association between the test and the disorder. They are essentially related to both the test result and the outcome. For example, in studying whether the symptom fatigue is predictive for a low blood hemoglobin level, it is important to know which study subjects have previously taken oral iron, as this can improve the fatigue symptoms and enhance the hemoglobin level as well. A confounder can only be controlled for if it is considered beforehand and measured, which requires insight into relevant external influences. In diagnostic research, the term "confounding variable" is used in a different, more pragmatic sense than in etiologic research, as consistent diagnostic correlations do not need to be fully causally understood to be useful.

Generally, according to Bayes's theorem, the pretest probability of the target disorder is seen as a basic determinant of the posttest probability, independent of the accuracy of the applied tests. However, the clinical spectrum of the disorder may be essentially different in high and low prevalence situations. Because the clinical spectrum can influence test accuracy (Chapters 1, 2, and 6), it is then crucial to separately measure spectrum characteristics, such as disease severity. Spectrum characteristics can then be analyzed as modifiers of test accuracy.

Good test reproducibility is a requirement for good accuracy in practice. Therefore, when the test under study is sensitive to inter- or intra-observer variability, documentation, and, if possible, reduction of this variability is important. Documentation can be achieved in a pilot study or in the context of the main study. For example, in a study of the accuracy and reproducibility of erythrocyte sedimentation rate (ESR) measurements in general practice centers, for measuring an identical specimen a clinically relevant range between practices from 4 to 40 mm/1 h was observed. The average coefficient of variation (CV: standard deviation as a percentage of the mean) was 37% between practices and 28% within practices.[19] Observer variability can be reduced by training. In the same ESR study, the average inter- and intrapractice CVs were reduced by training to 17% and 7%, respectively. The accuracy of a test can be evaluated in relation to the achieved reproducibility. This reproducibility must then, for practical purposes, be judged for its clinical acceptability and feasibility.

Outcome: the reference standard

Principles
Establishing a final and "gold standard" diagnosis of the target disorder is generally more invasive and expensive than applying the studied diagnostic test. It is exactly for this reason that good test accuracy (e.g., a very high sensitivity and specificity) would be useful in clinical practice to make a satisfactory diagnostic assessment without having to perform the reference standard. However, in performing diagnostic research, the central outcome variable – the presence or absence of the target disorder – must be measured, as it is the reference standard for estimating the test accuracy. A real gold – that is, perfect – standard test, with 100% sensitivity and specificity under all circumstances, is exceptional. Even pathological classification and MRI imaging are not infallible, and may yield false positive, false negative, and uninterpretable conclusions. Therefore, the term "reference standard" is nowadays considered better than "gold standard."

Box 3.4 The reference standard

Principles

  - to be applied on all included subjects
  - independent assessment of test and standard
  - standardized protocol

Possible problems with the reference standard

  - imperfect: classification errors
  - pathophysiological concept not well defined (independent from clinical presentation)
  - incorporation bias
  - too invasive
  - too complex

Possible solutions

  - pragmatic criteria
  - independent expert panel
  - clinical follow-up: delayed-type cross-sectional study
  - tailor-made standard protocol
  - prognostic criterion

The reference standard to establish the final diagnosis (outcome) should be applied for all included subjects. Applying different standard procedures for different patients may yield an inconsistent reference for the evaluated test, as each of the "standards" will have its own idiosyncratic error rate.

As a matter of principle, the results of the test for each patient should be interpreted without knowledge of the reference standard results. Similarly, the reference standard result should be established without knowing the outcome of the test under study. Where such blinding is not maintained, "test review bias" and "diagnosis review bias" may occur: nonindependent assessment of test and reference standard, mostly resulting in overestimation of test accuracy. The principle of blinding is especially important if subjective factors play a role in determining test results or the reference standard.[20]

The reference standard must be properly performed and interpreted using standardized criteria. Also this is especially important when the standard diagnosis depends on subjective interpretations, for example, by a psychiatrist, a pathologist, or a radiologist. In such cases, inter- and even intraobserver variability in establishing the standard can occur. For example, in evaluating the intraobserver variability of MRI assessment as the standard for nerve root compression in sciatica patients, the same radiologist repeatedly scored the presence of root compression as such consistently (κ: 1.0) but the site of root compression only moderately (κ: 0.60). In these situations, training sessions and permanent documentation of performance are important.[13]

Problems and solutions

Apart from the limitations in reaching a 100% perfect standard diagnosis because of classification error, meeting the requirements for a reference standard can be inherently problematic in various ways.

For many conditions, a reference standard cannot be measured on the basis of a well-defined pathophysiological concept, fully independent of the clinical presentation. Examples are sinusitis, migraine, depression, irritable bowel syndrome, and benign prostatic hyperplasia.[21] As, in such cases, information related to the test result (e.g., symptom status) is incorporated into the diagnostic criteria, "incorporation bias" may result in overestimation of test accuracy. Furthermore, a defined reference standard procedure may sometimes be too invasive for research purposes. For instance, when validating urinary flow measurement it would be unacceptable to apply invasive urodynamic studies to those with normal flow results.[22] And in studying the diagnostic value of nonacute abdominal pain in primary care for diagnosing intra-abdominal cancer, one cannot imagine that, as a definitive reference standard, all patients presenting with nonacute abdominal pain would be routinely offered laparotomy.[23] In addition, one may doubt whether such laparotomy, if it were to be performed, could always provide an accurate final diagnosis in the very early stage of a malignancy. Another problem can be that a complex reference standard might include a large number of laboratory tests, so that many false positive test results could occur by chance.

For these problems, practical solutions have been sought, as follows.

Pragmatic criteria

The absence of a well-defined pathophysiological concept can sometimes be overcome by defining consensus-based pragmatic criteria. However, if applying such reference standard criteria (such as a cut-off value on a depression questionnaire) is no more difficult than applying the test under study, evaluating and introducing the test will not be very useful.

Independent expert panel

Another method is the composition of an independent expert panel that, given general criteria and decision rules for clinical agreement, can assign a final diagnosis to each patient, based on the available clinical information. To achieve a consistent classification, the panel must be well prepared for its task, and a training session or pilot study using patients with an already established diagnosis is recommended. The agreement of the primary assessments of the individual panel members, before reaching to consensus, can be documented.

Clinical follow-up: delayed-type cross-sectional study

When applying a definitive reference standard is too invasive or otherwise inapplicable at the moment that the test should be predictive for the presence of the target disorder, a good alternative can be follow up of the clinical course during a suitable predefined period. Most diseases that are not self-limiting, such as cancers and chronic degenerative diseases, will usually become clinically manifest a period of months or a year or so after the first diagnostic suspicion (generally the moment of enrollment in the study) was raised. The follow-up period should not be too short to give early phase disorders the chance to become manifest and therefore to have a minimum number of "false negative" final diagnoses. Nor should it be too long to avoid the final diagnosis after follow-up being related to a new disease episode started after the baseline "cross section" (false positives).[23,24] In addition, it would be ideal to collect the decisive follow-up data for making the final diagnosis independently from and blinded to the health status and test results at time zero and also to blind the final outcome assessment for these test results.

One should take into account that "confounding by indication" can occur: management decisions during follow-up are possibly related to the health status at baseline and might therefore influence the clinical course and the probability of detecting the target disorder. This is especially a point of concern in studying target disorders with a rather variable clinical course, becoming clinically manifest dependent on management decisions.

It has to be acknowledged that the described method of clinical follow-up should not be considered as a "follow-up," or "cohort" study, as the focus is not on relating the time zero data to a subsequently developing (incident) disorder. In fact, the follow-up procedure is aimed at retrospectively assessing the (prevalent) health status at time zero, as a substitute for establishing the reference standard diagnosis of the target disorder immediately at time zero. Therefore, this design modification can be designated a "delayed-type cross-sectional study" instead of a follow-up study.[24,25]

The expert panel and the clinical follow-up can be combined in a composite reference standard procedure, in which the outcome after follow-up is evaluated and established by the panel.[23]

Tailor-made reference standard protocol

In some situations, for example, in diagnostic research on psychiatric illnesses, it can be difficult to separate test data at time zero (the presence of anxiety) from the information needed to make a final assessment (anxiety disorder). As mentioned earlier, in such situations, incorporation bias may be the result. If test data are indeed an essential part of the diagnostic criteria, one cannot avoid balancing a certain risk of incorporation bias against not being able to perform diagnostic research at all, or making a final diagnosis while ignoring an important element of the criteria. Often, one can find a practical compromise in considering that for clinical purposes it is sufficient to know to what extent the available diagnostic tests at time zero are able to predict the target disorder's becoming clinically manifest during a reasonably chosen follow-up period.[25] There is also the option to ask the expert panel to establish the final diagnosis first without the baseline test data and then to repeat it with these data incorporated. This can be done while adding an extra blinding step, such as randomly rearranging the order of anonymous patient records. If there then appear to be important differences in the research conclusions, this should be transparently reported and discussed as to the clinical implications.

When it is impossible to meet the principle that the reference standard should be similarly applied to all study subjects irrespective of their health or test result status, "next best" solutions can be considered. For example, to determine the accuracy of the exercise electrocardiogram (ECG) in primary care settings, it might be considered medically and ethically unjustified to submit those with a negative test result to coronary angiography. For these test negatives, a well-standardized clinical follow-up protocol (delayed-type cross-sectional study) might be acceptable. This option is particularly important when the focus is on the validity of exercise ECG in patients who have a relatively low prior probability of coronary heart disease. For this spectrum of patients, results of a study limited to those who would be clinically selected for coronary angiography would be clearly not applicable.[26,27,28] If so, one would still prefer an identical standard procedure for primary care patients, irrespective of previous test results, one could consider submitting all patients to the clinical follow-up standard procedure. To have some validation of this procedure, for the subgroup that had an angiography, one can compare the standard diagnoses based on the follow up with the angiography results.

In summary, although an identical and "hard" reference standard for all included study subjects is the general methodological paradigm, this is not always achievable. In such situations, given the described limitations and the suggested alternative approaches, a priori establishing a well-documented and reproducible reference standard protocol – indicating the optimal procedure for each type of patient – may be not only the best one can get but also sufficient for clinical purposes.

Prognostic criterion
Diagnostic testing should ultimately be in favor of the patient's health, rather than just an assessment of the probability of the presence of disease. In view of this, it is useful to incorporate prognosis or consequences for clinical management into the reference standard procedure.[29,30] It is then a starting point for further decision making (for example, whether treatment is useful or not) rather than a diagnostic endpoint. This is especially relevant in situations in which an exact nosological classification is impossible or not important, and when management is based primarily on the clinical assessment (e.g., in deciding about physiotherapy in low back pain or referral to a neurosurgeon in sciatica[13]). Sometimes making a final diagnosis is less important than a prognosis, in view of the clinical consequences (incidental fever) or the lack of a solid diagnostic consensus (pyriformis syndrome).

In establishing a "prognostic reference criterion," a pitfall is that prognosis can be influenced by interfering treatments. In this context, methods for unbiased assessment of the impact of testing on patient prognosis are important (Chapter 4). It is to be expected that with the progress of DNA testing for disease, prognostic relevance will increasingly be the reference standard, rather than just classifying.[31] Accordingly, "dia-prognostic" research, connecting diagnosis and prognosis as the basis for clinical decision making, will be high on the future research agenda.[32]

Standard shift as a result of new insights

At certain moments during the progress of pathophysiological knowledge on diagnosis, new diagnostic tests may be developed that are better than the currently prevailing reference standards. If this possibility is systematically ignored by reducing diagnostic accuracy research to just comparing new tests with traditional standards, possible new reference standards would never be recognized, as they would always seem less accurate than the traditional ones. Therefore, pathophysiological expertise should be involved in the evaluation of diagnostic accuracy. Examples of a shift in reference standard are the replacement of the clinical definition of tuberculosis by the identification of *Mycobacterium tuberculosis*, and of old imaging techniques by new ones (see also Chapter 1).

Specifying the study population

As in all clinical research, the study population for diagnostic research should be appropriately chosen, defined, and recruited. The selection of patients is crucial for the study outcome and its external (clinical) validity. As has already been emphasized, it is widely recognized that diagnostic accuracy is much dependent on the spectrum of included patients and the results of relevant tests performed earlier and may differ for primary care patients and patients referred to a hospital.[7,8,28]

After the test has successfully passed Phase I and Phase II studies (Chapter 2), the starting point is the clinical problem for which the test under study should be evaluated as to its diagnostic accuracy, taking the relevant health care setting into account. For example, the study can address the diagnostic accuracy of clinical tests for sciatica in general practice, the accuracy of ECG recording in outpatients with palpitations without a compelling clinical reason for immediate referral, or the diagnostic accuracy of the MRI scan in diagnosing intracerebral pathology in an academic neurological center. The study population should be representative for the "indicated," "candidate," or "intended" patient population, also called the target population, being clinically similar to the group of patients in whom the validated test is to be applied in practice (intention to test).[33,34] The "intention to diagnose" should be the key criterion for the study of newly presented clinical problems. For the evaluation of population screening of asymptomatic subjects, such as in the context of breast cancer screening or hypertension case finding, a study population similar to the target population "intended to be screened" is required.

Box 3.5 Study population

- In accordance with studied clinical problem
- Intention to test: "Intention to diagnose" or "intention to screen"
- Inclusion criteria corresponding with "indicated" population
- ("Iatrotropic") consecutive series or target population survey

---

The next step is generally straightforward: the specification of the relevant process of selection of patients for the study (corresponding with the clinical problem and the health care setting requirements), and the relevant inclusion criteria (in accordance with the indicated population and the relevant patient spectrum). Exclusion criteria may also be defined, identifying those patients for whom the reference standard procedure is too risky or too burdensome. The importance of explicitly formulated entry criteria is demonstrated by a study on the diagnostic value of reported collapse for the diagnosis of clinically relevant arrhythmias in general practice: if the inclusion was based on presented symptoms the odds ratio (OR) was 1.9, whereas for an inclusion based on coincidentally finding a pulse, <60 or >100 bpm or an irregular pulse, the OR was 10.1.[35] Investigators should include "indicated" patients, as long as there is no compelling reason not to do so in order to avoid that after the study a non-evidence-based testing practice will not be introduced or maintained for relevant parts of the "real-life" patient spectrum. In this context, it is emphasized that in the elderly, comorbidity in addition to the possible presence of the target disorder is often an important aspect of clinical reality.[36] For the clinical applicability of the study, measuring comorbidity and studying it as a modifier of diagnostic accuracy is the preferred approach, instead of excluding it.

In the section on study design, we discussed the choice between population survey and disorder- or test-oriented subject selection, covering the principal starting point of patient recruitment. In addition, the pros and cons of the various options for practical patient recruitment should be considered, as emphasized before. When problems presented to clinicians are studied, recruiting (a random sample of) a series of consecutively presenting patients who meet the criteria of the indicated population is most sensible for clinical validity purposes. This should preferably be supported by a description of the patient flow in health care before presentation. Sometimes, however, it may take too long to await the enrollment of a sufficiently large consecutive series – when the clinical problem or target disorder is very rare, or when a useful contribution to rapidly progressing diagnostic knowledge can only be made within a limited period. In such situations, active surveys of the target population or sampling from a patient register can be alternatives. However, it should be borne in mind that such methods may yield a population of study subjects with a different clinical spectrum. Also, for such subjects the indication to test is less clear than for patients who experienced an "iatrotropic" stimulus[4, 37] to visit a doctor at the very moment that they want their health problem to be solved.

Of course, for validating test procedures to be used in population screening, an active survey of a study population similar to the target population is the best approach.

In order to enhance external validity, it is essential to measure key demographic and clinical characteristics of the identified study population, and to evaluate nonresponse in relation to these characteristics. Furthermore, all important steps in the study protocol, with data on specific subgroups, including subgroup nonresponse, should be documented. This can be supported by a flow diagram.

Adverse effects of test and reference standard

Apart from its accuracy, the performance of a test has to be evaluated as to its (dis)comfort to both patient and doctor. In particular, a test should be minimally invasive and have a minimal risk of adverse effects and serious complications. Measuring these aspects in the context of a diagnostic accuracy study can add to the comparison with other tests as to their clinical pros and cons.

For the research community, it is also important to learn about the invasiveness and risks of the reference standard used. For example, if in the evaluation of the positive test results of hemoccult screening colonoscopy, sigmoidoscopy, or double-contrast barium enema were to be used, one might expect complications (perforation or hemorrhage) once in 300–900 subjects investigated.[38] Researchers can use the experience reported by colleagues studying similar problems to make an optimal choice of reference standard procedure, taking possible adverse events into consideration.

Statistical aspects

Box 3.6 Statistical aspects

- Sample size
- Bivariate and multivariable analysis
- Test accuracy or prediction of outcome
- Single test, comparing tests or strategies, additional testing
- Difference between diagnostic and etiologic data analysis

In the planning phase of the study, the required sample size is often not considered, although it is not less important than in any clinical epidemiological study.[39] To evaluate the relationship between a dichotomous test and the presence of a disorder, one can use the usual programs for sample size estimation. For example, for a case–referent study with equal group sizes, accepting certain values for type I and type II errors (e.g., 0.05 and 0.20, respectively) and using two-sided testing, one can calculate the number of subjects needed per group to detect a minimum sensitivity (proportion of test positives among the diseased, e.g., at least 0.60) assuming a certain maximum proportion of test positives among nondiseased (e.g., 0.20, implying a specificity of at least 0.80). For this example, the calculation using the program EPI-Info would yield a required number of 27 cases and 27 referents. Of course, when performing a cross-sectional study prospectively in a consecutive series with a low expected prevalence of the target disorder (i.e., unequal group sizes for disease status), the required sample will be much higher. Also, if a number of determinants is simultaneously included in the analysis, the required sample size is higher: as a rule of thumb, for each determinant at least 10 subjects with the target disorder are needed.[40]

Data analysis in diagnostic research follows the general lines of that in clinical epidemiological research. For single tests the first step is a bivariate analysis focused on one predictive variable only, for example in a 2×2 table in the case of a dichotomous test. It is possible to stratify for modifiers of accuracy, thereby distinguishing relevant clinical subgroups, and to adjust for potential confounding variables. In addition to point estimates, confidence intervals for the measures of diagnostic accuracy can be determined.[41] Subsequently, there are various options for multivariable analysis, taking multiple independent and various outcome variables into account simultaneously. Multiple logistic regression is especially useful for analyzing accuracy data.[17,18,19,42] The data analytical challenges in diagnostic research are discussed in detail in Chapters 7 and 8.

It is important to distinguish the analytical approach focusing on the accuracy of individual tests from the analysis where an optimal prediction of the presence of the studied disorder in patients is at stake. In the first, the dependent variable may even be test accuracy itself, as a function of various determinants. In the latter, a diagnostic prediction model can be derived with disease probability as the dependent variable, and with various tests, demographic, and clinical covariables as independent variables.[43,44,45]

When a number of tests are applied, there are various analytical options. First, the accuracy of all tests can be determined and compared. Furthermore, using multivariable analysis such as multiple logistic regression, the combined predictive power of sets of test variables can be determined. Moreover, starting from the least invasive and most easily available test (such as history taking), it can be evaluated whether adding more invasive or more expensive tests contributes to the diagnosis. For example, the subsequent contributions of history, physical examination, laboratory testing, and more elaborate additional investigations can be analyzed, supported by displaying the ROC curves (with areas under the curve) of the respectively extended test sets (see Chapters 7 and 8).[12,35,46]

It must be acknowledged that data analysis in diagnostic research is essentially different from etiologic data analysis. The principal difference is that etiologic analysis usually focuses on the effect of a hypothesized etiologic factor adjusted for the influence of possible confounders, thereby aiming at a causal interpretation. In diagnostic research, the focus is on identifying the best correlates of the target disorder irrespective of causal interpretations. It is, in fact, sufficient if these correlates (tests) can be systematically and reproducibly used for diagnostic prediction. Whereas in etiologic analysis there is a natural hierarchical relation between the possible etiologic factor of interest and the covariables to be adjusted for, such a hierarchy is absent for the possible predictors in diagnostic research. This implies that diagnostic data analysis can be more pragmatic, seeking for the best systematic correlates.

External validation

Analyses of diagnostic accuracy in the collected data set, especially the results of multivariable analyses, may produce too optimistic results that may not be reproducible in clinical practice or similar study populations.[47,48] Therefore, while this is not always done,[49] it is advisable to perform one or more separate external validation studies in independent but clinically similar populations.

Box 3.7 External (clinical) validation

- Results based on study data may be too optimistic
- "Split-half" analysis is no external validation
- Repeated studies in other, similar populations are preferred
- First exploration: compare first included half with second half
- Role of systematic reviews and meta-analysis

Sometimes authors derive a diagnostic model in a random part of the research data set and test its performance in the other part (e.g., split-half analysis). However, this approach is not addressing the issue of external validation: in fact, it only evaluates the degree of random error at the cost of possibly increasing such error by reducing the available sample size, often by 50%.[43] Also, other methods using one and the same database do not provide a real external validation. An exploratory approximation, however, could be to compare the performance of the diagnostic model in the chronologically first enrolled half of the patients, with that in the second half. The justification is that the second half is not a random sample of the total but rather a subsequent clinically similar study population. However, totally independent studies in other, clinically similar settings will be more convincing. In fact, over time, various studies can be done in comparable settings, enabling diagnostic systematic reviews and meta-analyses to be performed or updated. This may yield a constantly increasing insight into the performance of the studied diagnostic tests, both in general and in relevant clinical subgroups (Chapter 10).

Concluding remarks

Compared to research into etiology, pathophysiology, and treatment effects, diagnostic accuracy research has relatively recently been established as a specific domain of scientific interest.[50] This is an important development, as optimizing clinical decision making, health care provision, and patients' outcome largely depends on the quality of diagnostic performance.

As in any research, investigating the accuracy of diagnostic testing starts from the research question. It is based on the clinical problem under study, the test contrast to be evaluated, and the current state of knowledge, and is the key to the most appropriate research design. The elaborated research protocol should include the design type; the relevant determinants, encompassing the test(s) of interest, possible modifiers of test accuracy, and confounding variables; the reference standard procedure; inclusion criteria and a recruitment procedure that matches the clinical problem and the target population; a well-motivated sample size; and a suitably planned statistical analysis. These key elements should also be clearly reflected in the reporting of diagnostic accuracy studies in scientific journals, supported by the STARD guidelines (Chapter 9).[51] External (clinical) validation will generally require a new study in one or more independent, similar populations and justify separate publication, also to feed systematic reviews and meta-analyses.[52] Sometimes reviewers and editors do not well understand this if they ask that the primary diagnostic accuracy report should already include an external validation study, while they would never require such a "double study" in the case of a randomized therapy trial.

In view of the close relation between diagnosis, prognosis, and clinical decision making, it is important to connect accuracy research with the evaluation of prognostic impact. This will be further elaborated in the next chapter.

References

1. van den Akker M, Buntinx F, Metsemakers JF, et al. Multimorbidity in general practice: prevalence, incidence, and determinants of co-occurring chronic and recurrent diseases. *J Clin Epidemiol.* 1998;**51**:367–75.
2. Feinstein AR. Misguided efforts and future challenges for research on "diagnostic tests." *J Epidemiol Community Health.* 2002;**56**:330–32.
3. van den Bruel A, Cleemput I, Aertgeerts B, et al. The evaluation of diagnostic tests: various study designs are needed. *J Clin Epidemiol.* 2007;**60**(11):1116–22.
4. Feinstein AR. *Clinical epidemiology: the architecture of clinical research.* Philadelphia: W.B. Saunders; 1985.
5. Sackett DL, Haynes RB, Guyatt GH, et al. *Clinical epidemiology: a basic science for clinical medicine.* Boston: Little, Brown; 1985.
6. Lijmer JG, Mol BW, Heisterkamp S, et al. Empirical evidence of design-related bias in studies of diagnostic tests. *JAMA.* 1999;**282**:1061–66.
7. Ransohoff DF, Feinstein AR. Problems of spectrum and bias in evaluating the efficacy of diagnostic tests. *N Engl J Med.* 1978;**299**:926–30.
8. Knottnerus JA, Leffers P. The influence of referral patterns on the characteristics of diagnostic tests. *J Clin Epidemiol.* 1992;**45**:1143–54.

9. Moons KGM, Es GA van, Deckers JW, et al. Limitations of sensitivity, specificity, likelihood ratio, and Bayes's theorem in assessing diagnostic probabilities: a clinical example. *Epidemiology.* 1997;**8**:12–17.

10. Bossuyt PM, Irwig L, Craig J, et al. Comparative accuracy: assessing new tests against existing diagnostic pathways. *BMJ.* 2006;**332**:1089–92.

11. Sackett DL, Haynes RB. The architecture of diagnostic research. *BMJ.* 2002; **324**:539–41.

12. Stoffers HEJH. *Peripheral arterial occlusive disease: prevalence and diagnostic management in general practice.* PhD dissertation, Maastricht University, Maastricht: Datawyse; 1995.

13. Vroomen PCAJ. *The diagnosis and conservative treatment of sciatica.* PhD dissertation, Maastricht University, Maastricht: Datawyse, 1998.

14. Knottnerus JA, Knipschild PG, Van Wersch JWJ, et al. Unexplained fatigue and hemoglobin, a primary care study. *Can Fam Physician.* 1986;**32**:1601–164.

15. Oostenbrink R, Moons KG, Bleeker SE, et al. Diagnostic research on routine care data: prospects and problems. *J Clin Epidemiol.* 2003;**56**:501–6.

16. Miettinen OS. *Theoretical epidemiology: principles of occurrence research in medicine.* New York: John Wiley & Sons; 1985.

17. Spiegelhalter DJ, Knill-Jones RD. Statistical and knowledge-based approaches to clinical decision support systems, with an application to gastroenterology. *J R Stat Soc.* 1984;**147**:35–76.

18. Chan SF, Deeks JJ, Macaskill P, et al. Three methods to construct predictive models using logistic regression and likelihood ratios to facilitate adjustment for pretest probability give similar results. *J Clin Epidemiol.* 2008;**61**(1):52–63.

19. Dinant GJ, Knottnerus JA, Van Aubel PGJ, et al. Reliability of the erythrocyte sedimentation rate in general practice. *Scand J Primary Health Care.* 1989;**7**:231–35.

20. Moons KG, Grobbee DE. When should we remain blind and when should our eyes remain open in diagnostic studies? *J Clin Epidemiol.* 2002;**55**:633–36.

21. Spigt MG, van Schayck CP, van Kerrebroeck PE, et al. Pathophysiological aspects of bladder dysfunction: a new hypothesis for the prevention of "prostatic" symptoms. *Med Hypotheses.* 2004;**62**:448–52.

22. Wolfs GGMC. *Obstructive micturition problems in elderly male, prevalence and diagnosis in general practice.* PhD dissertation, Maastricht University, Maastricht: Datawyse, 1997.

23. Muris JW, Starmans R. *Non acute abdominal complaints: diagnostic studies in general practice and outpatient clinic.* PhD dissertation, Maastricht University, Maastricht; 1993.

24. Warndorff DK, Knottnerus JA, Huijnen LG, et al. How well do general practitioners manage dyspepsia? *J R Coll Gen Pract.* 1989;**39**:499–502.

25. Knottnerus JA, Dinant GJ. Medicine based evidence, a prerequisite for evidence based medicine. *BMJ.* 1997;**315**:1109–10.

26. Green MS. The effect of validation group bias on screening tests for coronary artery disease. *Stat Med.* 1985;**4**:53–61.

27. Begg CB, Greenes RA. Assessment of diagnostic tests when disease verification is subject to selection bias. *Biometrics.* 1983;**39**:207–16.

28. Knottnerus JA. The effects of disease verification and referral on the relationship between symptoms and diseases. *Med Decis Making.* 1987;**7**:139–48.

29. Hunink MG. Outcome research and cost-effectiveness analysis in radiology. *Eur Radiol.* 1996;**6**:615–20.

30. Moons KGM. *Diagnostic research: theory and application.* PhD dissertation, Erasmus Medical Centre, Rotterdam, 1996.

31. Ransohoff DF. Challenges and opportunities in evaluating diagnostic tests. *J Clin Epidemiol.* 2002;**55**:1178–82.
32. Knottnerus JA. Challenges in dia-prognostic research. *J Epidemiol Community Health.* 2002;**56**:340–41.
33. Dinant GJ. *Diagnostic value of the erythrocyte sedimentation rate en general practice.* PhD dissertation, Maastricht University, Maastricht; 1991.
34. van der Schouw YT, Verbeek AL, Ruijs SH. Guidelines for the assessment of new diagnostic tests. *Invest Radiol.* 1995;**30**:334–40.
35. Zwietering P. *Arrhythmias in general practice, prevalence and clinical diagnosis.* PhD dissertation, Maastricht University, Maastricht: Datawyse, 2000.
36. Schellevis FG, van der Velden J, van de Lisdonk E, et al. Comorbidity of chronic diseases in general practice. *J Clin Epidemiol.* 1993;**46**:469–73.
37. Knottnerus JA. Between iatrotropic stimulus and interiatric referral: the domain of primary care research. *J Clin Epidemiol.* 2002;**55**:1201–6.
38. Towler BP, Irwig L, Glasziou P, et al. Screening for colorectal cancer using the faecal occult blood test, hemoccult. *Cochrane Database Syst Rev.* 2007;(1):CD001216.
39. Bachmann LM, Puhan MA, ter Riet G, et al. Sample sizes of studies on diagnostic accuracy: literature survey. *BMJ.* 2006;**332**:1127–29.
40. Harrell FE, Jr, Lee KL, Mark DB. Multivariable prognostic models: issues in developing models, evaluating assumptions and adequacy, and measuring and reducing errors. *Stat Med.* 1996;**15**:361–87.
41. Guyatt GH, Sackett DL, Haynes RB. Evaluating diagnostic tests. In: Haynes RB, Sackett DL, Guyatt GH, et al. *Clinical epidemiology: how to do clinical practice research.* Philadelphia: Lippincott, Williams & Wilkins; 2006.
42. Biesheuvel CJ, Vergouwe Y, Steyerberg EW, et al. Polytomous logistic regression analysis could be applied more often in diagnostic research. *J Clin Epidemiol.* 2008;**61**(2):125–34.
43. Knottnerus JA. Diagnostic prediction rules: principles, requirements and pitfalls. *Prim Care.* 1995;**22**:341–63.
44. Laupacis A, Sekar N, Stiell IG. Diagnosis: Clinical prediction rules: a review and suggested modifications of methodological standards. *JAMA.* 1997;**277**:488–94.
45. McGinn T, Guyatt G, Wyer P, et al. Clinical prediction rules. In: Guyatt J. and Rennie D. (eds.), *Users' guides to the medical literature,* pp 471–83 Chicago: AMA Press, 2004.
46. Hopstaken RM, Muris JW, Knottnerus JA, et al. Contributions of symptoms, signs, erythrocyte sedimentation rate, and C-reactive protein to a diagnosis of pneumonia in acute lower respiratory tract infection. *Br J Gen Pract.* 2003;**53**:358–64.
47. Starmans R, Muris JW, Fijten GH, et al. The diagnostic value of scoring models for organic and non-organic gastrointestinal disease, including the irritable-bowel syndrome. *Med Decis Making.* 1994;**14**:208–16.
48. Bleeker SE, Moll HA, Steyerberg EW, et al. External validation is necessary in prediction research: a clinical example. *J Clin Epidemiol.* 2003;**56**:826–32.
49. Van den Bruel A, Aertgeerts B, Buntinx F. Results of diagnostic accuracy studies are not always validated. *J Clin Epidemiol.* 2006;**59**:559–66.
50. Knottnerus JA, van Weel C, Muris JW. Evaluation of diagnostic procedures. *BMJ.* 2002;**324**:477–80.
51. Bossuyt PM, Reitsma JB, Bruns DE, et al. Towards complete and accurate reporting of studies of diagnostic accuracy: the STARD initiative. *Clin Radiol.* 2003;**58**:575–80.
52. Grobee DE, Hoes AW. Clinical Epidemiology. Principles, methods and applications for clinical research. Boston: Jones and Barlett, 2008.

CHAPTER 4

Diagnostic testing and prognosis: the randomized controlled trial in test evaluation research

Jeroen G. Lijmer and Patrick M. M. Bossuyt

Summary box

- Test evaluations should focus on the likelihood that tests detect clinical events of interest and the effect that tests can have on these events by the way in which test results affect subsequent management decisions.
- Randomized controlled trails of medical tests are feasible and several designs are possible.
- Randomized controlled trails of medical tests can be made more efficient by randomizing only patients with the test result of interest.
- A randomized controlled trail of medical tests should incorporate a prespecified link between test and treatment options to ascertain validity and generalizability.
- Sample-size calculations need special attention and have to include an estimation of the discordance rate.

Why bother about the prognostic impact of a diagnostic test?

For scientific purposes, it is worth knowing whether a result from a medical test corresponds to the truth. Can this value be trusted? Is this test result truly a sign of disease? These are the first questions that come to the mind in the evaluation of medical tests.

The Evidence Base of Clinical Diagnosis: Theory and Methods of Diagnostic Research. 2nd edition.
Edited by J. André Knottnerus and Frank Buntinx. © 2009 Blackwell Publishing,
ISBN: 978-1-4051-5787-2.

From a patient perspective, mere knowledge about the present, true state of things is in most cases not enough. They want to get better. In relieving their health problems, information will not always suffice. Patients mainly benefit from medical testing if the information generated by that test is correctly used in subsequent patient management decisions.

Medical tests can affect a patient's health in multiple ways. First, undergoing the test can have an impact. The adverse effects range from slight discomfort and temporary unpleasantness to lasting side effects or death. On the other side, undergoing an elaborate procedure can also have a nonspecific positive effect on patient complaints—regardless of the information that results from it. This can be called the "placebo" effect of testing. We know very little about the magnitude and modifying factors of this context effect.

In addition to the effects from the diagnostic procedure, the information generated by the test also influences patients. Providing information on the likely cause of one's health problems or other aspects of health status can have both a positive and a negative effect, albeit limited. As patients, we want to be informed about the origin of our complaints, even in the absence of a cure. Such information may enable us to find better ways of coping with the complaints, by developing strategies to limit their disabling impact on our daily activities.

However, the main effects of medical tests on patient outcome will be indirect, as the result of subsequent clinical decisions based on the test results. These results can lead to additional testing or to starting or withholding therapeutic interventions. In many cases, not only the present state of health that is of interest but also the future course of disease. It then follows that the value of information from diagnostic tests lies not only in the past (where did this come from) or the present (how is it) but also in the future. Hence, the relevance of diagnostic information is closely related to prognosis: the implications for the future course of the patient's condition.

The first section of this chapter discusses the evaluation of the prognostic impact of a single test, starting from an evaluation of its prognostic value and moving on to the consequences for treatment. It closes with a presentation of randomized designs for evaluating test–treatment combinations. The second section contains an elaboration of these methods for comparing and evaluating multiple test strategies, also including randomized clinical trials. The chapter ends with a discussion on practical issues.

How to measure prognostic impact of a test

A recent example of the assessment of the prognostic value of a test is an evaluation of the routine exercise treadmill testing after percutaneous coronary intervention, which showed no use for routine tests. A more extensive studied problem can be found in the literature on the management of carotid disease. Several studies have examined the need to perform duplex ultrasonography in patients with a cervical bruit without further symptoms of cerebrovascular

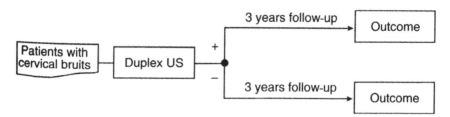

Figure 4.1 Prognostic study.

disease. To answer this question, an assessment has to be made of the value of duplex ultrasonography. Such an evaluation will often look at the amount of agreement between the index test (duplex ultrasonography) and the reference test (the best available method to reveal the true condition of the carotid arteries). In this case, the reference test will mostly likely be conventional angiography. If properly conducted, a 2 × 2 table can be constructed after the study is done and all indicators of diagnostic accuracy can be calculated. Unfortunately, many of the evaluation studies in diagnostic techniques for carotid stenosis performed so far did not meet the design requirements for an unbiased and useful evaluation.[1]

From a patient perspective, one could successfully argue that it is not so much the correspondence with "the truth" that should be of concern, especially not in asymptomatic patients. For these patients, the true value of the information should come from the strength of the association between data on the presence and the severity of carotid stenosis and the likelihood of vascular events in the near future. The appropriate reference standard for such an evaluation will not be an imaging procedure. Instead, one should look for clinical information collected through a meticulous follow-up of all patients subjected to the index test.

Figure 4.1 illustrates the general design of such a study. All patients with cervical bruits without previous cerebrovascular disease are eligible for the study. A duplex ultrasonography (US) of the right and left common and internal arteries is performed in all patients and the percentage of stenosis is measured. Ideally, none of the patients receives treatment. Subsequently, patients are followed by regular outpatient visits and telephone interviews. The following clinical indicators of poor outcome are recorded: transient ischemic attack (TIA), stroke, myocardial infarction, unstable angina, vascular deaths, and other deaths.

With data recorded in such a study, standard accuracy measures can be calculated to express the prognostic value of a test. Table 4.1, based on data published by Lewis et al.[2] shows a positive and negative predictive value of 47% and 80%, respectively, in predicting a poor outcome for a stenosis ≥80%, as detected on duplex. They also showed that the relative risk of a stenosis ≥50% for a TIA or stroke was 2.3. However, insufficient data were presented to reconstruct the 2×2 table for this cutoff point.

Table 4.1 Prognostic value of duplex ultrasonography

	Poor outcome	Favorable outcome	
Stenosis ≥ 80%	63 (47%)	72 (53%)	135
Stenosis <80%	113 (20%)	451 (80%)	564
Total	176	523	699

The study in Figure 4.1 can provide an answer to the question whether or not a test is able to discriminate between different risk categories for a specific event. Such prognostic information, although valuable to patients and health care professionals, does not answer whether there is an intervention that can improve the prognosis of these patients. To respond to the latter question, it is necessary to compare the prognosis for different treatment strategies.

Randomized designs for a single test

A slight modification of the design in Figure 4.1 allows us to measure the prognostic value of a test within the context of subsequent clinical decision making. Instead of treating all patients in an identical way, one can randomly allocate patients to one of the two treatment strategies, establishing the prognostic value of the test in each arm, in a way that is similar to the previous example.

A straightforward comparison of patient outcome in the two treatment arms provides an answer as to which treatment is the most effective for all patients included in the trial. Moreover, an analysis stratified by test result offers the possibility to compare the effectiveness of the treatment options for groups with identical test results.

This type of design and analysis can be illustrated with another example from the field of cerebrovascular disease. In the management of acute stroke patients, the role of intravenous anticoagulation and duplex ultrasonography of the carotid arteries is unclear. A large trial has been performed, with as its primary objective to document the efficacy of unfractionated heparin in the treatment of acute stroke. A secondary objective was an evaluation of the role of duplex ultrasonography in selecting patients for anticoagulation.[2–4] A simplified version of the design of this trial is outlined in Figure 4.2. Patients

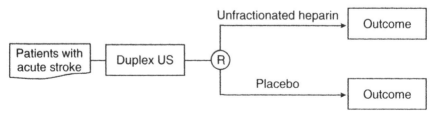

Figure 4.2 Basic RCT of a single diagnostic test.

Table 4.2 Analysis of a RCT of a single diagnostic test

a Unfractionated heparin	Poor outcome	Favorable outcome	
Stenosis ≥50%	38 (32%)	82 (68%)	120
Stenosis <50%	121 (23%)	400 (77%)	521
Total	159	482	641

b Placebo	Poor outcome	Favorable outcome	
Stenosis ≥ 50%	51 (47%)	58 (53%)	109
Stenosis <50%	116 (22%)	409 (78%)	525
Total	167	467	634

c Stenosis larger than 50% or occlusion	Poor outcome	Favorable outcome	
Unfract. heparin	38 (32%)	82 (68%)	120
Placebo	51 (47%)	58 (53%)	109
Total	89	140	229

d Stenosis Smaller than 50%	Poor outcome	Favorable outcome	
Unfract. heparin	121 (23%)	400 (77%)	521
Placebo	116 (22%)	409 (78%)	525
Total	237	809	1046

e Comparison of strategies	Poor outcome	Favorable outcome	
Duplex US	154 (24%)	491 (76%)	645
No duplex US	167 (26%)	467 (74%)	634
Total	321	958	1279

Duplex US: Decision whether to give UFH is based on duplex ultrasonography.
The odds ratios and their 95% CI (confidence interval) of a to e are 1.5 (0.99–2.4), 3.1 (2.0–4.8), 0.53 (0.31–0.90), 1.1 (0.80–1.4), and 0.88 (0.68–1.1). The relative odds ratio of a/b or c/d is 0.48.

with evidence of an ischemic stroke, with symptoms present for more than 1 hour but less than 24 hours, were eligible for the study. A duplex ultrasonography of the right and left common and internal arteries was performed in all included patients. Subsequently, patients were randomized to treatment with an unfractionated heparin or placebo and followed for 3 months. A favorable outcome after stroke was defined as a score of I (good recovery) or II (moderate disability) on the 5-point Glasgow Outcome Scale and a score of 12 to 20 on the modified Barthel Index.

Tables 4.2a and 4.2b show the prognostic value of Duplex ultrasonography in each trial arm. An odds ratio can be calculated for each table. These odds ratios can be interpreted as measures of the *natural prognostic value* (Table 4.2b) and the *prognostic value with intervention* (Table 2a), respectively. Another presentation of the same data gives us Tables 4.2c and 4.2d, which provide us with information on the treatment effect in both test result categories.

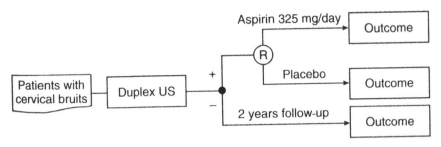

Figure 4.3 Randomizing abnormal test results.

We will call the odds ratios of the latter two tables *treatment effect in test normals* and *treatment effect in test abnormals*. In case the test discriminates well between patients that benefit from treatment and those that do not, the treatment effect in test abnormals will differ from the treatment effect in test normals. The ratio of the odds ratios of these two tables can therefore be used as a measure of the prognostic impact of the test.

The study in Figure 4.2 provides information on the treatment effect in all test result categories. In practice, it will not always be necessary or ethical to randomize all patients, as uncertainty may exist only for patients with a specific, say, abnormal, test result. This will be the case when there is information available that the prognosis for normal test results is good and that patients with such results need no intervention. A logical translation of such a question into a study design would be to randomize only patients with abnormal test results between the different treatment options.

Consider the first example of duplex ultrasonography in patients with cervical bruits. Such a trial could provide evidence that the natural history of patients with a stenosis of less than 50% have a good prognosis.

The trial outlined in Figure 4.3 can subsequently answer the question if therapy improves the prognosis of patients with a stenosis of 50% or more. As in the first example, all patients with cervical bruits without previous cerebrovascular disease are eligible for the study. A duplex ultrasonography of the right and left common and internal arteries is performed in all patients to measure the percentage of stenosis. Subsequently, if the stenosis is 50% or more, patients are randomly assigned to receive either aspirin 325 mg a day or placebo. The clinical endpoints, TIA, stroke, myocardial infarction, unstable angina, vascular deaths, and other deaths are recorded during follow-up.

Coté and colleagues performed such a trial in 1995. They randomized 372 neurologically asymptomatic patients with a carotid stenosis of 50% or more between aspirin and placebo. By comparing the outcomes in both treatment arms the effectiveness of treating patients with a stenosis of 50% or more with aspirin was evaluated (treatment effect in test abnormals). In 50 of the 188 patients receiving aspirin and 54 of the 184 patients receiving placebo a clinical event was measured during follow-up, yielding an adjusted hazard ratio (aspirin versus placebo) of 0.99 (95% confidence interval (CI), 0.67 to

Table 4.3 Analysis of a RCT, randomizing only abnormal test results

a Natural prognostic value				b Treatment effect in case of ≥50% stenosis			
	Poor outcome	Favorable outcome			Poor outcome	Favorable outcome	
Stenosis ≥50%*	54 (29%)	130 (71%)	184	Aspirin	50 (27%)	138 (73%)	188
Stenosis <50%	72 (22%)	255 (78%)	327	Placebo	54 (29%)	130 (71%)	184
Total	126	385	511	Total	104	268	372

RCT, randomized controlled trial.
*Random sample of patients with a stenosis ≥50%.

1.46). The authors concluded that aspirin did not have a significant long-term protective effect in asymptomatic patients with high-grade stenosis (more then 50%).

The trial in Figure 4.3 can also provide information on the accuracy of Duplex US in predicting the outcomes of interest (natural prognostic value). This can be done by comparing the outcome in patients in the placebo arm, who all had an abnormal test result, with the outcome in patients with a normal test result. A prerequisite for this comparison is that patient management in both of these arms is similar. Table 4.3a and 4.3b show the crude results and possible comparisons. Note that to calculate the diagnostic accuracy of Duplex US it is necessary to correct for the sampling rate of patients with a high-grade stenosis.

Alternative randomized designs

An alternative to the design in Figure 4.3 would be to move the point of randomization back in time, to the point where the test results are not yet known. This comes down to the randomization of all patients to either disclosure or nondisclosure of the results of the test.

The latter design was used to study the effect of MRI findings in patients with low back pain on patient outcome and to evaluate Doppler ultrasonography of the umbilical artery in the management of women with intrauterine growth retardation (IUGR).[5,6] In the latter study, 150 pregnant women with IUGR underwent Doppler ultrasonography and were subsequently randomized to disclosure or nondisclosure of the test results (Figure 4.4a). In the group in which the results of the test were revealed, women were hospitalized in case of abnormal flow and discharged with outpatient management in case of normal flow. In the nondisclosure group, all patients received the conventional strategy for women with IUGR of hospitalization, regardless of their test results. The trial compared perinatal outcome, neurological development, and postnatal growth between the two strategies. The trial design, depicted in Figure 4.4, allows us to determine the natural prognostic value

A

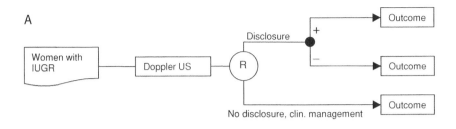

B

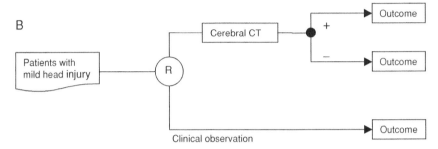

Figure 4.4 Alternative randomized designs.

and the treatment effect in test abnormals. Unfortunately, the authors did not report sufficient data to reconstruct the necessary 2×2 tables.

One could move the point of randomization further back in time, to the decision whether or not to perform the test. This was done in a large study evaluating the use of immediate computed tomography in patients with acute mild head injury.[7] The study is outlined in Figure 4.4B. Patients with mild head injury presenting at the emergency department were randomly allocated to two strategies. The first strategy consisted of applying the head CT scan in patients with mild head injury. In the case of a normal scan, patients were discharged home. In the case of an abnormal scan, treatment depended on the findings. In the second strategy, all patients were admitted for observation according to local standard practice guidelines. Subsequently, clinical outcome was measured after 3 months with the extended Glasgow coma scale questionnaire.

This design evaluates the effects of both the test and the treatment. It is not possible to distinguish the treatment effect from the prognostic value of the test. Similar outcomes in both arms will be observed if there is no difference in outcome with either home-care or clinical management in all patients satisfying the inclusion criteria for this trial. Any differences in outcome cannot be attributed to the test only. In case of a wrong choice of treatment, the outcome of the CT scan arm can turn out to be inferior to the conventional strategy, no matter how good or reliable the test actually is. This same line of reasoning can also be applied in case of a superior outcome in the CT scan arm. If there is a (sub)group of patients that is better off with home care, then the expected outcome in the patients allocated to immediate CT will always be superior, regardless of the intrinsic quality or accuracy of the test. Even a random test will then generate a benefit.

The study showed a slightly better outcome in the CT scan arm although nonsignificant. As the authors extensively monitored all clinical decisions, they concluded that this was due to early surgery in some patients with severe injury in the CT-scan group.

How to compare test strategies

In many clinical situations, there are multiple tests available to examine the presence of the target condition. When one wants to compare two competing tests, the first three designs introduced earlier for the evaluation of a single test have to be adapted slightly.

To compare the prognostic value of two tests, a straightforward translation of Figure 4.1 is to perform both tests in all patients and monitor the outcome of interest during a follow-up period. Such a design is outlined in Figure 4.5a.

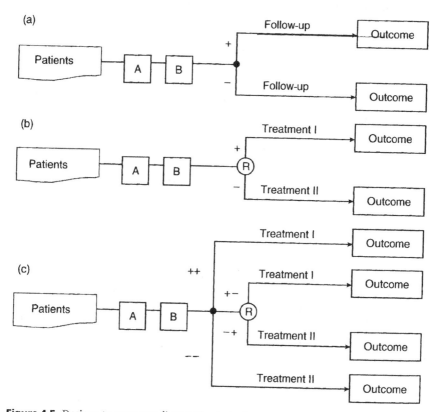

Figure 4.5 Designs to compare diagnostic strategies.

Table 4.4 A 4×2 table of the results of two dichotomous tests

		Outcome	
A	B	+	−
+	+		
+	−		
−	+		
−	−		
Total			

The data of such a study can be used to calculate and compare the prognostic value of each test, using conventional measures of test accuracy. One can also analyze the data by stratifying the results according to the possible test combinations. With two dichotomous tests, this will result in a 4×2 table (Table 4.4). Note that each possible combination of results on test A and test B is treated as a separate test result category, analogously to a single test with four possible result categories.

Subsequently, the predictive value or the likelihood ratio of each result category can be calculated as a measure of prognostic value.[8]

To examine both tests in the context of subsequent clinical decision making, it is possible to randomize all patients between two treatment strategies, similar to the design in Figure 4.2, regardless of their test results. Figure 4.5b shows an example of such a design: both tests are performed and all patients are randomly allocated to one of the two treatment options. This design allows one to explore the prognostic value of both tests in each treatment arm. In addition, the data of such a trial can be used to find the most effective treatment for all patients included in the trial. If statistical power allows it, subgroup analysis of the treatment effect in the four possible test result categories offers the possibility to identify the most effective treatment option for patients in the respective categories.

Although the previous design allows for a series of explorations, only some are relevant from a clinical perspective. When two tests are compared, one of them is often already used in clinical practice and decisions on subsequent management are made based on this test. Let us assume that, in clinical practice, test positive patients are treated and test negative patients are not. If future decisions are to be made under the guidance of the new test, patients who test positive on the new test will be treated and those who test negative will not. This means that the only patients that will be managed differently are the ones who test positive on the existing test but negative on the new one, and those who test negative on the existing test but positive on the new one.

As patients with concordant test results (++ or −−) will receive the same management, it is unnecessary and in some circumstances even unethical to

Table 4.5 Analysis of a RCT of two tests randomizing only discordant results

a Treatment effect A+B−		Poor outcome	Favorable outcome
A+	B−		
Treatment I			
Treatment II			
Total			

b Treatment effect A−B+		Poor outcome	Favorable outcome
A−	B+		
Treatment I			
Treatment II			
Total			

c Treatment		Poor outcome	Favorable outcome
A	B		
+	−		
−	+		
Total			

d No treatment		Poor outcome	Favorable outcome
A	B		
+	−		
−	+		
Total			

e Strategy based on A		Poor outcome	Favorable outcome
A	B		
+	−		
−	+		
Total			

f Strategy based on B		Poor outcome	Favorable outcome
A	B		
+	−		
−	+		

examine the treatment effect in these two subgroups. If a new test (B) is then examined with a goal to substitute the old, possibly more invasive and/or costly, test (A), the design in Figure 4.5c, randomizing only the discordant test results, is more efficient. Subsequently the treatment effect and the predictive values of the discordant result categories (A+B− and A−B+) can be examined (see Tables 4.5a–4.5d).

In gray are the outcomes of a treatment decision based on the results of test A, in white the outcomes based on test B.

By transposing these tables, it is possible to examine the effect of a clinical pathway based on test A or test B for patients with discordant test results (Tables 4.5e–4.5f). The difference in poor outcome rate between these two tables is, after correcting for the frequency of discordant results, equal to absolute risk difference of a clinical pathway based on test A compared to a pathway based on test B. To calculate the relative risk or the total risk of each strategy separately it is necessary to have information on the clinical event rate in each concordant group.

An alternative design, using the random disclosure principle, is outlined in Figure 4.6a. Both tests A and B are performed in all patients. Subsequently patients are randomized between a clinical pathway based on test A without

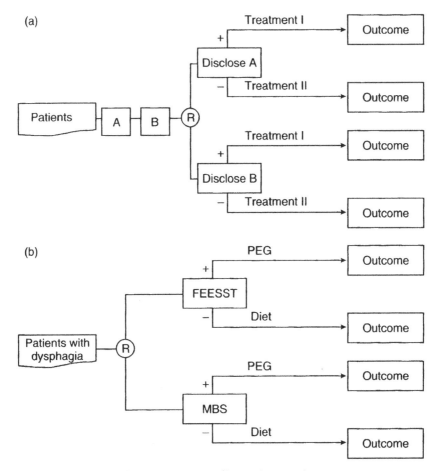

Figure 4.6 Alternative designs to compare diagnostic strategies.

disclosing the results of test B or a pathway based on test B with nondisclosure of the results of test A. The same measures and tables can be obtained from such a design as discussed for the design in Figure 4.5.

In some situations, one might want to let the point of randomization coincide with that of the clinical decision to choose either test A or test B and to act on the respective results. This design has to be chosen if there is a difference in the delay in obtaining the test results. An example is the evaluation of rapid diagnostic blood tests versus classic microscopic blood slide evaluation of outpatients suspected of malaria.[9] Another trial used this design to study two different diagnostic approaches for the management of outpatients with dysphagia.[10] Patients with dysphagia are at risk for aspiration pneumonia. Modified barium swallow test (MBS) and flexible endoscopic valuation of swallowing with sensory testing (FEESST) are supposed to distinguish patients who can benefit from behavioral and dietary management from those who will need a percutaneous endoscopic gastrostomy (PEG) tube.

For the discussion, we consider a simplified design as outlined in Figure 4.6b. Outpatients presenting with dysphagia were randomly allocated to either a strategy using MBS or a strategy using FEESST to guide subsequent management. During one year of follow-up, the occurrence of pneumonia was recorded in both trial arms. There were 6 cases of pneumonia in the 50 (12%) patients allocated to the FEEST strategy and 14 in the 76 (18%) patients allocated to the MBS strategy. The absolute risk difference was not significantly different from zero (risk difference 6%; 95% CI −6% to 19%). As no patient received both tests, it is not possible to distinguish the treatment effect from the prognostic value of the tests, nor is it possible to compare the outcome in the subgroups with discordant test results.

Often a new test is introduced to complement rather than to replace existing tests.[11] One example is where the new test is to be added to the diagnostic pathway before an existing test as a triage instrument. Patients with a particular test results (say, negative) on the new test will not be subjected to the existing test. Alternatively, the new test is added after the existing tests, making further refinement possible in diagnosis or treatment decisions.

If a test is added at the end of a diagnostic workup to further classify disease, all the designs, presented in Figures 4.2 to 4.4 for the single test evaluation can be used to evaluate this new classification. For example, to evaluate the prognostic impact of a genetic test for the classification of women with breast cancer in two different subgroups, one could use a design similar to the one in Figure 4.3. Women suspected of breast cancer are evaluated with the conventional diagnostic workup. Subsequently only women with breast cancer are eligible for the trial. In all these women genetic tests are performed. Depending on tests results, they are subsequently randomly allocated to one of the two types of treatment.

In case the goal of a new test is to limit the amount of people undergoing the classic diagnostic workup (triage), designs in Figures 4.5b and 4.5c and 4.6a can be used to evaluate the prognostic impact of such a strategy. Using the principle that only patients with test results that will actually account for the difference are randomized, one could also adapt the design of Figures 4.5b, randomizing only patients with the pair of discordant test results that will be treated differently if the new strategy is adopted. Another option is drawn in Figure 4.7a.

As the difference between the two strategies comes from the group of patients who are not selected for the classic diagnostic workup, one can randomize only these patients to either the classic workup and treatment or management based on the results of the new test.

Many studies to evaluate the use of a test as a triage instrument have randomized all patients between the two different diagnostic workups.[12–14] Lassen *et al.* evaluating helicobacter pylori serology as a way to reduce the number of patients subjected to endoscopy used the trial design outlined in Figure 4.7b.

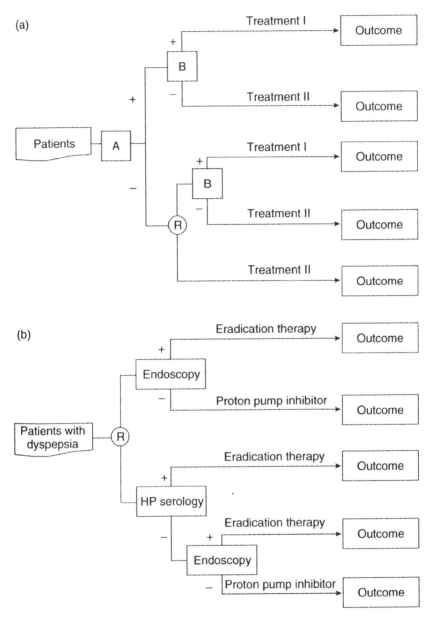

Figure 4.7 Designs to evaluate triage.

Patients presenting in primary care with dyspepsia were randomly assigned to either H Pylori and eradication therapy or prompt endoscopy. In case of a negative Helicobacter Pylori test. patients were still subjected to endoscopy. During a one-year follow-up, the symptoms were recorded on a Likert scale.

Table 4.6 Possible analyses of each randomized design

	1, 5a	2	3, 4a	5b	5c, 6a	4b, 6b, 7a, 7b
Natural prognostic value	X	X	X	X		
Prognostic value with intervention		X		X		
Treatment effect test abnormals		X	X	X		
Treatment effect test normals		X		X		
Treatment effect discordant tests					X	X
Strategy effect		X	X	X	X	X

Choice of design

Each of the designs discussed in Figures 4.1 to 4.7 has its own advantages and disadvantages. Depending on the clinical problem one wants to answer, the type of information needed, and the costs of tests or follow-up, one design can be preferred over another.

The outlined in Figures 4.2 to 4.4 can be used to evaluate a strategy with a new test compared to a classic strategy without such a test. In case of an add-on test, the classic strategy will consist of the classic diagnostic workup and treatment. In case of a replacement problem, any of the trial designs outlined in Figure 4.5b to 4.6b can provide an answer. The designs outlined in Figures 4.5b, 4.6a, 4.7a, and 7b can provide an answer in case of a triage problem.

Table 4.6 gives an overview of the information that can be deducted from the different designs.

The designs in Figures 4.2 and 4.5b, testing all patients and randomizing all between two treatment strategies, provide the most information. In addition to data on the effects of the two evaluated strategies, they can provide information on the treatment effect and, in the case in which one of the arms has no treatment (only follow-up), on the prognostic value of all possible test result categories. Yet these designs are not always ethical, as there is often evidence of one treatment being better for some of the test result categories. In that case, a better alternative are the designs outlined in Figures 4.3, 4.5c, and 4.7a in which only the group of patients are randomized: those for which there is uncertainty in the subsequent management. The designs in Figures 4.4b, 4.6b, and 4.7b have frequently been used in the medical literature, probably because of their pragmatic attractiveness. In these designs the point of randomization coincides with the decision to perform either test A or test B. From a cost-perspective these designs can be more be economical than the other designs, in case of an expensive test, as on average less patients receive tests, as compared to the other designs. In case follow-up is expensive designs randomizing only patients with the test category of interest (Figures 4.3, 4.5c, and 4.7) are more efficient, as less patients will be needed to achieve the same amount of statistical precision.[15] However, the latter designs are not feasible in case tests are compared that influence each other's performance.

For example, it is not possible to compare two surgical diagnostic procedures, mediastinoscopy and anterior mediastinomy, for the detection of mediastinal lymphomas by performing them both in all patients as suspected lymph nodes are removed.[16]

Practical issues

We have discussed the pros and cons of different designs to evaluate the prognostic impact of a single test or to compare different test strategies. In the design of a trial, there are several other issues that should be considered in advance. In all of the examples we have presented here there was a prespecified link between test results and management decisions. Test positive patients were to receive one treatment, test negative another. If such a link is absent, and physicians are free to select therapy for each test result, it will remain unclear to what extent poor results of the trial reflect deficiencies of the test itself, ineffective treatment options or, alternatively, incorrect management decisions. Detailed information on the treatment protocol is also necessary for others to implement the possible findings of the study. A clear specification of the treatment options and their relation with the different test results is an absolute necessity for any diagnostic study.[15]

As for each randomized controlled trial, methods to preserve allocation concealment and blinding deserve special attention. It has been shown empirically that inadequate concealment of allocation as well as inadequate blinding can lead to exaggerated estimates of a strategy's effectiveness.[17] One way to guard adequate allocation concealment is a central randomization procedure. In some situations the use of sealed opaque envelopes with monitoring of the concealment process may be more feasible.[18] Blinding of the outcome measurement for the randomization outcome is of greater importance for some outcomes than for others, but can be implemented with the same methods as developed for therapeutic trials. Blinding of the physician or patient to the allocation is more difficult. In case two different strategies are randomized (Figure 4.6b) one can imagine that the knowledge of the type of test influences subsequent management decisions of a physician, despite a prespecified link. For example an obstetrician might be more reassured with the results of a magnetic-resonance pelvimetry in breech presentation at term compared to manual pelvimetry, which will influence subsequent decisions to perform an emergency section.[19] One could choose a design that randomizes test results to overcome this problem. Alternatively, one could try to mask the physician by only presenting standardized test results without any referral to the type of test.

The a priori calculation of the necessary sample size for a randomized diagnostic study is not straightforward. When discussing Figure 4.5c, we showed that the expected difference in outcome between the two test strategies results from the expected difference in the category with discordant test results only. In trials in which patients are randomized to one of two test strategies

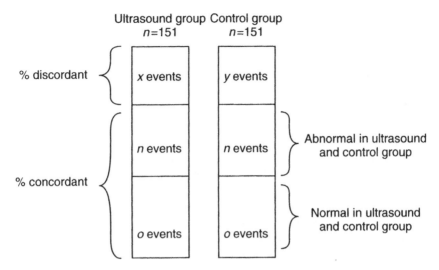

Figure 4.8 Sample size calculation.

(Figure 4.6b), a large group of participants will also not contribute to the final difference. Let us explain this with another randomized diagnostic trial from the literature in which ultrasonography was compared with clinical assessment for the diagnosis of appendicitis.[20] The authors report a power of 80% to detect a reduction in the nontherapeutic operation rate from 11% to 2%, by randomizing 302 patients. What are the nominator and denominator of these estimated rates?

Figure 4.8 shows the two trial arms. A large group of patients with abnormal results in the ultrasound group, indicating operation, would also have been detected at clinical examination. The same argument stands for a subgroup of patients with a normal ultrasound. The sum of these two groups forms the total with concordant test results. As patients with concordant test results will receive the same management, their event rates will be identical except for chance differences. The rate of 11% results from $(X + N + O)/151$. The rate of 2% results from $(Y + N + O)/151$. The rate difference, 9%, solely results from the events in the discordant group. By assuming a concordance rate of ultrasonography with clinical assessment of 80%, one can calculate the postulated rate difference in this discordant group: 9%/20% is 45%. This could result from a rate of nontherapeutic operations of 55% in patients with a positive clinical assessment and otherwise negative ultrasound, and a rate of 10% in patients with a positive ultrasound and otherwise negative clinical examination. (This implies that the event rate is 0% in the concordant group, which is not very likely as the authors already discuss in their introduction that 15%–30% of all operations are nontherapeutic.) With some extra calculations, we can show that the difference assumed by the authors implies a discordance rate of at least 80%. It would be very strange to expect such a high discordance rate in advance. This example shows that it is important to incorporate the discordance rate in sample size calculations of randomized trials of diagnostic tests.

Conclusions

In this chapter, we discussed the evaluation of the prognostic impact of tests. From a patient perspective, one could argue that it is not so much the correspondence with "the truth" that should be the focus of a diagnostic test evaluation but the likelihood that such a test detects events of clinical interest and the possibilities that exist to let test results guide subsequent clinical decision making to reduce the likelihood of these events occurring. The latter can be evaluated by evaluating a test–treatment combination in a clinical trial, for which several possible designs were discussed.

The examples of published randomized diagnostic trials in this chapter show that it is feasible to perform such a thorough evaluation of a diagnostic test. Recent examples include the evaluation of different diagnostic techniques for ventilation-assisted pneumonia and the comparison of multidetector row CT with digital substraction angiography,[21,22] additional examples can be found evaluating mediastinoscopy, cardiotocography, and MRI[12,23,24] and of a number of screening tests.[25–27] These date even back to 1975.[28]

In most of these trials, the point of randomization coincided with the clinical decision whether to perform the tests. This makes it impossible to differentiate between the treatment effect and the prognostic value of the test. Power analyses of any diagnostic trial should incorporate an estimation of the discordance rate, as differences in outcome can only be expected for patients that have discordant test results. In this chapter, we have shown that a design incorporating randomization of discordant test results is more efficient, provides more information, and is less prone to bias. Most important, all of these designs require a prespecified test–treatment link. This allows for application of study results in other settings and guards the internal validity of the study.

References

1. Rothwell PM, Pendlebury ST, Wardlaw J, et al. Critical appraisal of the design and reporting of studies of imaging and measurement of carotid stenosis. *Stroke*. 2000;**31**(6):1444–50.
2. Lewis RF, Abrahamowicz M, Cote R, et al. Predictive power of duplex ultrasonography in asymptomatic carotid disease. *Ann Intern Med*. 1997;**127**(1): 13–20.
3. Adams HP, Jr., Bendixen BH, Leira E, et al. Antithrombotic treatment of ischemic stroke among patients with occlusion or severe stenosis of the internal carotid artery: a report of the Trial of Org 10172 in Acute Stroke Treatment (TOAST). *Neurology*. 1999;**53**(1):122–25.

 4. Anonymous. Low molecular weight heparinoid, ORG 10172 (danaparoid), and outcome after acute ischemic stroke: a randomized controlled trial: the Publications Committee for the Trial of ORG 10172 in Acute Stroke Treatment (TOAST) Investigators. *JAMA.* 1998;**279**(16):1265–72.

 5. Nienhuis SJ, Vles JS, Gerver WJ, et al. Doppler ultrasonography in suspected intrauterine growth retardation: a randomized clinical trial. *Ultrasound Obstet Gynecol.* 1997;**9**(1):6–13.

 6. Modic MT, Obuchowski NA, Ross JS, et al. Acute low back pain and radiculopathy: MR imaging findings and their prognostic role and effect on outcome. *Radiology.* 2005;**237**(2):597–604.

 7. Geijerstam JL, Oredsson S, Britton M. Medical outcome after immediate computed tomography or admission for observation in patients with mild head injury: randomised controlled trial. *Br Med J.* 2006;**333**(7566):465.

 8. Simel DL, Samsa GP, Matchar DB. Likelihood ratios with confidence: sample size estimation for diagnostic test studies. *J Clin Epidemiol.* 1991;**44**(8):763–70.

 9. Reyburn H, Mbakilwa H, Mwangi R, et al. Rapid diagnostic tests compared with malaria microscopy for guiding outpatient treatment of febrile illness in Tanzania: randomised trial. *Br Med J.* 2007;**334**(7590):403.

10. Aviv JE. Prospective, randomized outcome study of endoscopy versus modified barium swallow in patients with dysphagia. *Laryngoscope.* 2000;**110**(4):563–74.

11. Bossuyt PM, Irwig L, Craig J, et al. Comparative accuracy: assessing new tests against existing diagnostic pathways. *Br Med J.* 2006;**332**(7549):1089–92.

12. Anonymous. Investigation for mediastinal disease in patients with apparently operable lung cancer. Canadian Lung Oncology Group. *Ann Thorac Surg.* 1995;**60**(5):1382–89.

13. Lassen AT, Hallas J, Schaffalitzky de Muckadell OB. Helicobacter pylori test and eradicate versus prompt endoscopy for management of dyspeptic patients: 6.7 year follow up of a randomised trial. *Gut.* 2004;**53**(12):1758–63.

14. Lassen AT, Pedersen FM, Bytzer P, et al. Helicobacter pylori test-and-eradicate versus prompt endoscopy for management of dyspeptic patients: a randomised trial. *Lancet.* 2000;**356**(9228):455–60.

15. Bossuyt P, Lijmer J, Mol B. Randomised comparisons of medical tests: Sometimes invalid, not always efficient. *Lancet.* 2000;**356**(9244):1844–47.

16. Elia S, Cecere C, Giampaglia F, et al. Mediastinoscopy vs. anterior mediastinotomy in the diagnosis of mediastinal lymphoma: a randomized trial. *Eur J Cardiothorac Surg.* 1992;**6**(7):361–65.

17. Schulz KF, Chalmers I, Hayes RJ, et al. Empirical evidence of bias: dimensions of methodological quality associated with estimates of treatment effects in controlled trials. *JAMA.* 1995;**273**(5):408–12.

18. Swingler GH, Zwarenstein M. An effectiveness trial of a diagnostic test in a busy outpatients department in a developing country: issues around allocation concealment and envelope randomization. *J Clin Epidemiol.* 2000;**53**(7):702–6.

19. van der Post JA, Maathuis JB. Magnetic-resonance pelvimetry in breech presentation. *Lancet.* 1998;**351**(9106):913.

20. Douglas C, Macpherson N, Davidson P, et al. Randomised controlled trial of ultrasonography in diagnosis of acute appendicitis, incorporating the Alvarado score. *Br Med J.* 2000;**321**:1–7.

21. A randomized trial of diagnostic techniques for ventilator-associated pneumonia. *N Engl J Med.* 2006;**355**(25):2619–30.

22. Kock MC, Adriaensen ME, Pattynama PM, et al. DSA versus multi-detector row CT angiography in peripheral arterial disease: randomized controlled trial. *Radiology.* 2005;**237**(2):727–37.
23. Dixon AK, Wheeler TK, Lomas DJ, et al. Computed tomography or magnetic resonance imaging for axillary symptoms following treatment of breast carcinoma? A randomized trial. *Clin Radiol.* 1993;**48**(6):371–76.
24. Strachan BK, van Wijngaarden WJ, Sahota D, et al. Cardiotocography only versus cardiotocography plus PR-interval analysis in intrapartum surveillance: a randomised, multicentre trial. FECG Study Group. *Lancet.* 2000;**355**(9202):456–59.
25. Anonymous. Controlled trial of universal neonatal screening for early identification of permanent childhood hearing impairment. Wessex Universal Neonatal Hearing Screening Trial Group. *Lancet.* 1998;**352**(9145):1957–64.
26. Kronborg O, Fenger C, Olsen J, et al. Randomised study of screening for colorectal cancer with faecal-occult-blood test *Lancet.* 1996;**348**(9040):1467–71.
27. Miller AB, To T, Baines CJ, Wall C. Canadian National Breast Screening Study-2: 13-year results of a randomized trial in women aged 50–59 Years. *J Natl Cancer Inst.* 2000;**92**(18):1490–99.
28. Morris DW, Levine GM, Soloway RD, et al. Prospective, randomized study of diagnosis and outcome in acute upper-gastrointestinal bleeding: endoscopy versus conventional radiography. *Am J Dig Dis.* 1975;**20**(12):1103–9.

CHAPTER 5

The diagnostic before–after study to assess clinical impact

J. André Knottnerus, Geert-Jan Dinant, and Onno P. van Schayck

Summary box

- The before–after design is more appropriate for evaluating the clinical impact of single or additional testing than comparing the impact of different diagnostic options.
- Demonstrating an effect of diagnostic testing on the patient's health outcome is more difficult than showing a change in the doctor's assessment and management plan.
- Whether and what specific blinding procedures have to be applied depends on the study objective.
- To optimize the assessment of the independent effect of the test information, performance of the test or disclosure of the test result can be randomized. This would change the before–after design in a randomized trial.
- The therapeutic consequences of the various test results can be standardized in the research protocol, provided that such therapy options are clinically rational and have a well-documented evidence base. The study will then evaluate the impact of the test result connected with a predefined therapeutic consequence, rather than the impact of the test result per se.
- If evaluating the doctor's assessment is the primary study objective, the assessment should preferably take place immediately after disclosure of the test result, with a minimal risk of interfering factors influencing the doctor's judgment.
- Because a rather long follow-up is mostly needed to estimate the impact of testing on the clinical course, the risk of interfering influences is substantial.

(*continued*)

The Evidence Base of Clinical Diagnosis: Theory and Methods of Diagnostic Research. 2nd edition. Edited by J. André Knottnerus and Frank Buntinx. © 2009 Blackwell Publishing, ISBN: 978-1-4051-5787-2.

> *(continued)*
> • Given that before–after studies can be carried out relatively fast, largely embedded in daily care, while randomized controlled trials (RCTs) are generally more complex or expensive, a well-designed before–after study may sometimes be used to explore whether and how a diagnostic RCT should be performed. If an RCT is impossible or infeasible, or ethically unacceptable, a well-designed before–after study can be the most suitable alternative.

Introduction

Apart from facilitating an accurate diagnosis, diagnostic testing is aimed at causing change: starting from a baseline situation, applying the test and interpreting its outcome should result in a new situation. In fact, the most important justification for diagnostic testing is that it is expected to make a difference, by influencing clinical management and ultimately benefiting the patient's well-being. Accordingly, performing a diagnostic test can be seen as an intervention that should be effective in bringing about a clinically relevant change.

In studying the clinical effect of a test result, the randomized controlled trial (RCT) is the strongest methodological design option,[1,2,3] as was dealt with in Chapter 4. However, although it is the paradigm for effectiveness research, an RCT cannot always be achieved.[4] This is, for example, the case if randomly withholding a test or test result from patients or doctors is considered medically or ethically unacceptable. Difficulties may also arise if the diagnostic test is integrated in the general skills of the clinician, so that performing it cannot be randomly switched on and off in his or her head, nor simply assigned to a different doctor. This is especially problematic if at the same time patients cannot be randomly assigned to a doctor. This situation may, for instance, occur in studying the impact of diagnostic reasoning skills in general practice. Also, when an RCT is complex and expensive, or will last too long to still be relevant when the results become available, one may wish to consider a more feasible alternative.

One alternative that may be considered is the diagnostic before–after study.[5] This approach seems attractive, as it fits naturally within the clinical process and is generally easier to perform than the randomized trial. Therefore, this chapter will discuss the potentials, limitations, and pitfalls of this design option.

The research question

Example

In a study to assess the diagnostic impact of erythrocyte sedimentation rate (ESR) in general practice, 305 consecutive patients with aspecific symptoms for whom general practitioners (GPs) considered ESR testing necessary were

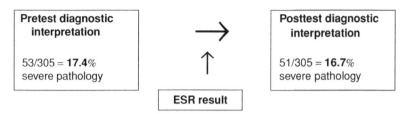

Figure 5.1 Pre- and posttest diagnostic assessment in studying the impact of ESR.

included.[6] Before testing, the GPs were asked to specify the most likely diagnosis in each patient, and to assess whether this diagnosis was severe in the sense of malignant or inflammatory disease for which further management would be urgently needed. Subsequently, the ESR was independently performed and the result was made available to the GPs, who then again specified their (revised) diagnostic assessment. After 3 months, based on all the available medical information, a clinical assessment was carried out for each patient by an independent clinician not knowing about the pre- and posttest assessments for each patient, in order to establish a final diagnosis (reference standard).[7]

In Figure 5.1 the percentage of patients most likely having severe pathology according to the GP is presented before and after disclosure of the ESR result. Overall, there seems to be no relevant pre- or posttest change. However, looking at Table 5.1, it is clear that there was a change in 32 individual patients: 17 from severe pathology to "other," and 15 from "other" to severe pathology.

Whether these changes had indeed resulted in a more accurate diagnostic assessment could be determined after correlating the GPs' pre- and posttest findings with the reference standard procedure. It appeared that the pretest accuracy of the GPs' assessment was 69% (that is, 69% of cases were correctly classified), whereas the posttest accuracy was 76%, implying an increase of 7%. Of the 32 patients with a diagnostic classification changed by the GP, nine with a positive (severe) posttest diagnosis proved to be "false positives," and two with a negative (other) posttest diagnosis were "false negatives."

The test characteristics of the ESR (cut-off value ≥ 27 mm/1h) could be also determined in relation to the reference diagnosis, yielding a sensitivity of 53%,

Table 5.1 Relation between pre- and posttest diagnostic assessments in studying the impact of ESR

Pretest interpretation	Posttest interpretation		
	Severe pathology	Other	Total
Severe pathology	36	17	53
Other	15	237	252
Total	51	254	305

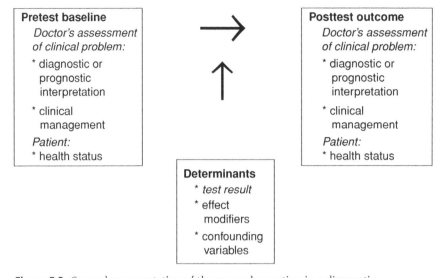

Figure 5.2 General representation of the research question in a diagnostic before–after study.

a specificity of 94%, a positive predictive value of 46%, and a negative predictive value of 91%.

The general model

The basic question in the diagnostic before–after study is whether applying a certain diagnostic procedure favorably influences the doctor's (a) diagnostic or (b) prognostic assessment of a presented clinical problem; (c) the further management; and, ultimately, (d) the patient's health. It essentially comprises the baseline (pretest) situation, a determinant (the test), and the outcome (posttest situation) (Figure 5.2).

The point of departure can be characterized by a clinical problem, with the doctor's assessment regarding the possible diagnosis, prognosis, or the preferred management option, and the patient's health status at baseline, without knowing the information from the test to be evaluated. The patient's health status at baseline is important, not only as a starting point for possible outcome assessment but also as a reference for generalizing the study results to similar patient groups.

The determinant of primary interest is performing the diagnostic test and disclosure of its result, which is in fact the intended intervention. Furthermore, it is often useful to consider the influence of effect modifying variables such as the doctor's skills and experience, and – as diagnostic classification is essentially involved with distinguishing clinically relevant subgroups – the patient's age and gender, and preexisting comorbidity. In addition, the effect of possible confounding variables should be taken into account. For example, extraneous factors such as reading publications or attending professional meetings may affect the clinician's assessment. But also the time needed to do the test and obtain its result may be important, as it may be used to think and study on the clinical problem, and this will independently influence the assessment. Moreover, the patient's health status may have changed as a result of the clinical course of the illness, by interfering comorbidity and related interventions, by environmental factors, or by visiting other therapists. The patient's symptom perception may have been influenced by information from family, friends, or the media, or by consulting the internet. Also, the patient may claim to have benefited from a diagnostic intervention because he does not wish to disappoint the doctor.

The key challenge for the investigator is now to evaluate the extent to which applying the diagnostic test has independently changed the doctor's diagnostic or prognostic assessment of the presented clinical problem, the preferred management option, or the patient's health status. The latter will generally be influenced indirectly, via clinical management, but can sometimes also be directly affected, for example, because the patient feels himself being taken more seriously by the testing per se. Moreover, patient self-testing,[8] which is becoming more common, can influence patient self-management.

At this point, two important limitations of the before–after design must be emphasized. First, the design is more appropriate to evaluate the impact of a single diagnostic procedures or "add on" technologies[5,9] (adding a new test to already existing tests) than to compare the impact of different diagnostic technologies or strategies. For the latter purpose, one could, in principle, apply both studied technologies, for example, colonoscopy and double-contrast barium enema, in randomized order, to all included patients, and then compare the impact of disclosing the test results, again in random order, on the clinicians' assessment. Another example would be to subject patients to both CT and MRI head scanning to study their influence on clinicians' management plans in those with suspected intracranial pathology. However, such comparisons are unrealistic, as the two tests would never be applied simultaneously in practice. Moreover, such studies are generally very burdensome for patients, not to say ethically unacceptable, and would make it virtually impossible to study the complication rate of each procedure separately.[10] When the various options are mutually exclusive, for example, when comparing diagnostic laparotomy with endoscopy in assessing intra-abdominal pathology as to their adverse effects, a before–after design is clearly inappropriate. In such situations, a randomized controlled trial is by far the preferred option. Only when the compared tests can be easily carried out together without any problem for the patient, these can be applied simultaneously. This can be done, for instance, when comparing the impact of different blood tests using the same blood sample. However, when the disclosure of the results of the compared tests to the clinicians is then randomized, which would be a good idea, we are in fact in the RCT option.

Second, demonstrating an effect of diagnostic testing on the patient's health outcome is much more difficult than showing a change in the doctor's assessment and management plan, as it usually takes quite some time to observe a health effect that might be ascribed to performance of the test. Controlling for the influence of the many possible confounders over time generally requires a concurrent control group of similar patients not receiving the test. However, a diagnostic before–after study could be convincing in case of: (1) studying a clinical problem with a highly predictable or even unavoidable outcome in the absence of testing (such as signs of an imminent rupture of an aneurysm of the aorta); (2) while adding specific diagnostic information (an appropriate imaging technique) leading to a specific therapeutic decision (whether and how to operate) (3), which is aimed at a clearly defined short-term effect, such as prevention of a rupture, and survival (followed by less specific long-term effects, e.g., rehabilitation). However, such opportunities are extraordinary. Besides, some clinicians would consider such clinical situations to be self-evident and not needing evaluation by research, while others may still see room for dispute as to what extent clinical events are predictable or unavoidable.

Working out the study

Pretest baseline
The study protocol follows the elements of the research question.

At baseline, the clinical problem and the study question are defined. The clinical problem could be aspecific symptoms as presented in primary care, for example, with the question being whether the ESR would contribute to the doctor's diagnostic assessment,[6,7] or sciatica, in order to study whether radiography would affect therapeutic decision making.

The health status of each patient to be included is systematically documented, using standardized measurement instruments for the presented symptoms, patient history, physical examination, and further relevant clinical data.

Overseeing all available patient data, the doctor makes a first clinical assessment of the probability of certain diagnoses or diagnostic categories. In primary care, for example, the probability of a severe organic malignant or inflammatory disorder can be assessed. This can be done for one specified diagnostic category, for a list of specified diagnoses, or in an open approach, just asking the differential diagnosis the doctor has in mind, with the estimated probability of each specific diagnostic hypothesis being considered.

Furthermore, the doctor is asked to describe the preferred diagnostic or therapeutic management plan, which can be done, again, according to a prepared list of items or as an open question.

At baseline, as earlier emphasized, possibly relevant effect modifying variables should be considered. Often the general clinical experience of the clinicians and their specific expertise regarding the test under study are important.

Furthermore, variables characterizing important clinical subgroups can be assessed, and potential confounding factors have to be measured to be able to take these into account in the data analysis. Recording of covariables is sometimes difficult, for example, for extraneous variables such as media exposure. Moreover, it cannot be excluded that important or even decisive factors are not identified or foreseen.

Diagnostic testing

In performing the diagnostic procedure under study and revealing its outcome after the baseline assessment, different options can be considered, depending on the specific study objective.

- If one wishes to assess the specific effect of the test information on the outcome, in addition to the pretest clinical information, the test result should be determined independently from the pretest information. This is especially relevant for test procedures with a subjective element in the interpretation of the result, such as patient interviews, auscultation, x-ray films, and pathological specimens. Accordingly, those who interpret the test should not be aware of the pretest information. However, when patient history itself is the test to be evaluated, this will generally not be feasible.

- If the investigator wishes to assess the diagnostic process as it is usually embedded in clinical practice, the interpretation of the test result can be carried out as usual without specific blinding procedures. However, particularly for tests with subjective elements in reading or interpretation of the results, this will imply that the independent contribution of the test cannot be determined.

- When it is important to limit possible confounding effects of a preoccupation of participating doctors with the expected relevance of a certain test, the investigator may wish to obscure the performing of the evaluated test itself. This can theoretically be achieved by not telling the doctor in advance about what specifically is being evaluated, and by disclosing the test result while also providing information on a number of other items irrelevant for the studied comparison. However, such masking is difficult and often not feasible, or may be so much in conflict with clinical reality that the findings will not be relevant for practice. Intentional obscuring of the specific research question will need the explicit approval of the medical ethics review board.

- To optimize the assessment of the independent effect of the test information, performance of the test or, even more precisely, disclosure of the test result, can be randomized so that half of the participants would and half would not get the result. In fact, this would change the before–after design into a randomized trial, which is discussed in Chapter 4.

Because tests are almost never perfect, applying it may produce misclassification. Even when most patients are more accurately classified if the clinician uses the test information, some patients with a correct pretest diagnosis may be incorrectly classified after testing, for example, because of a false positive or false negative result as has been shown in the ESR example. As this may have important negative consequences for those patients—for example, when a false positive mammography would lead to unnecessary surgery—it is recommended to include evaluation of the actual disease status in the context of the before–after study. This also enables the investigator to determine test accuracy by relating the test result cross-sectionally to the disease status, established according to an acceptable reference standard.[10] (see also Chapter 3)

Posttest outcome

The measurement of the final posttest outcome after disclosure of the test result (diagnostic assessment, preferred management plan, and/or patient health status) should follow the same procedure as the baseline measurement. In doing so, both the doctor and the patient will generally remember the baseline status, implying that the posttest assessment of the doctor's differential diagnosis and management options and the patient's symptom perceptions cannot be blinded for the pretest assessment. This has probably been the case in the example of the diagnostic impact of the ESR measurement.

When one is evaluating the impact of adding the test information to already known clinical information at baseline in order to make a comprehensive assessment, lack of blinding is not always a principal problem. In fact, it is clinically natural and supported by Bayes's theorem to study the impact of the test result in the light of the prior probability. However, when clinicians are more or less "anchored" to their initial diagnostic assessment, they are biased in that they do not sufficiently respond to the test information in revising their diagnostic assessment (Chapter 12). But even this can sometimes be acceptable for an investigator who deliberately aims to assess the impact of the test in clinical reality, where such anchoring is a common phenomenon.[11,12]

When the posttest outcome is patient status, objective assessment of this status independent of both pretest status and the doctor's interpretations is an important requirement. This is however not always easy to achieve, as has been outlined in the section on 'The research question.'

The clinical impact of testing will not be easily detected if there is no clear relationship between revision of the diagnostic classification based on the test information, and the revision of the management plan.[2] This relation can indeed be unclear when doctors ignore the test information, or when the same test result may lead to a variety of management decisions, including doing nothing. The latter can, for example, be the case when laboratory tests are carried out in asymptomatic patients. As a remedy, the therapeutic consequences of the various test results can be standardized in the research protocol, provided that such therapy options are clinically rational and have a well-documented evidence base. Accordingly, the study will then evaluate the impact of the test result connected with an already predefined therapeutic consequence, rather than the impact of the test result per se. On the other hand, when there is a lack of clarity beforehand as to the potential management consequences of

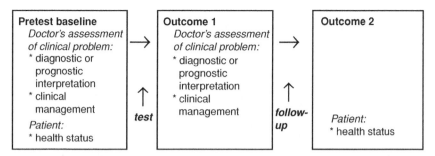

Figure 5.3 Separate posttest measurements of doctor's assessment (immediately) and patient health outcome (later).

performing a test, we should ask ourselves whether such testing should be evaluated or used at all.

If one evaluates a test which is already firmly accepted among the medical profession, the response of clinicians is in fact "programmed" by medical education, continuing medical education, or clinical guidelines. In such cases the investigator is studying the adherence to agreed guidelines rather than the independent clinical impact of the test result.

The time factor

The interval between the pre- and posttest assessments should be carefully chosen. Generally, the interassessment period should be short if evaluating the doctor's assessment is the primary study objective: the assessment should preferably take place immediately after disclosure of the test result, with a minimal risk of interfering factors influencing the doctor's judgment. Sometimes, however, this may take some time (e.g., bacterial culture or pathological specimen). As previously addressed, a rather long period until the final posttest assessment is mostly needed if estimating the impact of testing on the clinical course is the objective, although this longer period will be associated with an increased risk of interfering interventions and influences during follow-up. A combined approach can be chosen, with a pretest measurement, a posttest measurement of the clinician's assessment, and a longer follow-up period for measuring patient health outcome, respectively (Figure 5.3). In the analysis, then, the relation between the test's impact on the clinician's assessment and patient outcome could be studied if extraneous factors and changes in the clinical condition can be sufficiently controlled for. However, as outlined in the section on the research question, this is often impossible in the context of the before–after design. For the purpose of studying the test's impact on patient health, the randomized controlled trial is a more valid option.

Selection of the study subjects

Regarding the selection of the study subjects, similar methodological criteria to those discussed in Chapter 3 should be met: the study patient population should be representative for the "indicated," "candidate," or "intended" patient population, or target population, with a well-defined clinical problem, clinically similar to the group of patients in whom the diagnostic procedure would be applied in practice. Accordingly, the healthcare setting from where the patients come, the inclusion criteria, and the procedure for patient recruitment must be specified. Regarding the selection of participating doctors, the study objective is decisive. If the aim is to evaluate what the test adds to current practice, the pre- and posttest assessments should be made by clinicians representing usual clinical standards. However, if one wishes to ensure that the test's contribution is analyzed using a maximum of available expertise, top experts in the specific clinical field must be recruited.

Generally, in clinical studies a prospectively included consecutive series of patients with a clearly defined clinical presentation will be the most appropriate option with the lowest probability of selection bias. If one were to retrospectively select patients who had already had the test in the past, one would generally not be able to be certain whether those patients really had a similar clinical problem, and whether all candidate patients in the source population would have non-selectively entered the study population. Apart from this, a valid before–after comparison of the doctors' assessments (with the doctors first not knowing and subsequently knowing the test result) is not possible afterwards, as a change in diagnostic assessment and the planning of management cannot be reliably reconstructed post hoc.

Sample size and analysis

Sample size requirements for the before–after study design need to be met according to general conventions. Point of departure can be the size of the before–after difference in estimated disease probability or other effectiveness parameters (e.g., the decrease in the rate of [diagnostic] referrals) which would be sufficiently relevant to be detected. If the basic phenomenon to be studied is the clinical assessment of doctors, the latter are the units of analysis. When the consequences for the patients are considered the main outcome, their number is of specific interest.

The data analysis of the basic before–after comparison can follow the principles of the analysis of paired data. In view of the relevance of evaluating differences of test impact in various subgroups of patients, studying the effect of effect modifying variables and adjusting for confounding factors using multivariable analytical methods, will add to the value of the study. When the clinician and patient "levels" are to be considered simultaneously, multilevel analysis is to be used.

As it is often difficult to reach sufficient statistical power in studies with doctors as the units of analysis, and because of the expected heterogeneity in observational clinical studies, before–after studies are more appropriate to test the hypothesis of a substantial clinical impact than to find subtle differences.

Modified approaches

Given the potential sources of uncontrollable bias in all phases of the study, investigators may choose to use "paper" cases or clinical vignettes, audio- or video-recorded patients, interactive computer-simulated cases, or "standardized patients" especially trained to simulate a specific role consistently over time. Standardized (simulated) patients can consult the doctor even without being recognized as "non-real."[13,14] Furthermore, the pre- and posttest assessments can also be done by an independent expert panel in order to ensure that the evaluation of the clinical impact is based on best available clinical knowledge. The limitations of such approaches are that they do not always sufficiently reflect clinical reality, are less suitable (vignettes) for an interactive diagnostic work up, cannot be used to evaluate more invasive diagnostics (standardized patients), and do not allow additionally assessing diagnostic accuracy.

A before–after comparison in a group of doctors applying the test to an indicated patient population can be extended with a concurrent observational control group of doctors assessing indicated patients, without receiving the test information (quasi-experimental comparison). However, given the substantial risk of clinical and prognostic incomparability of the participating doctors and patients in the parallel groups compared, and of possibly incorrect able extraneous influences, this will often not strengthen the design substantially. If a controlled design is considered, a randomized trial is to be preferred (Chapter 4).

Concluding remarks

As Guyatt *et al.*[3] have pointed out, in considering a before–after design to study the clinical impact of diagnostic testing, two types of methodological problem must be acknowledged. First, we have to deal with problems for which, in principle, reasonable solutions can be found in order to optimize the study design. In this chapter, some of these "challenges" have been discussed. Examples are appropriate specifications of the clinical problem to be studied and the candidate patient population, and the concomitant documentation of test accuracy. Second, the before–after design has inherent limitations that cannot be avoided nor solved. If these are not acceptable, another design should be chosen. The most important of these limitations are (1) the before–after design is especially appropriate for evaluating a single diagnostic procedure or additional testing, rather than comparing two essentially different (mutually exclusive) diagnostic strategies; (2) the reported pretest management options may be different from the real strategy the clinicians would have followed if the test had not been available, or if they would not have known that there is a second (posttest) chance for assessment; (3) the pre- and posttest assessments by the same clinicians for the same patients are generally not independent; and (4) an unbiased evaluation of the impact of testing on the patients' health status can often not be achieved.

Acknowledging the large number of difficulties and pitfalls of the before–after design, as outlined in previous sections, we conclude that the design can have a place especially if the pre- and posttest assessment interval can be relatively short (evaluation of the test's impact on the doctor's assessment), and if the relation between the diagnostic assessment, the subsequent therapeutic decision making, and therapeutic effectiveness is well understood. If impact on patient outcome is studied, it is important that the clinical course of the studied problem in the absence of testing is well known and highly predictable.

Given the various limitations for studying the clinical impact of diagnostic tests, the randomized controlled trial design, if feasible, will in most cases be superior. However, given that before–after studies can be carried out relatively fast, largely embedded in daily care, whereas RCTs are often more complex or expensive, a well-designed before–after study may be useful to explore whether a diagnostic RCT could be worthwhile, or how it should be performed. In addition, if an RCT is impossible or infeasible, or ethically unacceptable, a before–after study may be the most suitable alternative. Other options, which could provide a more uniform clinical presentation and a better control of interfering variables, are before–after studies using written patient vignettes, interactive computer simulations, or standardized patients. The specific potentials and limitations (e.g., representing less clinical reality and impossibility of additional assessment of diagnostic accuracy) of these alternative approaches will then have to be taken into account.

References

1. Alperovitch A. Controlled assessment of diagnostic techniques: methodological problems. *Eff Health Care*. 1983;**1**:187–90.
2. Knottnerus JA, van Weel C, Muris JW. Evaluation of diagnostic procedures. *BMJ*. 2002;**324**:477–80.
3. Guyatt GH, Sackett DL, Haynes RB. Evaluating diagnostic tests. In: Haynes RB, Sackett DL, Guyatt GH, et al. *Clinical epidemiology: how to do clinical practice research*. Philadelphia: Lippincott, Williams & Wilkins; 2006.
4. Bossuyt PM, Lijmer JG, Mol BW. Randomised comparisons of medical tests: sometimes invalid, not always efficient. *Lancet*. 2000;**356**:1844–47.
5. Guyatt GH, Tugwell PX, Feeney DH, et al. The role of before–after studies in the evaluation of therapeutic impact of diagnostic technology. *J Chronic Dis*. 1986;**39**:295–304.
6. Dinant GJ, Knottnerus JA, van Wersch JWJ. Diagnostic impact of the erythrocyte sedimentation rate in general practice: a before–after analysis. *Fam Pract*. 1992;**9**:28–31.
7. Dinant GJ. Diagnostic value of the erythrocyte sedimentation rate in general practice. PhD dissertation. Maastricht University: Maastricht, 1991.
8. Deutekom M, Bossuyt PM. The increased availability of self-tests for medical analyses. Ned Tijdschr Geneesk 2007;**151**; 901–4 (abstract in English).
9. Bossuyt PM, Irwig L, Craig J, et al. Comparative accuracy: assessing new tests against existing diagnostic pathways. *BMJ*. 2006;**332**:1089–92.

10. Guyatt G, Drummond M. Guideline for the clinical and economic assessment of health technologies: the case of magnetic resonance. *Intl J Health Tech Assess Health Care*. 1985;**1**:551–66.
11. Tversky A, Kahneman D. Judgment under uncertainty: heuristics and biases. *Science* 1974;**185**:1124–31.
12. Elstein AS, Shulman LS, Sprafka SA. *Medical problem solving: an analysis of clinical reasoning*. Cambridge, MA: Harvard University Press; 1978.
13. Rethans JJ, Sturmans F, Drop R, et al. Assessment of the performance of general practitioners by the use of standardized (simulated) patients. *Br J Gen Pract*. 1991;**41**:97–909.
14. Bullens J, Rethans JJ, Goedhuys J, et al. The use of standardised patients in research in general practice. *Fam Pract*. 1997;**14**:431–35.

CHAPTER 6

Designing studies to ensure that estimates of test accuracy will travel

Les M. Irwig, Patrick M. M. Bossuyt, Paul P. Glasziou, Constantine Gatsonis, and Jeroen G. Lijmer

Summary box

- There may be genuine differences between test accuracies in different settings, such as primary care or hospital, in different types of hospital, or between countries.
- Deciding whether estimates of test accuracy are transferable to other settings depends on an understanding of the possible reasons for variability in test discrimination and calibration across settings.
- The transferability of measures of test performance from one setting to another depends on which indicator of test performance is to be used.
- Real variation in the performance of diagnostic tests (such as different test types, or a different spectrum of disease) needs to be distinguished from artifactual variation resulting from study design features. These features include the target condition and reference standard used, the population and the clinical question studied, the evaluated comparison, and the way the index test was performed, calibrated, and interpreted.
- In preparing studies on diagnostic accuracy, a key question is how to design studies that carry more information about the transferability of results.
- To ensure that estimates of diagnostic accuracy will travel, before starting to design a study the following questions must be answered:

The Evidence Base of Clinical Diagnosis: Theory and Methods of Diagnostic Research. 2nd edition.
Edited by J. André Knottnerus and Frank Buntinx. © 2009 Blackwell Publishing,
ISBN: 978-1-4051-5787-2.

- How are the target condition and reference standard defined?
- Is the objective to estimate global test performance or to estimate probability of disease in individuals?
- What is the population and clinical problem?
- Is the test being considered as a replacement or incremental test?
- To what extent do you want to study the reasons for variability of the results within your population?
- To what extent do you want to study the transferability of the results to other settings?
- Designing studies with heterogeneous study populations allows exploration of the transferability of diagnostic performance in different settings. This will require larger studies than have generally been carried out in the past for diagnostic tests.

Introduction

Measures of test accuracy are often thought of as fixed characteristics that can be determined by research and then applied in practice. Yet even when tests are evaluated in a study with adequate quality—including features such as consecutive patients, a good reference standard, and independent, blinded assessments of tests and the reference standard[1]—diagnostic test performance in one setting may vary from the results reported elsewhere. This has been explored extensively for coronary artery disease[2,3,4,5] but has also been shown for a variety of other conditions.[6,7,8] This variability is not only due to chance. There may be genuine differences between test accuracy in different settings, such as primary care or hospital, different types of hospital, or the same type of hospital in different countries. As a consequence, the findings from a study may not be applicable to the specific decision problem for which the reader has turned to the literature.

We suggest that deciding whether the estimates of test accuracy from studies are transferable to other settings depends on an understanding of the possible reasons for variability in test discrimination and calibration across settings. Variability may be due to artifactual differences (e.g., different design features of studies in different settings) or true differences (such as different test types, or a different spectrum of disease). To decide on the transferability of test results, we are concerned with true differences, after artifactual differences have been addressed.[9,10,11]

This chapter is divided into two main sections. The first is concerned with the reasons for true variability in accuracy; it explores conceptual underpinnings. The second section is a pragmatic guide for those interpreting and designing studies of diagnostic tests. It is based on the view that value can be added to studies of diagnostic tests by exploring the extent to which we can characterize the reasons for variability in diagnostic performance between patients in different settings, and examining how much variability remains unexplained.

Reasons for true variability in test accuracy: conceptual underpinnings

Measures of diagnostic test performance: discrimination and calibration

There are many measures of test accuracy. Broadly speaking, we can think of them as falling into one of the following categories.

1 *Global measures of test accuracy assess only discriminatory power.* These measures assess the ability of the test to discriminate between diseased and nondiseased individuals. Common examples are the area under the receiver operating characteristic curve, and the odds ratio, sometimes also referred to as the diagnostic odds ratio. They may be sufficient for some broad health policy decisions, for example, whether a new test is in general better than an existing test for that condition.

2 *Measures of test performance to estimate the probability of disease in individuals require discrimination and calibration.* These measures are used to estimate probabilities of the target condition in individuals who have a particular test result. An example is the predictive value: the proportion of people with a particular test result who have the disease of interest. To be useful for clinical practice, these estimates should be accompanied by other relevant information. For example, fracture rates in people with a particular result of a test for osteoporosis differ between people depending on their age, sex, and other characteristics. It is clumsy and difficult to estimate disease rates for all categories of patient who may have different prior probabilities. Therefore, the estimation is often done indirectly using Bayes's theorem, based on the patient-specific prior probability and some expression of the conditional distributions of test results: the distribution of test results in subjects with and without the target condition. Examples are the sensitivity and specificity of the test, and likelihood ratios for test results. These measures of test performance require more than the *discrimination* assessed by the global measures. They require tests to be *calibrated*. As an example of the difference between discrimination and calibration, consider two tests with identical odds ratios (and ROC curves) which therefore have the same discriminatory power. However, one test may operate at a threshold that gives a sensitivity of 90% and a specificity of 60%, whereas the other operates at a threshold that gives a sensitivity of 60% and a specificity of 90%. Therefore, they differ in the way they are calibrated.

Features that facilitate transferability of test results

The transferability of measures of test performance from one setting to another depends on which indicator of test performance is to be used. The possible

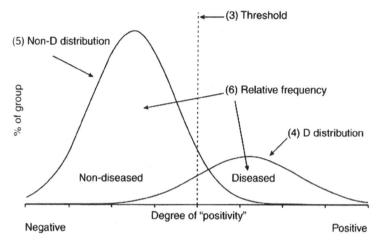

Figure 6.1 Distribution of test results in individuals with the disease of interest (D) and those without it (non-D). Numbers refer to assumptions for transferability of test results as explained in the text and Table 6.1.

assumptions involved in transferability are illustrated in Figure 6.1. Table 6.1 indicates the relationship between these assumptions and the transferability of the different measures of test performance.

The main assumptions in transferring tests across settings are as follows:

1 *The definition of disease is constant.* Many diseases have ambiguous definitions. For example, there is no single reference standard for heart failure, Alzheimer's disease, or diabetes. Reference standards may differ because conceptual frameworks differ between investigators, or because it is difficult to apply the same framework in a standardized way.

2 *The same test is used.* Although based on the same principle, tests may differ—for example over time, or if made by different manufacturers.

3 *The thresholds between categories of test result (e.g., positive and negative) are constant.* This is possible with a well-standardized test that can be calibrated across different settings. However, there may be no accepted means of calibration: for example, different observers of imaging tests may have different thresholds for calling an image "positive." The effect of different cut points is classically studied by the use of an ROC curve. In some cases, calibration may be improved by using category specific likelihood ratios, rather than a single cut point.

4 *The distribution of test results in the disease group is constant in shape and location.* This assumption is likely to be violated if the spectrum of disease changes: for example, a screening setting is likely to include earlier disease, for which test results will be closer to a nondiseased group (hence a lower sensitivity).

5 *The distribution of test results in the nondisease group is constant in shape and location.* This assumption is likely to be violated if the spectrum of nondisease

Table 6.1 Assumptions for transferring different test performance characteristics. More important assumptions are marked **X** and those that are less crucial are marked *X*

Measures of test Discriminatory power	Assumption*				Comment
	3	4	5	6	
Odds ratio	X	X	X		Both of these measures are used for global assessment of discriminatory power and are transferable if the assumptions are met. Neither of them is concerned with calibration and therefore cannot be used for assessing the probability of disease in individuals. Strictly speaking, assumptions 4 and 5 are sufficient but not necessary for the transferability of the area under the ROC curve
Area under ROC		X	X		
Measures of discriminatory power and calibration	3	4	5	6	
Predictive value		X	X	X	X	Directly estimates probability of disease in individuals
Sensitivity	X	X		*X*	
Specificity	X		*X*	*X*	These three measures can be used to estimate the probability of disease in individuals using Bayes's theorem
Likelihood ratios for a multi-category test	X	X	X		

*Assumptions are numbered as described in the text.

changes: for example, the secondary care setting involves additional causes of false positives due to comorbidity, not seen in primary care.

6 *The ratio of disease to nondisease (pretest probability) is constant.* If this were the case, we could use the posttest probability ("predictive" values) directly. However, this assumption is likely to be frequently violated: for example, the pretest probability is likely to be lowest in screening and greatest in referral settings. This likely nonconstancy is the reason for using Bayes's theorem to "adjust" the posttest probability for the pretest probability of each different setting.

All the measures of test performance need the first two assumptions to be fulfilled. The extent to which the last four assumptions are sufficient is shown in Table 6.1, although they may not be necessary in every instance; occasionally the assumptions may be violated, but, because of compensating differences, transferability is still reasonable.

Lack of transferability and applicability of measures of test performance

We need first to distinguish artifactual variation from real variation in diagnostic performance. Artifactual variation arises when studies vary in the extent to which they incorporate study design features, such as whether consecutive patients were included, or whether the reference standard and the index test were read blind to each other. Once such artifactual sources of variation have been ruled out, we may explore the potential sources of true variation.[12] The issues to consider are similar to those for assessing interventions. For interventions, we consider patient, intervention, comparator, and outcome (PICO).[13,14] For tests, the list is as follows, but with the target condition (equivalent to outcome in trials) shifted to the beginning of the list: (1) The target condition and reference standard used to assess it; (2) the population/clinical question; (3) the comparison; and (4) the index test. We now look at each of these in turn.

The target condition and the reference standard used to assess it

Test accuracy in any population will depend on how we define who has the target condition(s) that the test aims to detect. Clearly, the stage and spectrum of the target disease will influence the accuracy of the index test, as described later. However, even within a fixed spectrum and stage, there may be different definitions of who is "truly" diseased or not. Depending on the purpose of the study, the target conditions may be defined on grounds of clinical relevance, oriented to management decisions or prognosis, or defined on the grounds of pathological diagnosis. The definition of the target condition is therefore an active choice to be made by the investigator and its relevance interpreted by the reader of the study in the light of how they want to use the information. For example, should myocardial infarction include (a) "silent" myocardial infarction (with no chest pain)? (b) coronary thrombosis reversed by thrombolytic treatment, which then averts full infarction? This issue of the definition of the target condition and its method of ascertainment will clearly affect the apparent accuracy of the index test. For example, in parallel to considerations in clinical trials, the closer the reference standard is to a patient-relevant measure, the more this will help decisions about clinical applicability. Often reference standards that are considered objective and free of error are surrogates for (predictors of) natural history, which could be measured directly. Consider the reference standard for a test for appendicitis. The "objective" reference standard for a new test of appendicitis is often considered to be histology (arrow 2 on Figure 6.2.) In fact, conceptually, follow up of natural history is a far more useful reference standard than histology (Figure 6.2, arrow 1). It is patient- relevant: those people who would have been found to have abnormal histology but whose condition resolves without operation can be considered false positives of the histological reference standard (Figure 6.2, arrow 3). In practice, the data for arrow 3 cannot be established, and we need to use a combined reference standard that we would consider as natural

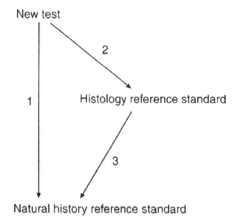

Figure 6.2 Choosing a relevant reference standard.

history when available and histology when not, rather than (as it is usually conceptualized) histology when available and natural history when not.

The usual presentation deals with a dichotomous definition of the target condition: it is either present or absent. In most cases, the possibility of multiple conditions is more plausible. If these are known in advance, the polytomous nature can be taken into account.[15,16,17]

Misclassification of the reference standard will tend to result in underestimation of test accuracy if the errors in the reference standard and test are uncorrelated. The degree of underestimation is prevalence dependent in a nonlinear way. Sensitivity is underestimated most when the prevalence of the target condition is low, whereas specificity is underestimated most when the prevalence of the target condition is high.[18,19] The odds ratio is underestimated most when prevalence is at either extreme. Therefore, error in the reference standard may cause apparent (rather than real) effect modification of test discrimination in subgroups in which the target condition has different prevalences.[20,21] This is shown in Table 6.2 where the same hypothetical test and reference standard are applied to a population in which disease prevalence is 50% (top half of table) and about 9% (bottom half). Sensitivity is reduced more in the population with 9% prevalence of disease, and specificity more in the population at 50% prevalence. The odds ratio is reduced most in the population at 9% prevalence. If errors in the reference standard are correlated with test errors, then the effect will be more difficult to predict. Correlated errors may result in overestimation of test accuracy.

The population and the clinical question

The population/clinical question are concerned not only with what disease is being tested for, but with what presentation of symptoms, signs and other information has prompted the use of the test. Test performance may vary in

Table 6.2 Reference standard misclassification results in underestimation of test accuracy and apparent effect modification of different prevalences

If reference standard has sensitivity = 0.9 and specificity = 0.8

Test	True disease			Test	Reference standard		
	Present	Absent	Total		Present	Absent	Total
Positive	80	30	110	Positive	78	32	110
Negative	20	70	90	Negative	32	58	90
Total	100	100	200	Total	110	90	200
Sensitivity = 0.80		OR = 9.3		Sensitivity = 0.71		OR = 4.4	
Specificity = 0.70				Specificity = 0.64			

If reference standard has sensitivity = 0.9 and specificity = 0.8

Test	True disease			Test	Reference standard		
	Present	Absent	Total		Present	Absent	Total
Positive	80	300	380	Positive	132	248	380
Negative	20	700	720	Negative	158	562	720
Total	100	1000	1100	Total	290	810	1100
Sensitivity = 0.80		OR = 9.3		Sensitivity = 0.46		OR = 1.9	
Specificity = 0.70				Specificity = 0.69			

different populations and with minor changes in the clinical question. There are three critical concepts that help in understanding why this occurs. These are the spectrum of disease, the referral filter, and the incremental value of the test.

• *Spectrum of disease and nondisease.* Many diseases are not on/off states, but represent a spectrum ranging from mild to severe forms of disease.[22] Tumors, for example, start small, with a single cell, and then grow, leading eventually to symptoms. The ability of mammography, for example, to detect a breast tumor depends on its size. Therefore, test sensitivity will generally differ between asymptomatic and symptomatic persons. If previous tests have been carried out the spectrum of disease in tested patients may be limited, with patients who have very severe forms of disease or those with very mild forms being eliminated from the population. For example, in patients with more severe urinary tract infection, as judged by the presence of more severe symptoms and signs, the sensitivity of dipstick tests was much higher than in those with minor symptoms and signs.[6]

Likewise, patients without the target condition are not a homogeneous group. Even in the absence of disease, variability in results is the norm rather than the exception. For many laboratory tests, normal values in women differ from those in men. Similarly, values in children differ from those in adults, and values in young adults sometimes differ from those in the elderly.

Commonly, the "nondiseased" group consists of several different conditions, for each of which the test specificity may vary. The overall specificity will depend on the "mix" of alternative diagnoses: the proportion of people in each of the categories that constitute the nondiseased; for example, prostate specific antigen may have a lower specificity in older people or those with prostatic symptoms, as it is elevated in men with benign prostatic hypertrophy.[23] In principle, patients without that target condition could represent a wide range of other conditions. However, the decision to use a test is usually made because of the presenting problem of the patient and the route by which they reached the examining clinician. Hence, the actual range of variability in patients without the target condition will depend on the mechanism by which patients have ended up in that particular situation. As an example, consider a group of ambulant outpatients presenting with symptoms of venous thromboembolism without having this disease compared to a group of inpatients suspected of venous thromboembolism but actually having a malignancy. The specificity of a d-dimer test in outpatients will be lower than that in inpatients.[24]

• *Referral filter.* The discriminatory power of tests often varies across settings because patients presenting with a clinical problem in one setting—for example primary care—are very different from those presenting to a secondary care facility with that clinical problem.[25,26] Patients who are referred to secondary care may be those with a more difficult diagnostic problem, in whom the usual tests have not resolved the uncertainty. These patients have been through a referral filter to get to the tertiary care center.

This concept can best be considered using the hypothetical results of a diagnostic test evaluation in primary care (Table 6.3). Imagine that patients are referred from this population to a source of secondary care, and that all the test positive patients are referred, but only a random half of the test negative patients. As shown in Table 6.4, the overall test discrimination, as reflected in the odds ratio, has not changed. However, there appears to be a shift in threshold, with an increased sensitivity and a decreased specificity.

Of course, it is unlikely that test negatives would be referred randomly; rather, it may be on the grounds of other clinical information that the practitioner is particularly concerned about those test negatives. If the practitioner is

Table 6.3 Accuracy of a test in primary care

| Test | Disease | | |
	Present	Absent	Total
Positive	60	40	100
Negative	40	60	100
Total	100	100	200

Sensitivity = 0.60   OR = 2.25
Sensitivity = 0.60

Table 6.4 Test accuracy if a random sample of test negatives are referred for verification

| | Disease | | |
Test	Present	Absent	Total
Positive	60	40	100
Negative	20	30	50
Total	80	70	150
Sensitivity = 0.75 OR = 2.25			
Specificity = 0.43			

Table 6.5 Diagnostic performances vary by setting because of selective patient referral

| | Disease | | |
Test	Present	Absent	Total
Positive	60	40	100
Negative	25	25	50
Total	85	65	150
Sensitivity = 0.71 OR = 1.5			
Specificity = 0.38			

correct in identifying patients about whom there is an increased risk of disease, the table could well turn out like Table 6.5.

In this case, because of the clinician's skill and the use of other information, the test threshold not only appears to be shifted but also the overall test performance of the test in secondary care has been eroded, as shown by the reduced odds ratio. The more successfully the primary care practitioner detects cases that are test negative but which nevertheless need referral for management of the disease of interest, the more the performance of the test in secondary care is eroded.

• *To what prior tests is the incremental value of the new test being assessed?* In many situations, several tests are being used and the value of a particular test may depend on what tests have been done before,[27] or simple prior clinical information.[28,29] In Table 6.6, two tests are cross-classified within diseased and nondiseased people. The sensitivity and specificity of each test is 0.6, and they remain 0.6 if test B is used after test A, that is, the test performance characteristics of B remain unaltered in categories of patients who are A positive and those who are A negative.

However, if the tests are conditionally dependent or associated with each other within diseased and nondiseased groups, for example because they both measure a similar metabolite, then the overall test performance of B is eroded,

Table 6.6 Incremental value when tests A and B are conditionally independent

	Have disease			No disease		
	A+	A−	Total	A+	A−	Total
B+	36	24	60	16	24	40
B−	24	16	40	24	36	60
Total	60	40	100	40	60	100

Notes: "Crude" sensitivity and specificity of both A and B = 0.6 and odds ratio = 2.25. If A is + or −, SnB = 0.6, SpB = 0.6, and OR = 2.25.

as judged by the OR changing from 2.25 to 2.00 (Table 6.7 and Figure 6.3). In addition, there appears to be a threshold shift: the test is more sensitive but less specific in patients for whom A is positive than in those for whom A is negative. In other words, not only is the *discrimination* of the new test (B) less if done after the existing test (A), as judged by the odds ratio, but the *calibration* appears to differ depending on the result of the prior test. In fact, the threshold has not altered but there has been a shift in the distribution of test results in diseased and nondiseased groups, conditional on the results of test A.

An example is provided by Mol and colleagues,[30] who evaluated the performance of serum hCG (human chorionic gonadotrophin) measurement in the diagnosis of women with suspected ectopic pregnancy. Several studies have reported an adequate sensitivity of this test.[30] However, the presence of an

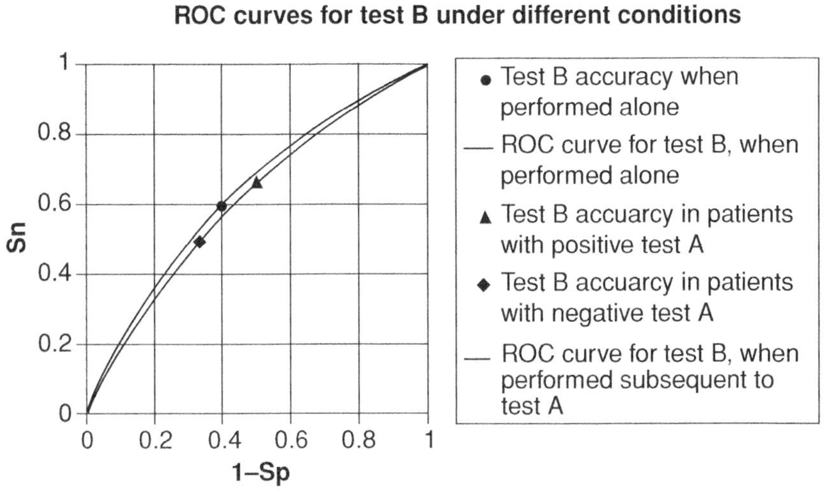

ROC curves for test B under different conditions

- Test B accuracy when performed alone
- ROC curve for test B, when performed alone
- Test B accuarcy in patients with positive test A
- Test B accuarcy in patients with negative test A
- ROC curve for test B, when performed subsequent to test A

Figure 6.3 Test characteristics for test B alone and in those with positive and negative test A.

Table 6.7 Incremental value when tests A and B are conditionally dependent

	Have disease			No disease		
	A+	A−	Total	A+	A−	Total
B+	40	20	60	20	20	40
B−	20	20	40	20	40	60
Total	60	40	100	40	60	100

Notes: "Crude" sensitivity and specificity of both A and B = 0.6. Odds ratio = 2.25. If A+, SnB = 0.67, SpB = 0.50 and OR = 2.00. If A−, SnB = 0.50, SpB = 0.67 and OR = 2.00.

ectopic or intrauterine pregnancy can also be diagnosed with ultrasound. Mol *et al.* reported the sensitivity of hCG to be significantly different in patients with signs of an ectopic pregnancy (adnexal mass, or fluid in the pouch of Douglas) on ultrasound, compared to those without signs on ultrasound. As a consequence, an uncritical generalization of the "unconditional" sensitivity will overestimate the diagnostic performance of this test if it is applied after an initial examination with ultrasound, as is the case in clinical practice.[30]

Categories of patients for whom new tests are most helpful are worth investigating. For example, whole-body positron emission tomography (PET) contributed most additional diagnostic information in the subgroup of patients in whom prior conventional diagnostic methods had been equivocal.[31]

The comparison: replacement or incremental test
A new test may be evaluated as a *replacement* for the existing test, rather than being done after the existing test, in which case the *incremental* value is of interest. For assessment of replacement value, the cross-classification of the tests is not necessary to obtain unbiased estimates of how the diagnostic performance of the new test differs from that of the existing one. However, information about how they are associated from a cross-classification will provide extra useful information and improve precision.[32]

Readers may have noticed that the issue of incremental value and the decreased test performance if tests are conditionally dependent is related to the prior issue of decreased test performance if the primary care clinician is acting as an effective referral filter. In our previous example, imagine that the test being evaluated is B. The clinician may be using test A to alter the mix of A+ and A−s that get through to secondary care, and the test performance of B reflects the way in which this mix has occurred.

The test
• *Discriminatory power.* Information about the test is relevant to both discriminative power and calibration. Discrimination may differ between tests that bear the same generic name but which, for example, are made by different

manufacturers. Tests may be less discriminatory when produced in "kit" form than in initial laboratory testing.[33] When tests require interpretative skill, they are often first evaluated in near-optimal situations. Special attention is usually devoted to the unambiguous and reproducible interpretation of test results. This has implications for the interpretation and generalizability of the results. If the readers of images are less than optimal in your own clinical setting, test accuracy will be affected downward.[34,35,36]

The usual presentation deals with a two-way definition of test results, into positive and negative. In many cases, *multiple categories of test results* is more plausible. In addition, there may be a category of uninterpretable test results that needs to be considered. The polytomous nature of tests should be taken into account, for which several methods are available. Rather than a simple positive–negative dichotomy and the associated characteristics sensitivity and specificity, likelihood ratios for the multiple categories and ROC curves can be calculated (see Chapter 7). In all cases, a more general $n \times n$ table can be used to describe test characteristics, and several likelihoods can be calculated.[16]

- *Calibration.* If the purpose of the study is clinical decision making, in which information is being derived to estimate probabilities of disease, then a second major issue is the calibration of test results. A continuous test may have equivalent ROCs and diagnostic ORs in two different settings, but very different likelihood ratios (LRs). For example, machine calibration may be different in the two settings, so that one machine may show results considerably higher than another. Likewise, even if two readers of radiographs have similar discriminative power, as shown by similar ROCs, the threshold they use to differentiate positive from negative tests (or adjacent categories of a multicategory test) may vary widely.[37,38,39,40,41]

In summary, variability in the discriminative power and calibration of the same test used in different places is the rule rather than the exception. When we strive for parsimony in our descriptions, we run the risk of oversimplification. In the end, the researcher who reports a study, as well as the clinician searching the literature for help in interpreting test results, has to bear in mind that test performance characteristics are never just properties of the test itself: they depend on several factors, including prior clinical and test information, and the setting in which the test is done.

Implications of variation in discriminative power and calibration of tests: questions to ask yourself before you start designing the study

1 What are the target condition and the reference standard?
2 Is the objective to estimate test performance using a global measure, or a measure that will allow estimation of the probability of disease in individuals?
3 What is the population and clinical problem?

4 Is the test being considered as a replacement or incremental test?

5 To what extent do you want to study the reasons for variability of the results within your population?

6 To what extent do you want to study the transferability of the results to other settings?

In what follows, we assume that the usual criteria for adequate design of an evaluation of a diagnostic test have been fulfilled. The issue is then: How do we design a study which will also help to ensure that its transferability can be determined? Based on the concepts in the first part of this chapter, we suggest that investigators ask themselves the following questions to help ensure that readers have the necessary information to decide on the transferability of the study to their own setting. These considerations are also reflected in the STARD checklist for reporting the results of diagnostic evaluation studies.[42]

What are the target condition and reference standard?

The target condition and reference standard need to be chosen to reflect the investigator's requirements. Is the choice appropriate to whether the investigator is doing the study to assist with predicting prognosis, deciding as the need for intervention, or researching pathological processes? For example, in a study of tests to assess stenosis of the carotid artery, it would be sensible to choose the reference standard as angiographic stenosis dichotomized around 70%, if this is the level of angiographic abnormality above which, on currently available evidence, the benefits of treatment outweigh the harm. On the other hand, if the study is being done by researchers whose interest is in basic science, they may wish to compare the test with stenosis assessed on surgically removed specimens at a different threshold, or across a range of thresholds.

Error in the reference standard is a major constraint on our ability to estimate test accuracy and explore reasons for variability of test characteristics.[18,19,43] Therefore, researchers should consider methods of minimizing error in the reference standard, for example, by using better methods or multiple assessments. Any information about the test performance characteristics of the reference standard will help interpretation, as will several different measures of the target condition, which can be combined. Multiple measures of the reference standard or multiple different tests also allow the use of more sophisticated analyses, such as latent class analysis, to minimize the potential for bias in estimates of test accuracy or factors that affect it.[21,44] Because the effects of misclassification in the reference standard have different effects in populations of different prevalence, as shown in Table 6.2, one may choose to assess a test in a population where any residual effects of error in the reference standard are minimized. For the odds ratio, this is at about 50% prevalence. For sensitivity, it is when prevalence is high, and for specificity when prevalence is low. However, when using this strategy, consider whether the spectrum of disease may also vary with prevalence. If so, you will need to judge whether reference standard misclassification is a sufficiently important problem to outweigh the potential for spectrum bias induced by choosing a study in a population with specified prevalence.

Is the objective to estimate test performance using a global measure (discrimination) or a measure that will allow estimation of the probability of disease in individuals (discrimination and calibration)?

Global assessment of the discriminatory power of the test requires measures such as the area under the ROC curve, or the diagnostic odds ratio. These may be sufficient for some purposes, for example if a policy decision needs to be made about alternative tests of equivalent cost, or to decide whenever a test has sufficient accuracy to warrant further calibration. For estimating the probability of disease in individuals, likelihood ratios (or sensitivity and specificity) are needed, with additional information on how tests were calibrated. Information about calibration should be provided in papers for readers to be able to use the result of your study. Access to selected example material, such as radiographs of lesions, will help readers understand what thresholds have been used for reading in your study.

What is the population and clinical problem?

This question defines how the inception cohort should be selected for study, although the breadth of the group selected will also be determined by the extent to which you wish to address the following questions. For example, a new test for carotid stenosis could be considered for all patients referred to a surgical unit. However, ultrasound is reasonably accurate at quantifying the extent of stenosis, and so investigators may choose to restrict the study of a more expensive or invasive test to patients in whom the ultrasound result is near the decision threshold for surgery. A useful planning tool is to draw a flow diagram of how patients reach the population/clinical problem of interest. This flow diagram includes what clinical information has been gathered and what tests have been done, and how the results of those tests determine entry into the population and clinical problem of interest. For example, in the flow diagram in Figure 6.4 the clinical problem is suspected appendicitis in children presenting to a hospital emergency service. The decisions based sequentially on clinical evidence and ultrasonography are shown. The flow diagram helps to clarify that computed tomography (CT) is being assessed only in patients in whom those prior tests had not resolved the clinical problem. Also as shown in the figure, in addition to being helpful at the design stage, publishing such flow diagrams, with numbers of patients who follow each step, is very helpful to readers.[45]

Is the test being considered as a replacement or incremental test?

As outlined earlier, the population and the clinical problem define the initial presentation and referral filter. In addition, a key question is whether we are

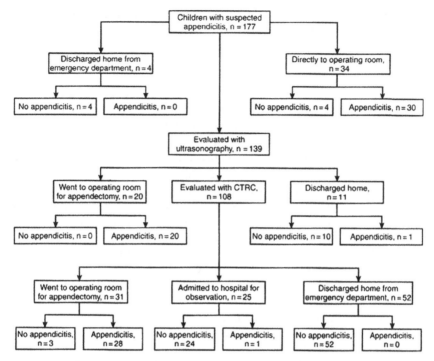

Figure 6.4 A flow diagram to formulate a diagnostic test research question. Study profile flow diagram of patients with suspected appendicitis. (From Garcia Pena BM *et al.* Ultrasonography and limited computed tomography in the diagnosis and management of appendicitis in children. *JAMA* 1999;**282**:1041–46. Reproduced with permission from the American Medical Association.[45])

evaluating the test to assess whether it should replace an existing test (because it is better, or just as good and cheaper) or to assess whether it has value when used in addition to a particular existing test. This decision will also be a major determinant of how the data will be analysed.[46,47,48]

To what extent do you want to study the reasons for variability of the results within your population?

How much variability is there between readers/operators?
Data should be presented on the amount of variability between different readers or test types and tools to help calibration, such as standard radiographs,[39,40] or laboratory quality control measures. The extent to which other factors, such as experience or training, affect reading adequacy will also help guide readers of the study. Assessment of variability should include not only test discriminatory power but also calibration, if the objective is to provide study results that are useful for individual clinical decision making.

Do the findings vary in different (prespecified) subgroups within the study population?

Data should be analyzed to determine the influence on test performance characteristics of the following variables, which should be available for each individual.

• *The spectrum of disease and nondisease, for example by estimating "specificity" within each category of "nondisease."* These can be considered separately by users or combined into a weighted specificity for different settings. The same approach can be used for levels (stage, grade) in the "diseased" group.

• *The effect of other test results.* This follows the approach often used in clinical prediction rules. It should take account of logical sequencing of tests (simplest, least invasive, and cheapest are generally first). It should also take account of possible effect modification by other tests. In some instances people would have been referred because of other tests being positive (or negative), so that the incremental value of the new test cannot be evaluated. In this case, knowing the referral filter and how tests have been used in it (as in Figure 6.4) will help interpretation. For example, a study by Flamen[31] has shown that the major value of PET for recurrent colorectal adenocarcinoma is in the category of patients in whom prior (cheaper) tests gave inconclusive results. It would therefore be a useful incremental test in that category of patients, but would add little (except cost) if being considered as a replacement test for all patients, many of whom would have the diagnostic question resolved by the cheaper test. This suggests that PET is very helpful in this clinical situation.[31]

• *Any other characteristics, such as age or gender.*

There are often a vast number of characteristics that could be used to define subgroups in which one may wish to check whether there are differences in test performance. The essential descriptors of a clinical situation need to be decided by the researcher. As for subgroup analysis in randomized trials,[49] these characteristics should be prespecified, rather than decided at analysis stage. The decision is best made on the basis of an understanding of the pathophysiology of the disease, the mechanism by which the test assesses abnormality, an understanding of possible referral filters, and knowledge of which characteristics vary widely between centers. Remember that variability between test characteristics in subgroups may not be due to real subgroup differences if there is reference standard misclassification and the prevalence of disease differs between subgroups, as shown in Table 6.2. Modeling techniques can be used to assess the effect of several potential predictors of test accuracy simultaneously.[50,51,52,53,54]

To what extent do you want to study the transferability of the results to other settings?

To address this question, you need to perform the study in several populations or centers, and assess the extent to which test performance differs, as has been done for the General Health Questionnaire[55] and predictors of coma.[56] The extent to which observed variability is beyond that compatible with random sampling variability can be assessed using statistical tests for heterogeneity. Predictors (as discussed above) should also be measured to assess the extent to which within-population variables explain between-population variability. Because of the low power of tests of heterogeneity, this is worth doing even if tests for heterogeneity between centers or studies are not statistically significant. The more the measured variables explain between-population differences, the more they can be relied on when assessing the transferability of that study to the population in the reader's setting. Between-site variability can also be explored across different studies using meta-analytical techniques.[57,58,59]

Sites for inclusion in the multicentered comparison should be selected as being representative of the sorts of populations in which the results of the diagnostic study are likely to be used. The more the variability in site features can be characterized—and indeed taken account of in the sampling of sites for inclusion in studies—the more informative the study will be. Data should be analyzed to determine the influence on results of the within-site (individually measured) patient characteristics mentioned above. They should also explore the following sources of between-site variability that are not accounted for by the within-site characteristics:

- Site characteristics, for example primary, secondary, or tertiary care.
- Other features, such as country.
- Prevalence of the disease of interest.

Residual heterogeneity between sites should be explored to judge the extent to which there is inexplicable variability that may limit test applicability.

Explanatory note about prevalence

The inclusion of "prevalence" in the above list may seem unusual, as it is not obviously a predictor of test performance. However, there are many reasons why prevalence should be included in the list of potential predictors, in an analogous way to the exploration of trial result dependence on baseline risk.[60,61] First, many of the reasons for variation between centers may not be easy to characterize, and prevalence may contain some information about how centers differ that is not captured by other crude information, for example whether the test is evaluated in primary, secondary or tertiary care centers. Second, it is a direct test of the common assumption that test performance characteristics such as sensitivity and specificity are independent of prevalence. Third, non-linear prevalence dependence is an indication that there is misclassification of the reference standard.

In summary, designing studies with heterogeneous study populations has merit. This will allow exploration of the extent to which diagnostic performance depends on prespecified predictors, and how much residual heterogeneity exists. The more heterogeneity there is in study populations, the greater the potential to explore the transferability of diagnostic performance to other settings, as shown in Table 6.8.

Table 6.8 The value of designing studies that enable the exploration of predictors of heterogeneity of diagnostic accuracy

Heterogeneity in diagnostic accuracy	Heterogeneity in study population	
	Yes	No
Yes	To what extent is heterogeneity in accuracy explained by predictors? If not, transferability is limited	Transferability limited
No	Highly transferable	Design does not allow exploration of transferability

Concluding remarks

There is good evidence that measures of test accuracy are not as transferable across settings as is often assumed. This chapter outlines the conceptual underpinnings for this and suggests some implications for how we should be designing studies that carry more information about the transferability of results. Major examples are examining the extent to which test discrimination and calibration depend on prespecified variables, and the extent to which there is residual variability between study populations which is not explained by these variables. This will require larger studies than have generally been done in the past for diagnostic tests. Improvements in study quality and designs to assess transferability are needed to ensure that the next generation of studies on test accuracy are more able to meet our needs.

Acknowledgments

We thank Petra Macaskill, Clement Loy, André Knottnerus, Margaret Pepe, Jonathan Craig, and Anthony Grabs for comments on earlier drafts. Clement Loy also provided Figure 6.3. We thank Barbara Garcia Pena for permission to use a figure from her paper as our Figure 6.4.

References

1. Begg C. Biases in the assessment of diagnostic tests. *Stat Med*. 1987;**6**:411–23.
2. Molarius ASJ, Sans S, Tuomilehto J, et al. Varying sensitivity of waist action levels to identify subjects with overweight or obesity in 19 populations of the WHO MONICA Project. *J Clin Epidemiol*. 1999;**52**:1213–24.
3. Detrano R, Janosi A, Lyons KP, et al. Factors affecting sensitivity and specificity of a diagnostic test: the exercise thallium scintigram. *Am J Med*. 1988;**84**:699–710.

4. Hlatky M, Pryor D, Harrell FE, Jr, et al. Factors affecting sensitivity and specificity of exercise electrocardiography. *Am J Med.* 1984;**77**:64–71.
5. Rozanski ADG, Berman D, Forrester JS, et al. The declining specificity of exercise radionuclide ventriculography. *N Engl J Med.* 1983;**309**:518–22.
6. Lachs MS, Nachamkin I, Edelstein PH, et al. Spectrum bias in the evaluation of diagnostic tests: lessons from the rapid dipstick test for urinary tract infection. *Ann Intern Med.* 1992;**117**:135–40.
7. Molarius ASJ, Sans S, Tuomilehto J, et al. Varying sensitivity of waist action levels to identify subjects with overweight or obesity in 19 populations of the WHO MONICA Project. *J Clin Epidemiol.* 1999;**52**:1213–24.
8. Starmans R, Muris JW, Fijten GH, et al. The diagnostic value of scoring models for organic and non-organic gastrointestinal disease, including the irritable-bowel syndrome. *Med Decis Making.* 1994;**14**:208–16.
9. Glasziou P, Irwig L. An evidence-based approach to individualising treatment. *BMJ.* 1995;**311**:1356–59.
10. National Health and Medical Research Council. How to use the evidence: assessment and application of scientific evidence. Handbook series on preparing clinical practice guidelines. Canberra, Commonwealth of Australia; 2000. Available from: http://www.health.gov.au/nhmrc/publicat/synopses/cp65syn.htm
11. Justice AC, Covinsky KE, Berlin JA. Assessing the generalizability of prognostic information. *Ann Intern Med.* 1999;**130**:515–24.
12. Gatsonis C, McNeil BJ. Collaborative evaluations of diagnostic tests: experience of the Radiology Diagnostic Oncology Group. *Radiology.* 1990;**175**:571–75.
13. Sackett D, Straus S, Richardson WS, et al. *Evidence-based medicine: how to practice and teach EBM.* Edinburgh: Churchill Livingstone; 2000.
14. Richardson W, Wilson M, Nishikawa J, et al. The well-built clinical question: a key to evidence-based decisions. *ACP J Club.* 1995;**123**:A12.
15. Brenner H. Measures of differential diagnostic value of diagnostic procedures. *J Clin Epidemiol.* 1996;**49**:1435–39.
16. Sappenfield RW, Beeler MF, Catrou PG, et al. Nine-cell diagnostic decision matrix. A model of the diagnostic process: a framework for evaluating diagnostic protocols. *Am J Clin Pathol.* 1981;**75**:769–72.
17. Taube A, Tholander B. Over- and underestimation of the sensitivity of a diagnostic malignancy test due to various selections of the study population. *ACTA Oncol.* 1990;**29**:1–5.
18. Buck A, Gart J. Comparison of a screening test and a reference test in epidemiologic studies. I. Indices of agreement and their relation to prevalence. *Am J Epidemiol.* 1966;**83**:586–92.
19. Gart J, Buck A. Comparison of a screening test and a reference test in epidemiologic studies. II. A probabilistic model for the comparison of diagnostic tests. *Am J Epidemiol.* 1966;**83**:593–602.
20. Kelsey JL, Whittemore AS, Evans AS, Thompson WD. *Methods in observational epidemiology.* 2nd ed. New York: Oxford University Press; 1996.
21. Walter SD, Irwig L, Glasziou PP. Meta-analysis of diagnostic tests with imperfect reference standards. *J Clin Epidemiol.* 1999;**52**:943–51.
22. Ransohoff DF, Feinstein AR. Problems of spectrum and bias in evaluating the efficacy of diagnostic tests. *N Engl J Med.* 1978;**299**:926–30.
23. Coley C, Barry M, Fleming C, et al. Early detection of prostate cancer. I. Prior probability and effectiveness of tests. *Ann Intern Med.* 1997;**126**:394–406.

24. van Beek EJR, Schenk BE, Michel BC. The role of plasma d-dimer concentration in the exclusion of pulmonary embolism. *Br J Haematol.* 1996;**92**:725–32.

25. Knottnerus J, Leffers P. The influence of referral patterns on the characteristics of diagnostic tests. *J Clin Epidemiol.* 1992;**45**:1143–54.

26. van der Schouw YT, van Dijk R, Verbeek AL. Problems in selecting the adequate patient population from existing data files for assessment studies of new diagnostic tests. *J Clin Epidemiol.* 1995;**48**:417–22.

27. Katz IA, Irwig L, Vinen JD, et al. Biochemical markers of acute myocardial infarction: strategies for improving their clinical usefulness. *Ann Clin Biochem.* 1998;**35**:393–99.

28. Whitsel E, Boyko E, Siscovick DS. Reassessing the role of QT in the diagnosis of autonomic failure among patients with diabetes: a meta-analysis. *Arch Intern Med.* 2000;**23**:241–47.

29. Conde-Agudelo A, Kafury-Goeta AC. Triple-marker test as screening for Down's syndrome: a meta-analysis. *Obstet Gynecol Surv.* 1998;**53**:369–76.

30. Mol B, Hajenius P, Engelsbel S. Serum human chorionic gonadotrophin measurement in the diagnosis of ectopic pregnancy when transvaginal sonography is inconclusive. *Fertil Steril.* 1995;**70**:972–81.

31. Flamen PSS, van Cutsem E, Dupont P, et al. Additional value of whole-body positron emission tomography with fluorine-18-2-fluoro-2-deoxy-d-glucose in recurrent colorectal cancer. *J Clin Oncol.* 1999;**17**:894–901.

32. Decode Study Group. Glucose tolerance and mortality: comparison of WHO and American Diabetes Association diagnostic criteria. *Lancet.* 1999;**354**:617–21.

33. Scouller K, Conigrave KM, Macaskill P, et al. Should we use CDT instead of GGT for detecting problem drinkers? A systematic review and meta-analysis. *Clin Chem.* 2000;**46**:1894–902.

34. West OC, Anbari MM, Pilgram TK, et al. Acute cervical spine trauma: diagnostic performance of single-view versus three-view radiographic screening. *Radiology.* 1997;**204**:819–23.

35. Scheiber CMM, Dumitresco B, Demangeat JL, et al. The pitfalls of planar three-phase bone scintigraphy in nontraumatic hip avascular osteonecrosis. *Clin Nucl Med.* 1999;**24**:488–94.

36. Krupinski EA, Weinstein RS, Rozek LS. Experience-related differences in diagnosis from medical images displayed on monitors. *Telemed J.* 1996;**2**:101–8.

37. Egglin TK, Feinstein AR. Context bias: a problem in diagnostic radiology. *JAMA.* 1996;**276**:1752–55.

38. Irwig L, Groeneveld HT, Pretorius JP, Itnizdo E. Relative observer accuracy for dichotomized variables. *J Chronic Dis.* 1985;**28**:899–906.

39. D'Orsi C, Swets J. Variability in the interpretation of mammograms. *N Engl J Med.* 1995;**332**:1172.

40. Beam C, Layde P, Sullivan DC. Variability in the interpretation of screening mammograms by US radiologists. Findings from a national sample. *Arch Intern Med.* 1996;**156**:209–13.

41. Warren R, Hayes C, Pointon L, Hoff, et al. A test of performance of breast MRI interpretation in a multicentre screening study. *Magn Reson Imaging.* 2006;**24**:917–29.

42. Bossuyt PM, Reitsma JB, Bruns DE, et al. Towards complete and accurate reporting of studies of diagnostic accuracy: the STARD initiative. *BMJ.* 2003;**326**:41–44.

43. Valenstein PN. Evaluating diagnostic tests with imperfect standards. *Am J Clin Pathol.* 1990;**93**:252–8.

44. Walter S, Irwig L. Estimation of test error rates, disease prevalence and relative risk from misclassified data: A review. *J Clin Epidemiol.* 1988;**41**:923–37.

45. Garcia Pena BM, Mandl KD, Kraus SJ, et al. Ultrasonography and limited computed tomography in the diagnosis and management of appendicitis in children. *JAMA.* 1999;**282**:1041–46.

46. Marshall R. The predictive value of simple rules for combining two diagnostic tests. *Biometrics.* 1989;**45**:1213–22.

47. Biggerstaff B. Comparing diagnostic tests: a simple graphic using likelihood ratios. *Statistics Med* 2000;**19**:649–63.

48. Chock C, Irwig L, Berry G, et al. Comparing dichotomous screening tests when individuals negative on both tests are not verified. *J Clin Epidemiol.* 1997;**50**:1211–17.

49. Oxman A, Guyatt G. A consumer guide to subgroup analyses. *Ann Intern Med.* 1992;**116**:78–84.

50. Tosteson ANA, Weinstein MC, Wittenberg J, et al. ROC curve regression analysis: the use of ordinal regression models for diagnostic test assessment. *Environ Health Perspect.* 1994;**102**(Suppl 8):73–78.

51. Toledano A, Gatsonis C. Ordinal regression methodology for ROC curves derived from correlated data. *Stat Med.* 1996;**15**:1807–26.

52. Pepe M. An interpretation for the ROC curve and inference using GLM procedures. *Biometrics.* 2000;**56**:352–59.

53. Leisenring W, Pepe M. Regression modelling of diagnostic likelihood ratios for the evaluation of medical diagnostic tests. *Biometrics.* 1998;**54**:444–52.

54. Leisenring W, Pepe M, Longton G. A marginal regression modelling framework for evaluating medical diagnostic tests. *Stat Med.* 1997;**16**:1263–81.

55. Furukawa T, Goldberg DP. Cultural invariance of likelihood ratios for the General Health Questionnaire. *Lancet.* 1999;**353**:561–62.

56. Zandbergen EGJ, de Haan RJ, et al. Prognostic predictors of coma transferable from one setting to another in SR. *Lancet.* 1998;**352**:1808–12.

57. Irwig L, Tosteson ANA, Gatsonis C, et al. Guidelines for meta-analyses evaluating diagnostic tests. *Ann Intern Med* 1994;**120**:667–76.

58. Rutter C, Gatsonis C. A hierarchical regression approach to meta-analysis of diagnostic test accuracy evaluations. *Stat Med.* 2001;**20**(19):2865–84.

59. Harbord RM, Deeks JJ, Egger M, et al. A unification of models for meta-analysis of diagnostic accuracy studies. *Biostatistics.* 2007;**8**(2):239–51.

60. Schmid C, Lau J, McIntosh MW, et al. An empirical study of the effect of the control rate as a predictor of treatment efficacy in meta-analysis of clinical trials. *Stat Med.* 1998;**17**:1923–42.

61. Boyko EJ. Comment on "Meta-analysis of Pap test." *Am J Epidemiol.* 1996;**143**(4):406–7.

CHAPTER 7

Analysis of data on the accuracy of diagnostic tests

*J. Dik F. Habbema, René Eijkemans, Pieta Krijnen, and
J. André Knottnerus*

Summary box

- Neither sensitivity nor specificity is a measure of test performance on its own. It is the combination that matters.
- The statistical approach for analyzing variability in probability estimates of test accuracy is the calculation of confidence intervals.
- The magnitude of the change from pretest to posttest probability (predictive value) reflects the informativeness of the diagnostic test result.
- The informative value of a test result is determined by the likelihood ratio: the ratio of the frequencies of occurrence of this result in patients with and patients without the disease.
- The odds ratio summarizes the diagnostic value of a dichotomous test but does not tell us the specific values of sensitivity and specificity and the likelihood ratios.
- A measure of performance for a continuous test is the area under the receiver operating characteristic (ROC) curve. This varies between 0.5 for a totally uninformative test and 1.0 for a test perfectly separating diseased and nondiseased.
- Bayes's theorem implies that "posttest odds equals pretest odds times likelihood ratio."
- One can derive the optimal cutoff from the relative importance of false positives and false negatives.
- A sensitivity analysis is important for getting a feeling for the stability of our conclusions.

The Evidence Base of Clinical Diagnosis: Theory and Methods of Diagnostic Research. 2nd edition.
Edited by J. André Knottnerus and Frank Buntinx. © 2009 Blackwell Publishing.
ISBN: 978-1-4051-5787-2.

- Bayes's theorem can also be formulated as a logistic regression equation. For the analysis of combination of tests, one needs multiple logistic regression
- When starting a data analysis, one must be confident that the research data have been collected with avoidance of important bias and with acceptable generalizability to the target population.

Introduction

After the painstaking job of collecting, computerizing, and cleaning diagnostic data, we enter the exciting phase of analyzing and interpreting these data and assessing the clinical implications of the results. It would be a pity if all the effort put into the research were not to be crowned with a sound analysis and interpretation. It is the purpose of this chapter to help readers to do so.

We will study the classic test performance measures introduced in Chapter 1: sensitivity, specificity, positive and negative predictive value, likelihood ratio, and error rate, first for dichotomous tests and later for continuous tests, including the possibility of dichotomization, with its quest for cutoff values. Receiver operating characteristic (ROC) curves are part of this.

Next, Bayes's theorem for the relationship between pretest and posttest probability of disease is discussed, followed by decision analytical considerations. For generalization of the one-test situation to diagnostic conclusions based on many diagnostic test results, there will be a discussion on logistic regression and its link with Bayes's theorem.

The strengths and weaknesses of study designs, possible biases, and other methodological issues have been discussed in previous chapters and will not be repeated here, although the discussion will provide some links between biases and analysis results.

We will refer to software for performing the analysis. Also, we will include appendices with tables and graphs, which can support you in the analysis.

Clinical example

Renal artery stenosis in hypertension

We use data from a study on the diagnosis of renal artery stenosis (RAS). In about 1% of all hypertensive patients, the hypertension is caused by a constriction (stenosis) of the renal artery. It is worth identifying these patients because their hypertension could be cured by surgery, and consequently their risk of myocardial infarction and stroke could be reduced. Moreover, renal failure could be prevented by relieving the stenosis. The definitive diagnosis of renal artery stenosis is made by renal angiography. This diagnostic reference test should be used selectively because it is a costly procedure that can involve serious complications. Thus, clinicians need a safe, reliable, and inexpensive screening test to help them select patients for angiography.

Table 7.1 The first three and last three patients of 8 × 437 data array from a study on diagnostics in possible renal artery stenosis (RAS)

Patient code	Age	Gender	Atherosclerotic vascular disease	Abdominal bruit	Creatinine (micromole)	Abnormal renogram	RAS on angiography
1	62	F	No	Yes	87	No	Yes
2	52	M	No	No	146	Yes	Yes
3	49	F	No	No	77	No	No
...	...	...	...	...	...	...	...
...	...	...	...	...	...	...	...
435	36	M	No	No	84	No	No
436	51	M	Yes	No	74	No	No
437	55	M	No	No	83	No	No

The diagnostic tests that we will use in this chapter are clinical characteristics suggestive of renal artery stenosis, and renography; angiography serves as the reference standard test for stenosis. The clinical characteristics used as examples are symptoms and signs of atherosclerotic vascular disease, the presence of an abdominal bruit and the serum creatinine concentration. Renography is a noninvasive test for detecting asymmetry in renal function between the kidneys, which also is suggestive of renal artery stenosis.

The data, listed as indicated in Table 7.1, are from a Dutch multicenter study aiming to optimize the diagnosis and treatment of renal artery stenosis. The study included 437 hypertensive patients aged 18–75 years, who had been referred for unsatisfactory blood pressure control or for analysis of possible secondary hypertension.

Diagnostic questions and concepts

One can ask a number of questions concerning this diagnostic problem. Some are mentioned below, with the diagnostic concept concerned in parentheses.

• How good is my diagnostic test in detecting patients with RAS (sensitivity)?
• How good is my diagnostic test in detecting patients without RAS (specificity)?
• How well does a positive/abnormal test result predict the presence of RAS (positive predictive value)?
• How well does a negative/normal test result predict the absence of RAS (negative predictive value)?
• What is a reasonable estimate for the pretest probability of RAS (prevalence of RAS)?
• How many false conclusions will I make when applying the diagnostic test (error rate)?
• How informative is my positive/negative test result (likelihood ratio)?
• How do I summarize the association between a dichotomous test and the standard diagnosis (diagnostic odds ratio)?

Table 7.2 A 2 × 2 table for analyzing the diagnostic value of renographic assessment in predicting renal artery stenosis

	Angiography		
Renography	Stenosis	No Stenosis	Total
Abnormal	71	33	104
Normal	29	304	333
	100	337	437

- What is an optimal cutoff level when I want to dichotomize a continuous test (ROC curve)?
- To what extent does the test result change my pretest belief/probability of RAS (Bayes's theorem)?
- How are the above concepts applied to a number of diagnostic tests simultaneously (logistic regression)?

Sensitivity and specificity for a dichotomous test

We will illustrate the dichotomous test situation by assessing how well renography is able to predict arterial stenosis. Therefore, we construct from our database the 2 × 2 table with, as entries for renographic assessment, "abnormal/ normal," and for angiography, "stenosis/no stenosis" (Table 7.2).

The generic table with the corresponding symbolism is given in Table 7.3, with N = total number of patients, N_{T+} = number of patients with positive test results, N_{T-} = number of patients with negative test results,

Together, *sensitivity* (the probability of a positive test result in diseased subjects, P(T+|D+) and *specificity* (the probability of a negative test result in nondiseased subjects, P(T−|D−), characterize the dichotomous test for the clinical situation at hand. Neither is a measure of test performance on its own: it is the combination that matters.[1]

Table 7.3 Generic 2 × 2 table representing possible classifications for the relationship between a diagnostic test and a diagnosis (reference test)

	Diagnosis		
Test	+	−	
+	TP	FP	N_{T+}
−	FN	TN	N_{T-}
	N_{D+}	N_{D-}	N

N_{D-}, number of patients without the disease, N_{D+}, the number of patients with the disease, TP, number of true positives, TN, number of true negatives, FP, number of false positives, and FN, number of false negatives.

For the example in Table 7.2, we can calculate:

Sensitivity $= TP/N_{D+} = 71/100 = 71\%$

Specificity $= TN/N_{D-} = 304/337 = 90\%$

In the next section, we will see the degree of variability with which these estimates are associated.

Sampling variability and confidence intervals for probabilities

Confidence intervals

A main challenge in the analysis of diagnostic data is to assess how confident we can be about the test characteristics as observed in our patients. This may sound strange because an observed proportion, for example the sensitivity of renography in Table 7.2 of 71%, is a fact. However, it is unlikely that we will again find exactly 71% for sensitivity in a new series of 437 similar patients. An indication of the limits of what can reasonably be expected is therefore important (even when the same patients would have been reexamined in the same or another setting, other data will be obtained because of inter- and intraobserver variability).

The statistical method for analyzing the variability in estimates of sensitivity, and of all other probability estimates that we will discuss, is confidence intervals.[2] The probability level of the confidence interval can be chosen. A higher level of confidence corresponds to a larger interval in terms of number of percentiles covered. Throughout the chapter, we will – conventionally – work with 95% confidence intervals. The interpretation of a *95% confidence interval* for an observed proportion, that is, a probability estimate, is as follows: when the data sampling is repeated many times, the 95% confidence interval calculated from each sample will, on average, contain the "true" value of the proportion in 95% of the samples. Variability in sensitivity estimates is illustrated in Table 7.4. In part(a) of this table, the 100 stenosis patients of our study are subdivided into four groups of 25 consecutive patients. It is seen that the four subgroup sensitivities range enormously, from 48% to 88% (tables and formulas for the confidence interval will be discussed later). Part(b) illustrates what sensitivities we would have obtained if we had finished the study earlier, that is, after observing the first 5, 10, 25, 50, and 100 stenosis patients of the present study.

As you see from Table 7.4(a), the 95% confidence intervals of the highest and lowest estimates of sensitivity of 0.88 and 0.48 just touch each other. Table 7.4(b) shows that the width and the confidence interval become smaller with increasing sample size, as you would expect. For confidence intervals, and more generally for the accuracy of statistical estimates, the square root rule applies: when one makes the sample size A times as large, the confidence interval will be a factor $\sqrt{A}$ smaller. For example, for a two-times smaller confidence interval one needs four times as many patients. You can check the (approximate) validity of the square root rule in Table 7.4(b).

Table 7.4 Analysis of diagnostic data of patients with possible renal artery stenosis (RAS): confidence intervals for sensitivity of renography in diagnosing RAS; (a) variability in sensitivity between equal numbers of RAS patients, and (b) smaller confidence intervals with larger sample size, as cumulated during the study

	TP	N_{D1}	Sensitivity	95% confidence interval
(a)	18	25	0.72	0.51–0.88
	22	25	0.88	0.69–0.97
	19	25	0.76	0.55–0.91
	12	25	0.48	0.28–0.69
(b)	3	5	0.60	0.15–0.95
	7	10	0.70	0.35–0.93
	18	25	0.72	0.51–0.88
	40	50	0.80	0.66–0.90
	71	100	0.71	0.61–0.80

The confidence interval for the 71% sensitivity estimate for the total study runs from 61% to 80% (bottom line in Table 7.4). Table 7.5 gives confidence intervals for a number of confidence levels, with wider intervals for higher levels.

For the specificity of renography in diagnosing RAS, we get the following confidence interval around the 90% estimate for the total number of 337 nondiseased subjects: from 87% to 93%. As you can see, the confidence interval is roughly half the size of the confidence interval for the sensitivity, which reflects about four times as high the number of observations on which the estimate is based (square root rule!).

Some theory and a guide to the tables in the Appendix

The theory of calculating confidence intervals for proportions is based on the binomial distribution and requires complicated calculations. In general, the confidence interval is asymmetrical around the point estimate of the sensitivity

Table 7.5 Confidence interval for the 71% (71 out of 100) sensitivity estimate of renography in diagnosing RAS, for different confidence levels

Confidence level (%)	Confidence interval (%)
50	67–74
67	66–76
80	64–77
90	63–78
95	61–80
99	58–82
99.9	54–84

because of the "floor" and "ceiling" effects implied by the limits of 0 and 1 to any probability.

Fortunately, when the numbers are not small the 95% confidence interval becomes approximately symmetrical and the upper and lower limits can be calculated by adding or subtracting $1.96 \times$ *standard error*, with the standard error calculated by:

$$\sqrt{\frac{\hat{p}(1 - \hat{p})}{N}}$$

where $\hat{p}$ stands for the proportion or probability estimate, and N for the number of observations on which the proportion is based (in practice, multiplication by 2 instead of the more tedious 1.96 works well). Thus, the standard error has to be multiplied by 4 to obtain the width of the 95% confidence interval.

For other confidence levels, the multiplication factor 1.96 should be replaced by other values (see Appendix A.3).

Appendix Tables A.1 and A.2 give confidence levels for situations with small sample sizes where you need the tedious binomial calculations. Table A.3 gives the confidence interval for a number of situations in which the above formula for the standard error works well. In cases not covered by the tables, the standard error can be calculated using the formula. The reader can now verify the correctness of the confidence intervals presented in this section.

The formula can be used for calculating the required sample size in case a desired width of the confidence interval can be specified, and the order of magnitude of the value of the test characteristic can be quantified:

$$N = 16\,p(1 - p)/w^2$$

For example, when one would like to have a confidence interval of $\pm 10\%$ and when it is estimated that the sensitivity could well be around 80%, the study population should include about 270 persons with the disease ($16 \times 0.8 \times 0.2/0.01$).

Positive and negative predictive value: pre- and posttest probability of disease

The *positive predictive value* (PPV) is the probability that the patient has the disease when the test result is positive. This "posttest probability" is easily derived from Table 7.2. For the probability of RAS in case of abnormal renography, it is:

$$PPV = P(D+\,|T+) = TP/N_{T+} = 71/104 = 68\%$$

The confidence interval (CI) can be estimated using the formula on page 137 or Table A.3.: the 95% confidence interval for PPV runs from 59% to 77%.

The *negative predictive value* (NPV), that is, the probability that the patient does not have the disease if the test result is negative, translates in our case to the probability of no stenosis in case of normal renography. We get:

$$NPV = P(D- |T-) = TN/N_{T-} = 304/333 = 91\%$$

with 95% CI from 88% to 94% (see Table A.3).

The probabilities of no stenosis for an abnormal renogram and of stenosis for a normal renogram, and their CIs, are obtained as 100% minus PPV and 100% minus NPV, respectively because the probabilities of stenosis and no stenosis have to add up to 100%:

$$P(D- |T1) = 1 - P(D+ |T+) = 32\% \quad (95\% \text{ CI: } 23\% \text{ to } 41\%)$$
$$P(D+ |T2) = 1 - P(D- |T+) = 9\% \quad (95\% \text{ CI: } 6\% \text{ to } 12\%)$$

The PPV and NPV are *posttest* probabilities, that is, they are the updated probabilities given the information provided by the positive and negative test results, respectively. Before the test, we have the *pretest* probabilities of presence and absence of disease, which for our RAS example are:

$$P(D+) = 100/437 = 23\% \quad (95\% \text{ CI: } 19\% \text{ to } 27\%)$$
$$P(D-) = 337/437 = 77\% \quad (95\% \text{ CI: } 73\% \text{ to } 81\%)$$

The magnitude of the change from pre- to posttest probability reflects the informativeness of the diagnostic test result. In our case, the pretest probability of stenosis of 23% changes to 68% in case of an abnormal renogram, and to 9% in case of a normal renogram.

Error rate

How well does our diagnostic test discriminate between patients with and without stenosis, or, more generally, how well does the test discriminate between the two disease categories? So far, we have only looked at partial measures of performance, such as sensitivity, specificity, and predictive values. None of these concepts on its own gives an assessment of the performance of the test.

The most straightforward measure expresses how many errors we make when we diagnose patients with an abnormal test result as diseased, and those with a normal test result as nondiseased. This concept is known as the *error rate*. For our example, the error rate is easily calculated from Table 7.1. There are 29 false negative results, as the test was negative when stenosis was present, and 33 false positive results, with the test being abnormal when there was no stenosis. Thus, in total there are 62 errors, from 437 patients.

This gives the following calculations for the error rate and its confidence interval, the latter being derived from Table A.3 (the closest entry is 60 out of 500, with a half-CI size of 0.028; interpolation to 70 and 300 shows that ±3% is indeed the correct CI):

$$\text{Error rate(ER)} = 62/437 = 14\% \quad (95\% \text{ CI: } 11\% \text{ to } 17\%)$$

The error rate is a weighted average of errors among persons with the disease (the false negatives) and among those without the disease (the false positives), as is seen from the following equation:

$$ER = P(T- |D+) \times P(D+) + P(T + |D-) \times P(D-)$$

For our stenosis example, we can easily verify this expression for the error rate:

$$ER = (29/100) \times (100/437) + (33/337) \times (337/437) = 62/437 = 14\%$$

The weights in this formula are 23%, being the pretest probability of disease, and 77% for the probability of no disease.

This equation enables us to investigate what the error rate would be if the pretest probability of disease were different. For example, if the pretest probability of disease were 50% instead of 23%, the error rate would be calculated as:

$$ER = 29/100 \times 0.5 + 33/337 \times 0.5 = 19.4\%$$

Using this formula, we can speculate about the performance of the test in situations that differ from the original context (the assumption is that false positive and false negative rates do not change. This is unfortunately not always valid; see Chapters 1, 2, and 6).

Information in a diagnostic test result: the likelihood ratio

The informative value, or weight of evidence, of a test result is determined by the frequency of occurrence of this result in patients with the disease compared to those without the disease. If, for example, a certain test result occurs twice as often in patients with the disease, this result gives an evidence factor of 2 in favor of the disease. If, on the other hand, a test result occurs twice as often in patients without the disease, it gives an evidence factor of 2 in favor of nondisease, that is, a factor 2 against the disease (or a factor 1/2 in favor of disease).

This important probability ratio is called the likelihood ratio (LR). Each test result X has its own likelihood ratio $LR(X) = P(X|D+)/P(X|D-)$.

For dichotomous tests, we have only two test results, T+ and T−, and therefore also only two likelihood ratios:

the LR of a positive test result: $LR(T+) = P(T+ |D+)/P(T+ |D-)$
$$= Se/(1 - Sp)$$
the LR of a negative test result: $LR(T-) = P(T- |D+)/P(T- |D-)$
$$= (1 - Se)/Sp$$

For our example of renal artery stenosis, we obtain the following values for the likelihood ratio of an abnormal and a normal renogram, respectively:

$LR(T+) = 0.71/0.10 = 7.1$ with 95% CI: 5.1 to 10.3
$LR(T-) = 0.29/0.90 = 0.32$ with 95% CI: 0.24 to 0.44.

Thus, an abnormal renogram provides a factor of 7 in favor of stenosis, whereas a normal renogram yields a factor of 3 (i.e., $1/0.32$) in favor of no stenosis.

The following approximate formula has been used to calculate the 95% confidence interval for the likelihood ratio:

$$\exp\left(In\frac{p_1}{p_2} \pm 1.96\sqrt{\frac{1-p_1}{p_1 n_1} + \frac{1-p_2}{p_2 n_2}} \right)$$

in which $p_1 = P(X|D+)$ is based on sample size n_1 and $p_2 = P(X|D-)$ on sample size n_2.[3]

Diagnostic odds ratio

For a dichotomous test, it is possible to summarize the association between the test and the diagnosis (reference standard) presented in the 2×2 table in one measure: the diagnostic odds ratio (OR), which is equivalent to the cross-product of the table. Looking at the example of renal artery stenosis (Table 7.2):

$$OR = (71/33)/(29/304) = (71 \times 304)/(33 \times 29) = 22.6, \text{ with } 95\% \text{ CI: } 12.4 \text{ to } 41.3$$

The OR is equivalent to the ratio of LR(T+) and LR(T−), as can be easily checked in the table. The 95% confidence interval of the OR is provided by the software recommended in the references with this chapter.

The advantage of the OR is that it summarizes in one figure the diagnostic association in the whole table. However, this summary measure does not tell us the specific values of the likelihood ratios of the two test results, nor those of sensitivity and specificity. These measures have to be calculated as described earlier.

Continuous tests and their dichotomization and trichotomization

Another test for investigating the presence or absence of renal artery stenosis is the serum creatinine concentration. This test has a continuous range of possible test results. For analysis, results can best be grouped in classes of sufficient size (Table 7.6). Each class has its own evidence for and against stenosis, as expressed in the likelihood ratio.

The theory thus far has concerned only dichotomous tests, but the specific concepts for the dichotomous test situation can be translated into more general concepts for tests with an ordinal outcome scale or continuous tests, which are subdivided into more than two categories. The probabilities of observing a test result for stenosis and nonstenosis patients are given in Table 7.6. The likelihood ratio is a concept linked to a specific test result, and so also applies to multicategory tests. For example, the likelihood ratio for a test result in the

Table 7.6 Probability of test results and diagnostic information of serum creatinine concentration in relation to renal artery stenosis

Serum creatinine (micromoles/L)	Stenosis	No stenosis	All	Likelihood ratio (95% CI)
≤ 60	1 (1%)	19 (6%)	20 (5%)	0.18 (0.02–1.31)
61–70	4 (4%)	36 (11%)	40 (9%)	0.37 (0.14–1.03)
71–80	13 (13%)	67 (20%)	80 (18%)	0.65 (0.38–1.13)
81–90	12 (12%)	71 (21%)	83 (19%)	0.57 (0.32–1.01)
91–100	17 (17%)	71 (21%)	88 (20%)	0.81 (0.50–1.30)
101–110	15 (15%)	41 (12%)	56 (13%)	1.23 (0.71–2.13)
111–120	7 (7%)	10 (3%)	17 (4%)	2.33 (0.92–6.04)
121–130	9 (9%)	9 (3%)	18 (4%)	3.33 (1.37–8.26)
131–150	11 (11%)	8 (2%)	19 (4%)	4.58 (1.92–11.20)
>150	11 (11%)	5 (1%)	16 (4%)	7.33 (2.64–20.84)
All	100 (100%)	337 (100%)	437 (100%)	

category 61–70 micromoles can be calculated as the ratio of the likelihood of this test result in diseased and the likelihood of this result in nondiseased, that is: $(4/100)/(36/337) = 0.37$. As expected, the likelihood ratio increases with higher serum creatinine levels. Values <100 are evidence against stenosis (LR < 1) and values exceeding 100 are evidence for stenosis (LR > 1). The irregularity in this increasing trend in the 81–90 class reflects sampling variation, and not an underlying biological phenomenon.

We will now analyze the relationship between the multicategory test of serum creatinine described in Table 7.6 and its possible simplification to a dichotomous test. *Dichotomization* can take place at any category boundary. This is done in Table 7.7, which gives in each row the corresponding dichotomous test data. For example, based on a cutoff level of 80 the number of patients with and without stenosis over the value of 80 is 82 and 215, respectively, resulting in a sensitivity of 82% and a specificity of 36%. Likelihood ratios can again be calculated, now for the two results of the dichotomized test. As can be seen, much information is lost by the dichotomization. All results above and below the threshold are aggregated, and the likelihood ratio after dichotomization becomes an average of the likelihood ratios of the individual classes above and below this threshold. Also, the question of the choice of the cutoff value is a difficult one, especially when patients require a different amount of evidence in deciding for or against a certain further action. In our case, it could well be that some patients with a history that more clearly corroborates renal artery stenosis only need limited further evidence in order to decide for surgical intervention, whereas others need high likelihood ratios for the same decision.

The sensitivity–specificity pairs obtained for different cutoff values can be connected in a graph, yielding the so-called *ROC curve* (Figure 7.1). The more

Table 7.7 Probability of test results and diagnostic information of dichotomized serum creatinine concentration values for nine possible cutoffs between high and low values

Serum creatinine (Micromols)	Stenosis Se	No stenosis 1 − Sp	All	LR+	LR−
>60	99 (99%)	318 (94%)	417 (95%)	1.05	0.18
>70	95 (95%)	282 (84%)	377 (81%)	1.14	0.31
>80	82 (82%)	215 (64%)	297 (68%)	1.29	0.50
>90	70 (70%)	144 (43%)	114 (49%)	1.64	0.52
>100	53 (53%)	73 (22%)	126 (29%)	2.44	0.60
>110	38 (38%)	32 (9%)	70 (16%)	4.00	0.69
>120	31 (31%)	22 (7%)	53 (12%)	4.77	0.74
>130	22 (22%)	13 (4%)	35 (8%)	5.64	0.81
>150	11 (11%)	5 (1%)	16 (4%)	7.33	0.90
Total	100 (100%)	337 (100%)	437 (100%)		

the ROC curve moves toward the left upper corner, which represents a perfect dichotomous test with 100% sensitivity and 100% specificity, the better the test is. The steepness of the slope between two adjoining cutoff points represents the likelihood ratio of an observation falling in between these two

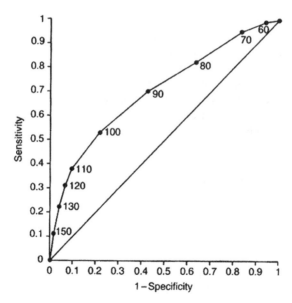

Figure 7.1 Receiver operating characteristic (ROC) curve for serum creatinine concentration in diagnosing renal artery stenosis. For each cutoff value of the serum creatinine, the probability of finding a higher value in stenosis (Se) and in nonstenosis patients (1 − Sp) is plotted. The area under the ROC curve is 0.70 (95% CI 0.64–0.76)

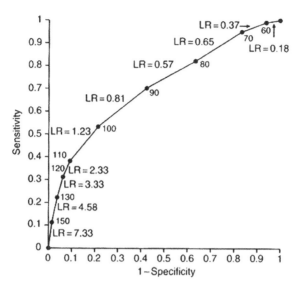

Figure 7.2 Receiver operating characteristic (ROC) curve for serum creatinine concentration in diagnosing renal artery stenosis, with the likelihood ratio for stenosis for each class of serum creatinine values.

points. This is shown in Figure 7.2. The likelihood ratios in Figure 7.2 are the same as those in Table 7.6.

A measure of performance for the test is the *area under the ROC curve*.[4] This varies between 0.5 for a totally uninformative test with a likelihood ratio of 1 for all its cutoff values (the diagonal of Figure 7.1), and 1 for a test that perfectly separates diseased and nondiseased (Se = Sp = 1.0). The serum creatinine has an area under the curve of 0.70 for differentiating between stenosis and nonstenosis patients. The interpretation of the value of 0.70 is as follows. Consider the hypothetical situation that two patients, drawn randomly from the stenosis patients and the nonstenosis patients, respectively, are subjected to the serum creatinine test. If the test results are used to guess which of the two is the stenosis patient, the test will be right 70% of the time. The confidence interval can be calculated using a computer program (see software references).

If a continuous test such as serum creatinine has to be summarized in a few classes for further condensation of the results or for further decision making, it is often more useful to consider a trichotomization than a dichotomization. In Table 7.8, we have divided the serum creatinine value into three classes, one for values giving a reasonable evidence for stenosis (likelihood ratio greater than 2.0), one for results giving reasonable evidence against stenosis (likelihood ratio smaller than 0.5), and an intermediate class for rather uninformative test results. It is seen that serum creatinine gives informative test results

Table 7.8 Probability of test results and diagnostic information of serum creatinine concentration for a trichotomization of the test results

Serum creatinine (Micromoles/l)	Stenosis	No stenosis	All	Likelihood ratio
≤ 70	5 (5%)	55 (16%)	60 (14%)	0.31
71–110	57 (57%)	250 (74%)	307 (70%)	0.77
>110	38 (38%)	32 (10%)	70 (16%)	4.00
All	100 (100%)	337 (100%)	437 (100%)	

in about 30% of patients, whereas the test results are rather uninformative in the remaining 70%.

From pretest probability to posttest probability: Bayes's theorem

The formula for calculating how the pretest probability changes under the influence of diagnostic evidence into a posttest probability is known as Bayes's theorem. In words, this is as follows:

> If disease was A times more probable than no disease before carrying out a certain test, and if the observed test result is B times as probable in diseased as in nondiseased subjects, then the disease is $(A \times B)$ as probable compared to no disease after the test.

A, B and $A \times B$ are respectively the pretest odds, the likelihood ratio, and the posttest odds, and a technical formulation of Bayes's theorem is therefore: "posttest odds (O(X)) equals pretest odds (O) times likelihood ratio (LR(X))"; and in formula: $O(X) = O \times LR(X)$. An example: take the dichotomous renography test (Table 7.2). The pretest odds (A) are 100:337, or 0.30. Assuming a positive test result, the likelihood ratio B equals 7.1. Bayes's theorem tells us now that the posttest odds of disease are $0.30 \times 7.1 = 2.13$. This corresponds to a probability of $2.13/(2.13 + 1) = 0.68$, because of the relationship between probability P and odds O: $O = P/(1 - P)$, and therefore $P = O/(1 + O)$.

Another example: take the category 61–70 for serum creatinine (Table 7.6) with a likelihood ratio of 0.37. In the posttest situation, stenosis is $0.30 \times 0.37 = 0.11$ times as probable as no disease. This yields a probability of stenosis of $0.11/1.11 = 0.10$.

The formula of Bayes's theorem for directly calculating the posttest probability is as follows:

$$P(D+ \,|X) = \frac{P(D+) \times P(X|D+)}{P(D+) \times P(X|D+) + P(D-) \times P(X|D-)}$$

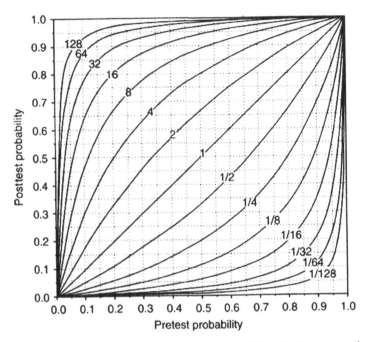

Figure 7.3 Graphical presentation in which the result of Bayes's theorem can be read for a number of likelihood ratios. Each curve represents one likelihood ratio. For example, a pretest probability of 0.7 and a likelihood ratio of 4 give rise to a posttest probability of about 0.90.

For dichotomous test we can express this formula in terms of sensitivity (Se) and specificity (Sp), and positive and negative predictive values (PPV and NPV), as can also be easily derived from the (2 × 2) Tables 7.2 and 7.3:

$$PPV = \frac{P(D+) \times Se}{P(D+) \times Se + P(D-) \times (1 - Sp)} \text{ and}$$

$$NPV = \frac{P(D-) \times Sp}{P(D-) \times Sp + P(D+) \times (1 - Se)}$$

Figure 7.3 gives a graphical presentation of Bayes's theorem and enables you to directly calculate the posttest probability from pretest probability and likelihood ratio. The two examples described earlier can be graphically verified with a pretest probability of stenosis of 23%: a likelihood ratio of 7.1 gives a posttest probability of 68%, and a likelihood ratio of 0.37 gives a posttest probability of 10% (these posttest probabilities can only be read approximately in the figure). For an alternative, nomogram type of representation of Bayes's theorem, see Chapter 2, Figure 2.1.

Table 7.9 Decrease in false positives and increase in false negatives when increasing the cutoff between high and low serum creatinine values by one class at a time. Eleven possible cutoffs are considered

Serum creatinine (micromoles/L)	No stenosis	Stenosis	FP decrease: FN increase per step	Approximate trade-off
>0	337	100	337:0	
>60	318	99	19:1	20:1
>70	282	95	36:4	10:1
>80	215	82	67:13	5:1
>90	144	70	71:12	5:1
>100	73	53	71:17	5:1
>110	32	38	41:15	3:1
>120	22	31	10:7	1:1
>130	13	22	9:9	1:1
>150	5	11	8:11	1:1
"Very high"	0	0	5:11	1:2
Total	337	100		

Decision analytical approach of the optimal cutoff value

The error rate is a good measure of test performance, as it gives the number of false positives and false negatives in relation to the total number of diagnostic judgments made. It should be realized that the error rate implicitly assumes that false positives and false negatives have an equal weight. This may not be reasonable: for example, a missed stenosis may be judged as much more serious than a missed nonstenosis. Here we enter the realm of decision science, where the loss of wrong decisions is explicitly taken into account. As an appetizer to decision analysis, look at Table 7.9. This is based on Table 7.7, but now with an indication of how many false positives are additionally avoided and how many additional false negatives are induced by increasing the threshold between positive and negative ("cutoff") with one class of serum creatinine values at a time.

With the (uninteresting) cutoff value of 0, we would have 337 false positives (FP) and 0 false negatives (FN). Increasing the threshold from 0 to 60 would decrease the FP by 19 and increase the FN by 1. A shift from 60 to 70 would decrease the FP by 36 and increase the FN by four, and so on, until the last step in cutoff from 150 to "very high" serum creatinine values, by which the last five FP are prevented but also the last 11 stenosis patients are turned into FN.

One can derive the optimal cutoff from the relative importance of false positives and false negatives. For example, if one false positive is judged to be four times more serious than a false negative, a good cutoff would be

100, because all shifts in cutoff between 0 and 100 involve a trade-off of at least five FN to one FP, which is better than the 4:1 judgment on the relative seriousness of the two types of error. A further shift from 100 to 110 is not indicated because the associated trade-off is three FN or less to one FP or more, which is worse than the 4:1 judgment. Note that for different pretest values of stenosis the FN:FP trade-offs will change, and therefore also the optimal threshold. For example, if the pretest probability were two times higher, the threshold would shift to 60 (calculations not shown).

For a further study of decision analytical considerations, the reader is referred to Sox *et al.*[5]

Sensitivity analysis

In a sensitivity analysis, we look at what would have happened to our conclusions in case of other, but plausible, assumptions. This is important for getting a feeling for the stability of the conclusions.

We saw an example of a sensitivity analysis in our discussion of the error rate, when we looked what the error rate would have been if the pretest probability of stenosis had been different from the 30% in the study.

Sensitivity analysis could also be conducted using Figure 7.3, the graphical representation of Bayes's theorem. Using the confidence intervals for the pretest probability and for the likelihood ratio, we can assess the associated uncertainty in the posttest probability. For example, when we have a confidence interval for the pretest probability between 0.5 and 0.7, and a confidence interval for the likelihood ratio of our test results between 4 and 8, Figure 7.3 tells us that values for the posttest probability between 0.8 and 0.95 are possible.

A third type of sensitivity analysis could be done using the relative seriousness of false positive and false negative results by checking how the threshold between positive and negative test results will shift when different values for this relative seriousness are considered.

The logistic regression formulation of Bayes's theorem

The analysis of a combination of several diagnostic tests is more complicated than the analysis of a single diagnostic test. There is, however, a standard statistical method, logistic regression analysis, that can be applied in this situation. Logistic regression is, in fact, a representation of Bayes's theorem, which can easily be extended to many diagnostic tests applied simultaneously. It is a general method for the analysis of binary outcome data, such as the presence or absence of disease.[6] The equivalence of the logistic formula and Bayes's theorem is best seen by using a logistic transformation, in order to have an additive instead of a multiplicative formula. Thus "posttest odds equals pretest odds times likelihood ratio," becomes, after taking the logarithm, "log posttest odds equals log pretest odds *plus* log likelihood ratio." Or, in formula form, with the L indicating "logarithm":

$O(X) = O \times LR$ becomes $LO(X) = LO + LLR(X)$

The corresponding logistic regression *formula* is as follows: the log odds of disease, (also called logit (LO)), given test result X, is a linear function of the test result:

$LO(X) = b_0 + b_1 X$

Usually, the natural logarithm (Ln) is used, as we will do in the remainder of this section. We will illustrate logistic regression by applying it to the renography test for renal artery stenosis, the results of which were depicted in Table 7.2.

We start with the situation before performing the test: our best estimate of stenosis is then the prior or pretest probability, based on the observation that we have 100 patients with and 337 patients without stenosis. The logistic formula in this case $LnO = b_0$, and contains only a constant b_0, because no tests have been performed yet. Thus b_0, the Ln pretest odds, which in this case is Ln $(100/337) = -1.21$.

Next the renography test is performed. The test result is coded as $X_1 = 0$ (normal) or $X_1 = 1$ (abnormal), and the logistic formula is $LnO(X_1) = b_0 + b_1 X_1$. We will derive the coefficients b_0 and b_1 by applying the log odds form of Bayes's theorem to both the normal and the abnormal test results. The logistic formula follows immediately from the results.

In case of a normal renogram ($X_1 = 0$) there are 29 patients with and 304 patients without stenosis in Table 7.2. Bayes's theorem tells that the log odds on stenosis for result $X_1 = 0$, $LnO(X_1 = 0) = Ln(29/304) = -2.35$, equals the Ln pretest odds of -1.21 plus the Ln likelihood ratio of a normal renogram, which is -1.14.

In case of an abnormal renogram ($X_1 = 1$) there are 71 patients with and 33 patients without stenosis, and $LnO(X_1 = 1) = Ln(71/33) = 0.77$, being the Ln pretest odds of -1.21 plus the Ln likelihood ratio 1.98 of an abnormal renogram. Combining the two applications of Bayes's theorem, we get:

$LnO(X_1) = -1.21 - 1.14$ (when $X_1 = 0$) $+ 1.98$ (when $X_1 = 1$).

This can be simplified to the logistic formula:

$LnO(X_1) = b_0 + b_1 X_1 = -2.35 + 3.12 X_1$.

Two remarks can be made: the coefficient b_1 (3.12) is precisely the Ln of the diagnostic odds ratio (22.6) of renography discussed earlier. And b_0 in the logistic formula can no longer be interpreted as a pretest log odds of stenosis, but as the $LnO(X_1 = 0)$. This completes the logistic regression analysis of one dichotomous test.

When more than one test is involved the calculations are extensions of the described single test situation, using the multiple logistic regression formula:
$Ln(X_1, X_2, \ldots, X_k) = b_0 + b_1X_1 + b_2X_2 + \ldots + b_kX_k$. Using this approach, the investigator can account for dependency and interaction between the various tests. However, such multivariable calculations are very troublesome to do by hand. In general, when many tests, including continuous tests, are involved, standard statistical software such as SPSS or SAS will have to be used. This software also provides 95% confidence intervals for $b_0, b_1, b_2, \ldots b_k$, and the corresponding odds ratios (e^b).

From multiple logistic regression analysis, one can not only learn about the predictive value of a combination of tests, but also what a certain test adds to other tests that have already been formed.

Concluding remarks

In this chapter, we have given an overview of the most important performance measures of diagnostic tests, illustrated with a clinical example. Also, the estimation of confidence intervals to account for sampling variability has been explained. Furthermore, decision analytical considerations and sensitivity analysis, as methods to deal with value judgments and uncertainties, have been introduced. Finally, the principles of logistic regression to analyze the predictive value of multiple tests, when applied simultaneously, have been outlined.

In applying the presented analysis techniques, it is presupposed that the research data have been collected with the avoidance of important bias (affecting internal validity) and with acceptable generalizability to the target population where the diagnostic test(s) are to be applied (external validity). These issues regarding the validity of the study design are dealt with in Chapters 1–6. In general, in the analysis phase, one cannot correct for shortcomings of the validity of the study design, such as bias resulting from an unclear or inappropriate process of selection of study subjects or from an inadequate reference standard. However, if potential factors that may affect test performance are measured during the study, these can be included as independent covariables in the analysis. An example may be age as a potential effect modifier of the performance of renography. The potential influence of other possible biases can be explored using sensitivity analysis.

In the past decade, new data analytical challenges have resulted from the need to synthesize a number of studies and to analyze the pooled data of those studies (meta-analysis). Also, in such a pooled analysis, the usual performance measures of diagnostic tests can be assessed, as is shown in Chapter 10. Finally, although it is always the aim to minimize the number of lost outcomes or not-performed tests, in most studies these will not be totally avoided. Although associated methodological problems are discussed in Chapter 2, there are various options for the analytical approach to such "missing values" on which professional biostatisticians can give advice.

References

1. Sackett DL, Haynes PB, Tugwell P. *Clinical epidemiology: a bisic science for clinical medicine.* Boston: Little, Brown and Co; 1985.
2. Altman DG, Machin D, Bryant TN, et al. *Statistics with confidence.* 2nd ed. London: BMJ Books; 2000 (includes software).
3. Simel DL, Samsa GP, Matchar DB. Likelihood ratios with confidence: sample size estimation for diagnostic test studies. *J Clin Epidemiol.* 1991;**44**:763–70.
4. Hanley JA, McNeil BJ. The meaning and use of the area under a receiver operating characteristic (ROC) curve. *Radiology.* 1982;**143**:29–36.
5. Sox HC, Jr, Blatt MA, Higgins MC, et al. *Medical decision making.* Stoneham, MA: Butterworths; 1988.
6. Hosmer DW, Lemeshow S. *Applied logistic regression.* New York: Wiley; 1989.

Software

- For the analysis of test results, including logistic regression for single and multiple tests and confidence intervals for the diagnostic odds ratio, standard statistical software such as SPSS, SAS, Stata, S-plus, R, or BMDP may be used. In SPSS, S-plus, R, and SAS analysis of the area under the ROC curve (plus confidence intervals) can be performed.
- Visual Bayes is a freely available program introducing basic methods for the interpretation and validation of diagnostic tests in an intuitive way. It may be downloaded from http://www.imbi.uni-freiburg.de/medinf.
- Treeage-DATA is a decision analysis program in which diagnostic tests and subsequent treatment decisions can be represented. Good opportunities for sensitivity analysis.

Appendix: Tables for confidence intervals for proportions

Tables A.1–A.2
Exact confidence intervals for proportions based on small N (Table A.1) or on small n (Table A.2).

Table A.3
Half 95% confidence intervals for proportions.

For all tables
N = number of observations (denominator), n = number of successes (numerator).

Table A.1
Example: In a group of five patients with renal artery stenosis, three were positive on diagnostic renography. The estimated sensitivity of renography is therefore 3/5, that is, 0.6 with 95% confidence interval (0.15–0.95).

Table A.2
Exact confidence intervals for small n. Because the binomial distribution is symmetric around $p = 0.5$, the table can also be used for small values of $N - n$: when using $N - n$ instead of n the resulting confidence interval changes to (1-upper limit, 1-lower limit).

Example for small n: A new screening test for a disease is required to have a very low false positive rate that is, high specificity. In a sample of 200 proven nondiseased subjects, only one had a positive test result. The false positive rate is estimated at $1/200 = 0.005$ and the exact 95% confidence interval is (0.000–0.028)

Example for small $N - n$: In the previous example, we can estimate the specificity as 199/20050.995, with 95% confidence interval (0.972–1.000).

Table A.3
The half 95% confidence interval for proportions, based on the normal approximation to the binomial distribution for large numbers of observations. With this approximation, the half 95% confidence interval for a proportion $\hat{p} = n/N$ is $1.96 \times$ SE, with SE being the standard error. The 95% confidence interval is constructed by subtracting (lower confidence limit) or adding (upper confidence limit) the number from the table to the estimate p. By symmetry, the values for n and for $N - n$ are the same. When the values of n and N are not given directly in the table, linear interpolation for n and/or N may be used.

Example
In a group of 333 patients with a negative renography, 29 nevertheless appeared to suffer from renal artery stenosis. The estimated negative predictive value (NPV) of renography is therefore (333–29)/333, that is, 0.91.

The value from the table is required for $N = 333$ and $N - n = 29$. We use linear interpolation for N. At $N = 300$, the table gives a value of 0.0335 and at $N = 500$ the value is 0.0205, for $N = 29$, taking the averages of the values for $n = 28$ and 30.

Linear interpolation at $N = 333$ requires:

$(\{\text{Value at } N = 333\} - 0.0355) : (0.0205 - 0.0335) = (333 - 300) : (500 - 300)$.
Thus $\{\text{Value at } N = 333\} = 0.03$.

The 95% confidence interval becomes $(0.91 - 0.03, 0.91 + 0.03) = (0.88 - 0.94)$.

Note 1
Instead of interpolation, the formula for SE could have been used directly:

$$\text{SE} = \sqrt{\frac{\hat{p}\,(1 - \hat{p})}{N}}, \text{ giving SE} = \sqrt{\frac{\dfrac{304}{333}\left(1 - \dfrac{29}{333}\right)}{333}} = 0.0154$$

Multiplying by 1.96 gives a value of 0.03 for the half 95% confidence interval.

Note 2

For other levels of confidence, the numbers in Table A.3 have to be multiplied by a factor. The following table gives multiplication factors for a few commonly used levels of confidence:

Confidence level (%)	Multiplication factor
50	0.34
67	0.49
80	0.65
90	0.84
95	1
99	1.31
99.9	1.68

Table A.1 Exact 95% confidence intervals for proportions n/N for N from 2 to 25

N	P	95%	CI	N	P	95%	CI	N	P	95%	CI
		N = 2				*N* = 8 (*cont.*)				*N* = 12 (*cont.*)	
0	0	0.00	0.78	5	0.63	0.24	0.91	4	0.33	0.10	0.65
1	0.5	0.01	0.99	6	0.75	0.35	0.97	5	0.42	0.15	0.72
2	1	0.22	1.00	7	0.88	0.47	1.00	6	0.5	0.21	0.79
		N = 3		8	1	0.69	1.00	7	0.58	0.28	0.85
0	0	0.00	0.63			*N* = 9		8	0.67	0.35	0.90
1	0.33	0.01	0.91	0	0	0.00	0.28	9	0.75	0.43	0.95
2	0.67	0.09	0.99	1	0.11	0.00	0.48	10	0.83	0.52	0.98
3	1	0.37	1.00	2	0.22	0.03	0.60	11	0.92	0.62	1.00
		N = 4		3	0.33	0.07	0.70	12	1	0.78	1.00
0	0	0.00	0.53	4	0.44	0.14	0.79			*N* = 13	
1	0.25	0.01	0.81	5	0.56	0.21	0.86	0	0	0.00	0.21
2	0.5	0.07	0.93	6	0.67	0.30	0.93	1	0.08	0.00	0.36
3	0.75	0.19	0.99	7	0.78	0.40	0.97	2	0.15	0.02	0.45
4	1	0.47	1.00	8	0.89	0.52	1.00	3	0.23	0.05	0.54
		N = 5		9	1	0.72	1.00	4	0.31	0.09	0.61
0	0	0.00	0.45			*N* = 10		5	0.38	0.14	0.68
1	0.2	0.01	0.72	0	0	0.00	0.26	6	0.46	0.19	0.75
2	0.4	0.05	0.85	1	0.1	0.00	0.45	7	0.54	0.25	0.81
3	0.6	0.15	0.95	2	0.2	0.03	0.56	8	0.62	0.32	0.86
4	0.8	0.28	0.99	3	0.3	0.07	0.65	9	0.69	0.39	0.91
5	1	0.55	1.00	4	0.4	0.12	0.74	10	0.77	0.46	0.95
		N = 6		5	0.5	0.19	0.81	11	0.85	0.55	0.98
0	0	0.00	0.39	6	0.6	0.26	0.88	12	0.92	0.64	1.00
1	0.17	0.00	0.64	7	0.7	0.35	0.93	13	1	0.79	1.00
2	0.33	0.04	0.78	8	0.8	0.44	0.97			*N* = 14	
3	0.5	0.12	0.88	9	0.9	0.55	1.00	0	0	0.00	0.19
4	0.67	0.22	0.96	10	1	0.74	1.00	1	0.07	0.00	0.34
5	0.83	0.36	1.00			*N* = 11		2	0.14	0.02	0.43
6	1	0.61	1.00	0	0	0.00	0.24	3	0.21	0.05	0.51
		N = 7		1	0.09	0.00	0.41	4	0.29	0.08	0.58
0	0	0.00	0.35	2	0.18	0.02	0.52	5	0.36	0.13	0.65
1	0.14	0.00	0.58	3	0.27	0.06	0.61	6	0.43	0.18	0.71
2	0.29	0.04	0.71	4	0.36	0.11	0.69	7	0.5	0.23	0.77
3	0.43	0.10	0.82	5	0.45	0.17	0.77	8	0.57	0.29	0.82
4	0.57	0.18	0.90	6	0.55	0.23	0.83	9	0.64	0.35	0.87
5	0.71	0.29	0.96	7	0.64	0.31	0.89	10	0.71	0.42	0.92
6	0.86	0.42	1.00	8	0.73	0.39	0.94	11	0.79	0.49	0.95
7	1	0.65	1.00	9	0.82	0.48	0.98	12	0.86	0.57	0.98
		N = 8		10	0.91	0.59	1.00	13	0.93	0.66	1.00
0	0	0.00	0.31	11	1	0.76	1.00	14	1	0.81	1.00
1	0.13	0.00	0.53			*N* = 12				*N* = 15	
2	0.25	0.03	0.65	0	0	0.00	0.22	0	0	0.00	0.18
3	0.38	0.09	0.76	1	0.08	0.00	0.38	1	0.07	0.00	0.32
4	0.5	0.16	0.84	2	0.17	0.02	0.48	2	0.13	0.02	0.40
				3	0.25	0.05	0.57	3	0.2	0.04	0.48

Table A.1

N	P	95%	CI	N	P	95%	CI	N	P	95%	CI
	N = 15 (cont.)				*N = 17 (cont.)*				*N = 19 (cont.)*		
4	0.27	0.08	0.55	12	0.71	0.44	0.90	16	0.84	0.60	0.97
5	0.33	0.12	0.62	13	0.76	0.50	0.93	17	0.89	0.67	0.99
6	0.4	0.16	0.68	14	0.82	0.57	0.96	18	0.95	0.74	1.00
7	0.47	0.21	0.73	15	0.88	0.64	0.99	19	1	0.85	1.00
8	0.53	0.27	0.79	16	0.94	0.71	1.00		*N = 20*		
9	0.6	0.32	0.84	17	1	0.84	1.00				
10	0.67	0.38	0.88					0	0	0.00	0.14
11	0.73	0.45	0.92		*N = 18*			1	0.05	0.00	0.25
12	0.8	0.52	0.96	0	0	0.00	0.15	2	0.1	0.01	0.32
13	0.87	0.60	0.98	1	0.06	0.00	0.27	3	0.15	0.03	0.38
14	0.93	0.68	1.00	2	0.11	0.01	0.35	4	0.2	0.06	0.44
15	1	0.82	1.00	3	0.17	0.04	0.41	5	0.25	0.09	0.49
				4	0.22	0.06	0.48	6	0.3	0.12	0.54
	N = 16			5	0.28	0.10	0.53	7	0.35	0.15	0.59
0	0	0.00	0.17	6	0.33	0.13	0.59	8	0.4	0.19	0.64
1	0.06	0.00	0.30	7	0.39	0.17	0.64	9	0.45	0.23	0.68
2	0.13	0.02	0.38	8	0.44	0.22	0.69	10	0.5	0.27	0.73
3	0.19	0.04	0.46	9	0.5	0.26	0.74	11	0.55	0.32	0.77
4	0.25	0.07	0.52	10	0.56	0.31	0.78	12	0.6	0.36	0.81
5	0.31	0.11	0.59	11	0.61	0.36	0.83	13	0.65	0.41	0.85
6	0.38	0.15	0.65	12	0.67	0.41	0.87	14	0.7	0.46	0.88
7	0.44	0.20	0.70	13	0.72	0.47	0.90	15	0.75	0.51	0.91
8	0.5	0.25	0.75	14	0.78	0.52	0.94	16	0.8	0.56	0.94
9	0.56	0.30	0.80	15	0.83	0.59	0.96	17	0.85	0.62	0.97
10	0.63	0.35	0.85	16	0.89	0.65	0.99	18	0.9	0.68	0.99
11	0.69	0.41	0.89	17	0.94	0.73	1.00	19	0.95	0.75	1.00
12	0.75	0.48	0.93	18	1	0.85	1.00	20	1	0.86	1.00
13	0.81	0.54	0.96								
14	0.88	0.62	0.98		*N = 19*				*N = 21*		
15	0.94	0.70	1.00	0	0	0.00	0.15	0	0	0.00	0.13
16	1	0.83	1.00	1	0.05	0.00	0.26	1	0.05	0.00	0.24
				2	0.11	0.01	0.33	2	0.1	0.01	0.30
	N = 17			3	0.16	0.03	0.40	3	0.14	0.03	0.36
0	0	0.00	0.16	4	0.21	0.06	0.46	4	0.19	0.05	0.42
1	0.06	0.00	0.29	5	0.26	0.09	0.51	5	0.24	0.08	0.47
2	0.12	0.01	0.36	6	0.32	0.13	0.57	6	0.29	0.11	0.52
3	0.18	0.04	0.43	7	0.37	0.16	0.62	7	0.33	0.15	0.57
4	0.24	0.07	0.50	8	0.42	0.20	0.67	8	0.38	0.18	0.62
5	0.29	0.10	0.56	9	0.47	0.24	0.71	9	0.43	0.22	0.66
6	0.35	0.14	0.62	10	0.53	0.29	0.76	10	0.48	0.26	0.70
7	0.41	0.18	0.67	11	0.58	0.33	0.80	11	0.52	0.30	0.74
8	0.47	0.23	0.72	12	0.63	0.38	0.84	12	0.57	0.34	0.78
9	0.53	0.28	0.77	13	0.68	0.43	0.87	13	0.62	0.38	0.82
10	0.59	0.33	0.82	14	0.74	0.49	0.91	14	0.67	0.43	0.85
11	0.65	0.38	0.86	15	0.79	0.54	0.94	15	0.71	0.48	0.89

(continued)

Table A.1 (*continued*)

N	P	95%	CI	N	P	95%	CI	N	P	95%	CI
N = 21 (cont.)				*N* = 23 (cont.)				*N* = 24 (cont.)			
16	0.76	0.53	0.92	4	0.17	0.05	0.39	15	0.63	0.41	0.81
17	0.81	0.58	0.95	5	0.22	0.07	0.44	16	0.67	0.45	0.84
18	0.86	0.64	0.97	6	0.26	0.10	0.48	17	0.71	0.49	0.87
19	0.9	0.70	0.99	7	0.3	0.13	0.53	18	0.75	0.53	0.90
20	0.95	0.76	1.00	8	0.35	0.16	0.57	19	0.79	0.58	0.93
21	1	0.87	1.00	9	0.39	0.20	0.61	20	0.83	0.63	0.95
				10	0.43	0.23	0.66	21	0.88	0.68	0.97
N = 22				11	0.48	0.27	0.69	22	0.92	0.73	0.99
0	0	0.00	0.13	12	0.52	0.31	0.73	23	0.96	0.79	1.00
1	0.05	0.00	0.23	13	0.57	0.34	0.77	24	1	0.88	1.00
2	0.09	0.01	0.29	14	0.61	0.39	0.80	*N* = 25			
3	0.14	0.03	0.35	15	0.65	0.43	0.84	0	0	0.00	0.11
4	0.18	0.05	0.40	16	0.7	0.47	0.87	1	0.04	0.00	0.20
5	0.23	0.08	0.45	17	0.74	0.52	0.90	2	0.08	0.01	0.26
6	0.27	0.11	0.50	18	0.78	0.56	0.93	3	0.12	0.03	0.31
7	0.32	0.14	0.55	19	0.83	0.61	0.95	4	0.16	0.05	0.36
8	0.36	0.17	0.59	20	0.87	0.66	0.97	5	0.2	0.07	0.41
9	0.41	0.21	0.64	21	0.91	0.72	0.99	6	0.24	0.09	0.45
10	0.45	0.24	0.68	22	0.96	0.78	1.00	7	0.28	0.12	0.49
11	0.5	0.28	0.72	23	1	0.88	1.00	8	0.32	0.15	0.54
12	0.55	0.32	0.76					9	0.36	0.18	0.57
13	0.59	0.36	0.79	*N* = 24				10	0.4	0.21	0.61
14	0.64	0.41	0.83	0	0	0.00	0.12	11	0.44	0.24	0.65
15	0.68	0.45	0.86	1	0.04	0.00	0.21	12	0.48	0.28	0.69
16	0.73	0.50	0.89	2	0.08	0.01	0.27	13	0.52	0.31	0.72
17	0.77	0.55	0.92	3	0.13	0.03	0.32	14	0.56	0.35	0.76
18	0.82	0.60	0.95	4	0.17	0.05	0.37	15	0.6	0.39	0.79
19	0.86	0.65	0.97	5	0.21	0.07	0.42	16	0.64	0.43	0.82
20	0.91	0.71	0.99	6	0.25	0.10	0.47	17	0.68	0.46	0.85
21	0.95	0.77	1.00	7	0.29	0.13	0.51	18	0.72	0.51	0.88
22	1	0.87	1.00	8	0.33	0.16	0.55	19	0.76	0.55	0.91
				9	0.38	0.19	0.59	20	0.8	0.59	0.93
N = 23				10	0.42	0.22	0.63	21	0.84	0.64	0.95
0	0	0.00	0.12	11	0.46	0.26	0.67	22	0.88	0.69	0.97
1	0.04	0.00	0.22	12	0.5	0.29	0.71	23	0.92	0.74	0.99
2	0.09	0.01	0.28	13	0.54	0.33	0.74	24	0.96	0.80	1.00
3	0.13	0.03	0.34	14	0.58	0.37	0.78	25	1	0.89	1.00

Table A.2 Exact 95% confidence intervals for proportions n/N for small n (0 – 7) and $N = 30, 35, \ldots, 70, 80, 90, 100, 120, 150, 200, 300, 500, 1,000, 2,000$

N	0		1		2		3		4		5		6		7	
30	0.000	0.095	0.001	0.172	0.008	0.221	0.021	0.265	0.038	0.307	0.056	0.347	0.077	0.386	0.099	0.423
35	0.000	0.082	0.001	0.149	0.007	0.192	0.018	0.231	0.032	0.267	0.048	0.303	0.066	0.336	0.084	0.369
40	0.000	0.072	0.001	0.132	0.006	0.169	0.016	0.204	0.028	0.237	0.042	0.268	0.057	0.298	0.073	0.328
45	0.000	0.064	0.001	0.118	0.005	0.151	0.014	0.183	0.025	0.212	0.037	0.241	0.051	0.268	0.065	0.295
50	0.000	0.058	0.001	0.106	0.005	0.137	0.013	0.165	0.022	0.192	0.033	0.218	0.045	0.243	0.058	0.267
55	0.000	0.053	0.000	0.097	0.004	0.125	0.011	0.151	0.020	0.176	0.030	0.200	0.041	0.222	0.053	0.245
60	0.000	0.049	0.000	0.089	0.004	0.115	0.010	0.139	0.018	0.162	0.028	0.184	0.038	0.205	0.048	0.226
65	0.000	0.045	0.000	0.083	0.004	0.107	0.010	0.129	0.017	0.150	0.025	0.170	0.035	0.190	0.044	0.209
70	0.000	0.042	0.000	0.077	0.003	0.099	0.009	0.120	0.016	0.140	0.024	0.159	0.032	0.177	0.041	0.195
80	0.000	0.037	0.000	0.068	0.003	0.087	0.008	0.106	0.014	0.123	0.021	0.140	0.028	0.156	0.036	0.172
90	0.000	0.033	0.000	0.060	0.003	0.078	0.007	0.094	0.012	0.110	0.018	0.125	0.025	0.139	0.032	0.154
100	0.000	0.030	0.000	0.054	0.002	0.070	0.006	0.085	0.011	0.099	0.016	0.113	0.022	0.126	0.029	0.139
120	0.000	0.025	0.000	0.046	0.002	0.059	0.005	0.071	0.009	0.083	0.014	0.095	0.019	0.106	0.024	0.116
150	0.000	0.020	0.000	0.037	0.002	0.047	0.004	0.057	0.007	0.067	0.011	0.076	0.015	0.085	0.019	0.094
200	0.000	0.015	0.000	0.028	0.001	0.036	0.003	0.043	0.005	0.050	0.008	0.057	0.011	0.064	0.014	0.071
300	0.000	0.010	0.000	0.018	0.001	0.024	0.002	0.029	0.004	0.034	0.005	0.038	0.007	0.043	0.009	0.047
500	0.000	0.006	0.000	0.011	0.000	0.014	0.001	0.017	0.002	0.020	0.003	0.023	0.004	0.026	0.006	0.029
1,000	0.000	0.003	0.000	0.006	0.000	0.007	0.001	0.009	0.001	0.010	0.002	0.012	0.002	0.013	0.003	0.014
2,000	0.000	0.001	0.000	0.003	0.000	0.004	0.001	0.004	0.001	0.005	0.001	0.006	0.001	0.007	0.001	0.007

Table A.3 Half 95% confidence intervals (=1.96 SE) of proportions n/N for N = 30, 35, ..., 70, 80, 90, 100, 120, 150, 200, 300, 500, 1,000, 2,000

										N									
N = n	30	35	40	45	50	55	60	65	70	80	90	100	120	150	200	300	500	1000	2000
8	0.158	0.139	0.124	0.112	0.102	0.093	0.086	0.080	0.075	0.066	0.059	0.053	0.045	0.036	0.027	0.018	0.011	0.006	0.003
9	0.164	0.145	0.129	0.117	0.106	0.098	0.090	0.084	0.078	0.069	0.062	0.056	0.047	0.038	0.029	0.019	0.012	0.006	0.003
10	0.169	0.150	0.134	0.121	0.111	0.102	0.094	0.088	0.082	0.072	0.065	0.059	0.049	0.040	0.030	0.020	0.012	0.006	0.003
11	0.172	0.154	0.138	0.126	0.115	0.106	0.098	0.091	0.085	0.075	0.068	0.061	0.052	0.042	0.032	0.021	0.013	0.006	0.003
12	0.175	0.157	0.142	0.129	0.118	0.109	0.101	0.094	0.088	0.078	0.070	0.064	0.054	0.043	0.033	0.022	0.013	0.007	0.003
13	0.177	0.160	0.145	0.132	0.122	0.112	0.104	0.097	0.091	0.081	0.073	0.066	0.056	0.045	0.034	0.023	0.014	0.007	0.004
14	0.179	0.162	0.148	0.135	0.124	0.115	0.107	0.100	0.094	0.083	0.075	0.068	0.057	0.047	0.035	0.024	0.014	0.007	0.004
15	0.179	0.164	0.150	0.138	0.127	0.118	0.110	0.102	0.096	0.086	0.077	0.070	0.059	0.048	0.037	0.025	0.015	0.008	0.004
16	0.179	0.165	0.152	0.140	0.129	0.120	0.112	0.105	0.098	0.088	0.079	0.072	0.061	0.049	0.038	0.025	0.015	0.008	0.004
17		0.166	0.153	0.142	0.131	0.122	0.114	0.107	0.100	0.090	0.081	0.074	0.062	0.051	0.039	0.026	0.016	0.008	0.004
18		0.166	0.154	0.143	0.133	0.124	0.116	0.109	0.102	0.092	0.083	0.075	0.064	0.052	0.040	0.027	0.016	0.008	0.004
19			0.155	0.144	0.135	0.126	0.118	0.111	0.104	0.093	0.084	0.077	0.065	0.053	0.041	0.028	0.017	0.009	0.004
20			0.155	0.145	0.136	0.127	0.119	0.112	0.106	0.095	0.086	0.078	0.067	0.054	0.042	0.028	0.017	0.009	0.005
22				0.146	0.138	0.129	0.122	0.115	0.109	0.098	0.089	0.081	0.069	0.057	0.043	0.029	0.018	0.009	0.005
24					0.138	0.131	0.124	0.117	0.111	0.100	0.091	0.084	0.072	0.059	0.045	0.031	0.019	0.009	0.005
26						0.132	0.125	0.119	0.113	0.103	0.094	0.086	0.074	0.061	0.047	0.032	0.019	0.010	0.005
28							0.126	0.120	0.115	0.105	0.096	0.088	0.076	0.062	0.048	0.033	0.020	0.010	0.005
30							0.127	0.121	0.116	0.106	0.097	0.090	0.077	0.064	0.049	0.034	0.021	0.011	0.005
32								0.122	0.117	0.107	0.099	0.091	0.079	0.066	0.051	0.035	0.021	0.011	0.005
34									0.117	0.108	0.100	0.093	0.081	0.067	0.052	0.036	0.022	0.011	0.006
36										0.109	0.101	0.094	0.082	0.068	0.053	0.037	0.023	0.012	0.006
38										0.109	0.102	0.095	0.083	0.070	0.054	0.038	0.023	0.012	0.006

40	0.110	0.103	0.096	0.084	0.071	0.055	0.038	0.024	0.012	0.006
45		0.103	0.098	0.087	0.073	0.058	0.040	0.025	0.013	0.006
50			0.098	0.088	0.075	0.060	0.042	0.026	0.014	0.007
55				0.089	0.077	0.062	0.044	0.027	0.014	0.007
60				0.089	0.078	0.064	0.045	0.028	0.015	0.007
70					0.080	0.066	0.048	0.030	0.016	0.008
80						0.068	0.050	0.032	0.017	0.009
90						0.069	0.052	0.034	0.018	0.009
100						0.069	0.053	0.035	0.019	0.010
120							0.055	0.037	0.020	0.010
140							0.056	0.039	0.022	0.011
160							0.056	0.041	0.023	0.012
180								0.042	0.024	0.013
200								0.043	0.025	0.013
300									0.028	0.016
400									0.030	0.018
500									0.031	0.019
1000										0.022

CHAPTER 8

Multivariable analysis in diagnostic accuracy studies: what are the possibilities?

Frank Buntinx, Bert Aertgeerts, Marc Aerts, Rudi Bruyninckx, J. André Knottnerus, Ann van den Bruel, and Jef van den Ende

---

Summary box

- Diagnostic research requires multivariable analytical approaches to take the contributions of different tests to a diagnosis simultaneously into consideration.
- Tree-building methods, logistic regression analysis, and neural networks can provide solutions to this challenge. Latent class analysis adds a method that can be used in situations without a normal reference standard.
- For each method, we provide a short description, an overview of advantages and disadvantages, and a real-life example.
- Researchers should concentrate on either logistic regression analysis or classification and regression tree (CART) type methods, try to master it in detail and consequently use it, always keeping in mind that alternatives are available, each with their own advantages and disadvantages.

Introduction

Individual signs, symptoms, or test results are seldom sufficient to reliably diagnose a disorder.[1] In most situations, various parts of information are needed and the diagnostic value of each part (each test) is not independent, but conditional upon what is known already. Age may be a bad predictor of an urological

---

The Evidence Base of Clinical Diagnosis: Theory and Methods of Diagnostic Research. 2nd edition.
Edited by J. André Knottnerus and Frank Buntinx. © 2009 Blackwell Publishing,
ISBN: 978-1-4051-5787-2.

cancer. However, in patients with gross hematuria, age above 60 increased the likelihood of an urological cancer (positive predictive value) from 17% (all ages) to 34%.[2]

This is not addressed by classic bivariably analyzed diagnostic studies. The analysis of the combined diagnostic value from a number of tests as well as the diagnostic value of a test conditional on (a series of) previous test results needs a multivariable approach. A number of solutions for this type of analysis are available. None of them, however, is perfect. Each has its own strengths, weaknesses, and problems. In this chapter, we describe some of the most appealing methods that have been used, in a way that is understandable for clinicians without formal statistical training. For more detailed and technical information, we refer to the book of Pepe[3] and to the papers that are mentioned in the literature section. Six methods are described with their advantages and their own problems: simple tree building and the more sophisticated classification and regression tree (CART) analysis as examples of tree-building methods, classical and "manipulated" logistic regression analysis, which are the most frequently used techniques, the less standard neural networks, and finally latent class analysis as a method of dealing with situations where no reference standard is available. In the Appendix, we will show one way of how the usual indicators of diagnostic accuracy can be calculated from the standard output of a multiple logistic regression analysis. This also narrows the distance between logistic regression analysis and the tree-building methods.

For each method, we provide a short description, some advantages and disadvantages (under characteristics) and a real life example.

Overview of the methods

Simple tree building

Sensitivity and specificity are calculated for all outcome categories of all relevant tests. The test with the best results according to a predetermined criterion (e.g., sensitivity) is retained. For each result of this first test, all remaining tests are reexamined. This is repeated as long as necessary, resulting in a decision tree. At each node of the tree sensitivity and specificity (or other indicators of diagnostic accuracy) are calculated for the total tree, adding up all true or false positives and negatives at that moment. This method is based on reaching a predetermined goal in terms of one or more diagnostic indicators and nodes visualize the different decisions. This goal can be, for example, further testing until for the whole study population a specificity of 0.80 is reached, in which case an endpoint is reached; or no further testing as soon as the sensitivity falls below 0.80. Any (combination of) diagnostic indicators (sensitivity, specificity, likelihood ratio, predictive value, or odds ratio) can be used as well as any cutpoint (for continuous results) as long as it is predetermined before the start of the analysis.

Characteristics

1 *Calculations* are straightforward and can be made by hand or using a simple Excel file. Everybody can see and understand what is happening. There is no black box phenomenon.

2 As the tree unfolds, *interactions* are taken into account.

3 In addition to the "prediction" of the presence or absence of one diagnosis ("this patient either has a myocardial infarction or not"), trees can be produced that have more than two *outcome categories* (this patient has a myocardial infarction or an unstable angina or something else). For practical reasons, the number of possible endpoints will generally be restricted to a maximum of two or three.

4 *The choice of the indicators and cut-points* can be based on the exact aims of the tests that are studied. Are you most interested in the as complete as possible detection of cases (maximize sensitivity) or in avoiding false positive cases (maximize positive predictive value)? Based on the work of Connell and Koepsell,[4] it has been suggested to use the sum of sensitivity and specificity as a general measure of gain in (additional) certainty.[1] The *asymmetry* in the diagnostic value of a positive and a negative test result (if a positive result of test T is highly predictive for the presence of disease D, this does not mean that a negative test result largely excludes the presence of disease D) that is inherent to most diagnostic tests is simply addressed as positive and negative test results are independently processed.

5 This technique is almost impossible with large numbers of tests, and for tests with continuous outcomes it is only applicable if they are categorized. The sequence of including test results can be manipulated. This permits taking into account the cost of a test (financially, but even more in terms of pain, threat or other type of burden for the patient), the use of common sense and the normal progression of a clinical approach. "Easy" tests, for example, age, sex, and initial complaint are used first. They can be followed by more detailed results of history taking and the basic physical examination, next by the answers to more difficult questions, questionnaires, or more complex examinations, by the results of additional technological tests and finally by the results of unpleasant, invasive or harmful examinations. Comparison of the results of two subsequent nodes permits to study the incremental gain of the additional test. The basic tree allows for each test to be used only once in a sequence. Calculations are possible, however, that also allow a test result that initially was rejected to be tested again and maybe included in a subsequent stage of the sequence.

6 Patient records including *missing values* have to be excluded as soon as the missing value has to be taken into account.

7 No measure of *imprecision* is generally used during tree building.

8 There is no way to *control* whether the rules are set previous to the analysis. This permits the researcher to change the rules of the game during the analysis, resulting in possible data dredging and overoptimistic fitting of the models. The choice of the cut-points is arbitrary.

Example

In a random sample of subsequent male patients visiting their GP, the GP's initial judgment, questionnaires, and laboratory tests were used to identify alcohol abusers, using the Diagnostic and Statistical Manual of Mental Disorders (DSM) criteria as operationalized in the Composite International Diagnostic Interview as the gold standard.[5] In a secondary analysis of the same data, all possible trees were constructed, allowing all combinations of tests except those in which laboratory tests preceded clinical information or questionnaire results. The repeated use of a test was not possible. At each node of the tree, sensitivity and specificity of the total available model up to that node were calculated, based on the results of all patients. The model searched for the highest sensitivity combined with a specificity at or above the specificity of the initial judgment of the GP.

Use of classification and regression tree (CART) software

This is a computationally strong extension of the first method in which a number of choices are predetermined.[6] Well-known examples are CART[7] or Quinlan's C4.5[8] software. The CART program (Classification and Regression Trees) produces decision trees using variables (coded signs and symptoms) directing to diagnostic categories. At each node of the tree, the program calculates which variable is the "most discriminating" and constructs at that node a bifurcation of two branches. In case of a continuous variable, an optimal cut-point is calculated and the variable is dichotomized. For each resulting branch, CART calculates the next most discriminating variable and continues in this way until either the size of the subgroups or the discriminating power become too small. A final statistical pruning technique results in an optimal tree where optimality is measured by various criteria.

Characteristics

1 Complex and specific software is required and the statistical calculations result in a black box phenomenon. However, CART software is *freely available* on the Internet (e.g., the r part package in R, see http://cran.r-project.org/). It is fully data driven and can handle complex high-dimensional datasets. The result is an easily interpretable tree.

2 The *sequence* of including test results can be manipulated, be it not as simple as in a hand written tree. Continuous test results are easily handled through calculation of the "best" cut-point by the software.

3 *Interactions* are automatically taken into account.

4 In addition to the "prediction" of the presence or absence of one diagnosis, trees can also result in more than two possible *diagnostic outcomes*.

5 Depending from the exact software package, most *indicators of diagnostic accuracy* are presented or can easily be calculated from the output. The *asymmetry* in the diagnostic value of a positive and a negative test result is addressed, as positive and negative test results are independently processed. Weights can be attributed to false negative and false positive results.

6 Procedures to deal with missing data are part of the CART software. One interesting procedure is based on the use of surrogate splits. The surrogate split approach attempts to utilize the information in the other predictors to assist in making the decision to send an observation to the left or the right daughter node. One looks for the predictor that is most "similar" to the original predictor in classifying the observations. Similarity is measured by a measure of association. It is not unlikely that in one or more observations the predictor that yields the best surrogate split may also be missing. Then we have to look for the second best, and so on. In this way, all available information is used.

7 As all possible interactions, for which patient information is available, are tested, the required sample size may be high.

8 Relatively simple final decision rules may be related to quite complex trees. In some software (e.g., CART), the complexity of a tree is penalized during the tree-building process. The models also tend to result in redundant branches of the tree, suggesting that some variables are important while they are not.[7]

9 Both a split half and a cross-validation procedure are routinely available for misclassification error estimation. However, an important disadvantage of CART remains its variability. Different datasets from the same setting can lead to quite different final trees. Methods which average different trees based on bootstrap samples (bagging and random forests), solve this problem at the cost of interpretability.[9]

Example
A group of general practitioners studied the diagnostic value of a list of signs and symptoms in identifying children with a serious infection (n = 31; 0.8%) out of a group of 3981 consecutive ill children. CART software provided a tree with a sensitivity of 96.8%, specificity of 88.5%, and positive and negative predictive value of 6.2% and 100%, using six steps and five tests, respectively.[10]

Logistic regression analysis
Computer software builds a model with the presence or absence of the disease as the dependent variable and all available diagnostic test results, with or without interaction terms, as the independent variables.

Characteristics
1 It is a complex, but reasonably fast, technique, resulting in a black box phenomenon. The required software is available in almost all standard statistical software packages.

2 Continuous test results are easily handled, with or without categorization. Categorization will be needed, however, to make it easier for clinicians to use the final model in daily life. The variables can be entered into the model building process together or they can be used one by one (stepwise procedure). In a forward stepwise procedure, the variable with the strongest significance will be entered first, followed one by one by the others in order of statistical significance, as far as they are still showing significance. Another option is the backward procedure, where the most complex model is gradually simplified by deleting the most nonsignificant variables one by one, until only significant variables are left in the model.

3 Interactions can be taken into account. If all possible interactions are taken into account, this generally results in very complex models that are difficult to explain to clinicians who have not been involved in the analysis. Interaction analysis is therefore usually only performed for a maximum of two or three terms. It is of course possible to calculate all predictive values from the computer output (see Appendix) and to present them as a tree.

4 In principle, logistic regression is restricted to the decision whether one specific diagnosis is present or not. Therefore, this is the use most people will be familiar with. Nevertheless, some techniques for polytomous logistic regression analysis are available and progressively gaining interest in diagnostic research.[11]

5 The diagnostic value of a test can be reported as an adjusted (or conditional) odds ratio for the relation of a positive versus negative test result and the presence or absence of the disease. The diagnosis can be predicted from the model on the basis of all test results for a specific patient or a group of patients with similar test results. The diagnostic value of the model can be expressed as the area under the (ROC, or receiver operating characteristic) curve (AUC). The AUC is the graphical representation of the sensitivity and specificity of the prediction model as a function of the cutoff point of the predicted posterior probability.

The use of an odds ratio for a test may suggest that the positive and negative results of a test are of a symmetrical nature; that is, that a test is equally strong for ruling in as for ruling out a diagnosis. Most tests, however, are intrinsically asymmetrical. A modeling technique has been proposed that enables the calculation of sensitivity and specificity in both one-test and multiple-tests situations. Each test variable x is transformed to $x - x_0$ before model building with x_0 being the (virtual) value of x for which posterior disease odds = prior disease odds.[1] In case of interaction, branch specific test characteristics can be calculated. The method is described in more detail in the Appendix. Alternative methods have been developed by Albert[12] and by Spiegelhalter and Knill-Jones.[13,14] A comparison of the three methods showed generally similar post-test probabilities.[15]

6 The presence of a missing value for one variable results in the exclusion of the whole patient record, unless an imputation technique is used.

7 The required sample size depends on the number of variables, including the number of interaction terms. As interactions are usually only partially analyzed, the required sample size is far less, compared to the tree-building methods.

8 The use of statistical significance to decide whether a test is included into the model is less intuitively understandable to clinicians. Results will therefore be less appealing to them. However, given statistical significance, also other criteria can be used, such as the maximal sum of sensitivity and specificity, invasiveness or cost.[1] This is highlighted in the next section.

Example
In their analysis on the diagnostic value of signs and symptoms for diagnosing pneumonia, Hopstaken *et al.*[16] identified three significant symptoms. They used backward logistic regression analysis to identify the independently significant symptoms, including interaction terms if significant (which was not the case). They reported both odds ratios and a prediction rule with the positive predictive value for each combination of test results.

Manipulated logistic regression analysis
In this variant, the order of including test results is manipulated by the researcher. This permits taking into account the cost of a test (financially, but even more in terms of pain, fear or other type of burden for the patient), the use of common sense and the normal progression of a clinical approach. Clusters of "easy" tests are presented first (e.g., age, sex, and initial complaint). They are followed by more results of additional history taking and the basic physical examination, next by the answers to more difficult questions, questionnaires or more complex examinations, by the results of additional technological tests and finally by the results of clearly unpleasant, invasive or harmful examinations. The researcher decides on the sequence of presenting the clusters to the software. "Statistics" decide which tests of a cluster are entered or rejected.

Characteristics
1 Instead of entering all possible test results together in the model, or entering them in a sequence dictated by statistical test results, the order in which tests are included in the model is dictated by indicators that are considered relevant by the researchers. However, this also means that the order in which the test results are entered into the model building procedure is more or less arbitrarily decided by the researcher or by a group advising him or her. As a result, two groups doing a similar study or even another analysis in the same dataset may use a different sequence and therefore reach a different final model. It is then important that the indicators used are specified and reported.
2 Other characteristics are similar to option 3.

Example
De Lepeleire *et al.* used this method to build a model for the early diagnosis of dementia in community dwelling elderly. The sequence of presenting different tests to the model was decided by a group of clinical experts. The final model included four signs and symptoms and reached an AUC of 0.93. Complex tests

with a high discriminative power in crude data analysis, did not add to this basic model.[17] Similarly, in a second part of their analysis on the diagnostic value of tests for diagnosing pneumonia, Hopstaken *et al.* added laboratory test results to the initial model including signs and symptoms only, as this was considered a logical second step in diagnostic reasoning. The C-Reactive Protein (CRP) proved to add significant information to the initial model.[16]

Neural networks

The central idea of the application of neural networks in diagnostic studies is to extract linear combinations of all diagnostic test results (the inputs) as so-called derived features, and then model the presence or absence of the disease (the target) as a nonlinear function of these features.[18]

Advantages

1 Neural networks are powerful *learning methods* developed separately in artificial intelligence and statistics; they have good predictive power. Software is readily available in statistical packages as S-PLUS (commercial) and its freeware counterpart R. A variety of additional commercial shareware and freeware software tools for neural networks are readily available at the Internet.
2 A neural network (for a binary target) can be seen as an extension of logistic regression.[9,19]
3 Dealing with interactions and with diagnostic asymmetry is an intrinsic part of the calculations.
4 Neural networks can easily deal with more than two diagnostic categories.
5 Neural networks have major difficulties in handling missing data.
6 Neural networks are especially effective in problems with a high signal-to-noise ratio and settings where prediction without interpretation is the goal. They are less effective for problems where the goal is to interpret the process that generated the data. It is a black box method. There are many variants and different implementations, making them hard to understand for nonexperts. For this reason, neural networks have been less used in medical applications.

Example

The presence of left bundle branch block (LBBB) in the electrocardiogram (ECG) increases the difficulty in recognizing an acute myocardial infarction (AMI). Various ECG criteria for the diagnosis of AMI have proved to be of limited value. Five hundred and eighteen ECGs, recorded at an emergency department, with an LBBB configuration, were used to compare the performance of neural networks to that of six sets of conventional ECG criteria and two experienced cardiologists. Of this sample, 120 patients had an AMI. Artificial neural networks of the feed-forward type were trained to classify the ECGs as AMI or not AMI. The neural network showed higher sensitivities than both the conventional criteria and the cardiologists when compared at the same levels of specificity.[20]

Latent class analysis

This is a method to be used when a real reference standard is absent. In this way, the method differs from what was discussed before. In a ward, or a population, we observe patterns of symptoms. So we might see patients with hemoptysis, fever and weight loss, patients with haemoptysis with no fever nor weight loss, others with fever and weight loss but without hemoptysis, and so on. We know that tuberculosis might, at least partly, account for these patterns. Direct microscopy and culture can help, but are not sensitive enough: we lack a reliable gold standard or "reference standard." Latent class analysis hypothesizes a "hidden" disease or condition, which might explain the "constellation" of symptom patterns.

The group of cases with a certain pattern would encompass both patients with and without the disease. The proportion of tuberculosis (the hypothetical condition) patients with all three symptoms would, in case of conditional independence of symptoms, be given by: [Prevalence × sens (hemoptysis) × sens (fever) × sens (weight loss)], where "sens" stands for the (yet unknown) sensitivity for each indicated symptom, while the proportion of patients, for example, without tuberculosis presenting with hemoptysis and weight loss but without fever would be given by:

[(1–prevalence) × (1–spec) (hemoptysis) × (1–spec) (weight loss) × spec (fever)], where spec stands for the (yet unknown) specificity. The presence of all possible combinations of test results in diseased and nondiseased can be summed up. There would be 2^3 patterns, from which seven disease characteristics are to be found: the prevalence, and the sensitivity and specificity of each of the three symptoms. Latent class analysis intends to offer an explanation for the "constellation of patterns" through the seven disease characteristics. Consecutive values are substituted for the disease characteristics, until through repetitive approximation the predicted distribution of the patterns comes close to the observed in the ward or the population. The closer, the better the model explains reality.

Characteristics

1 Results are given in sensitivity and specificity, allowing for asymmetry in test interpretation.
2 Current programs provide several indicators of model fit, prevalence of the condition, sensitivities and specificities of disease characteristics, Likelihood ratios, and post-test probabilities for all patterns.
3 Early versions of the software required conditional independence, but modern versions allow controlling for it. Moreover, clinicians can judge about the importance of a certain confounding/interaction term and correct for it or not in the model.[21]
4 The concept of "latent class" is difficult to explain, which does not add to trust in the methodology. Most explanations use quite complex formulas. In the absence of a gold standard (a reliable reference test), sensitivity and specificity can be estimated. However, the true nature of the latent condition

is not known. While tuberculosis is relatively easy to identify, since microscopy and culture strongly point to the disease, we might be identifying AIDS instead of tuberculosis. For other conditions like alcoholism, it may be even more difficult as no specific characteristic exists, hence doubt can remain on the nature of the disease we are looking at. As an example, we may be identifying depression in stead of alcoholism.

5 The number of variables is limited. As the number of combinations (patterns) doubles with every additive variable, and since "empty" patterns (no patients in this combination) should be avoided, the required sample size almost doubles with every extra variable.

6 Different models can explain the same constellation, and give quite different prevalences, sensitivities, and specificities.

Example
The true prevalence of tuberculosis in a certain population is unknown as the culture, the classical reference standard, lacks sensitivity. In a 300-patient cohort in Kigali, Rwanda, prevalence, sensitivity, and specificity of clinical and paraclinical data were studied. The estimated prevalence was 20% higher than predicted by culture, but the values for sensitivity and specificity were almost the same, except for sensitivity of direct microscopy. Posttest probability was given for different combinations of disease characteristics.

Additional methods
Experiments have been performed with Bayesian networks.[22,23] These are mathematically complex methods for which specific software is required. Most clinical researchers are insufficiently familiar with the theory behind and with the operationalization of the procedures. Also the translation of results into routine clinical practice can therefore be expected to be problematic. The black box problem is even larger than for regression modeling. Finally, the available experience at this moment is rather scarce. These problems are even more prominent with respect to support vector machines or boosting methods.

Problems shared by all methods

Validation
In all these procedures, the results that are reported are based on models or trees that are built on a certain datasets. Although exceptions exist,[24] models that are developed in one population, tend to behave worse as soon as they are tested in another, even similar population.[25,26,27] Before they gain any clinical value they therefore have to be confirmed in at least one second population. The optimal solution is to perform a validation study in which exactly the same model is tested in a new and independent, but clinically similar population.[24,29,30] As the model or tree proves to be reliable in an increasing number of independent populations, its generalizability and therefore also its clinical relevance progressively increase. An "intermediate" option is a

cross-validation procedure: The sample of patients is divided in two subsamples. The first one (sometimes called the "learning sample") is used to build the model or tree. The second subsample (the validation sample) is then used to confirm or validate the model or tree that was initially built. Such a procedure is routinely available, for example, in CART software.[7] It can easily be performed, however, in all situations that were discussed. This is heavily paid, however, as the statistical power for each of both subsamples drops. Moreover, this method does not represent a real external validation in a new and independent study population.

Performance of the final model

There is no formal rule to decide on how good a final model is. In case of a dichotomous result of both the prediction model and the reference standard, a classic 2×2 table can be constructed by using the diagnoses "predicted" by the model as a test result and comparing this with the reference standard result. Accuracy as well as the usual indicators of the diagnostic value of a test (sensitivity, specificity, predictive values, and likelihood ratios) can then be calculated for the model. Also ROC curves can be produced if different cut-points of the predicted posterior probability are subsequently used. In case of subsequent entering of various (clusters of) tests, the area under the curve (AUC) can be calculated after each step that is been taken. The increase in AUC after each step will teach you to what extent the model/tree is improving while progressively becoming more complex (Figure 8.1). On the basis of this increase in AUC and its statistical significance it can than be decided at which moment to stop.[16,17,30]

Overlapping subgroups

Handling of overlapping subgroups is only possible if the shared test characteristic comes first in the tree-building procedure. For example, patients with retrosternal chest pain (opposed to another localization on the chest) and no pain at palpation may be at high risk for myocardial infarction.[31] Another high-risk group may consist of patients with retrosternal chest pain and irradiation of the pain to the neck and mouth. The diagnostic value of pain localization is easily detected if the localization of the pain is addressed first by the tree-building procedure. It may be difficult to detect, however, whether the localization is only relevant after inclusion of one or both of the two other symptoms. Which of the symptoms comes first during tree building may depend on the results in a small number of patients and the consequences may be important as the second symptom may totally disappear from the model unless both symptoms are fixed to each other and commonly handled on the basis of pre-existing information. A related problem is the following: If two tests give results that are very near to each other, the first one (i.e., the test with the highest degree of statistical significance) will be selected and entered into the model. The second test will probably loose all additional significance (conditional upon the result of the first test) and be rejected by the

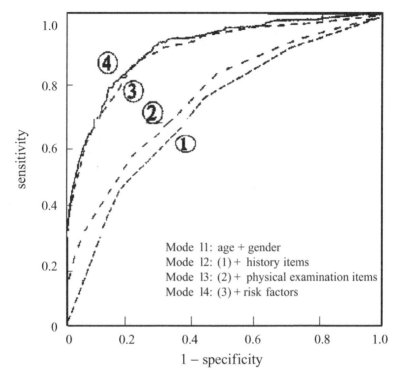

Figure 8.1 ROC curves of the four multiple logistic regression models for diagnosing peripheral arterial occlusive disease (N = 4,310 legs), evaluating the diagnostic value of four models with increased clinical complexity with inclusion of added variables with each step. Areas under the curve AUCs are, respectively, for model 1: 0.69; for model 2: 0.72; for model 3: 0.86; and for model 4: 0.87. Each subsequent logistic model was shown to be a significant improvement on its predecessor using likelihood ratio tests.[30]

model although it may be a very relevant test if used without the first one, for example if information is only available on the second and not on the first symptom.[1,29] As a medical example, one might think of the competition between the hemoglobin level and the hematocrit to be included in a predictive model, although each of these can have an important contribution especially in the absence of the other. The decision which test is the strongest may be based on the result in a small number of patients only.

Number of tests to be included

Some authors use a criterion for the maximal number and the choice of tests to be included in the multivariate model to be tested.[17] For example, it has been suggested that a total number of 1,000 subjects in the study would be sufficient to examine a three-test situation with all interactions.[1] Such rules can be helpful in a specific situation, but they are more or less arbitrary and do not provide robust guidance. In logistic regression analysis, not all possible interactions tend to be analyzed and the required sample size will then generally be less.

Selection of tests to be included
If a large number of test results are available, the resulting model may be very complex and very difficult to interpret. However, selecting possible tests on the basis of their behavior in bivariate analysis does not solve this problem: a test may be very effective in an unselected population, but fail to add relevant information if the results of previous tests are already available. However, this can be sorted out in the multivariable analysis. More problematic is the opposite: an initially weak test may be a strong confirmation test in a (by previous testing) highly selected population, and this will be missed in case of preselection by bivariate statistical significance. It has been suggested that tree building should be used for selecting the relevant tests. In a second stage, the model should then be refined by logistic regression analysis.[8]

Meta-analysis
Meta-analysis of the results of this kind of studies is at the moment practically impossible unless exactly the same models or trees are fit in different studies. Probably only methods based on individual patient data pooling will be able to do the job.[32] In the future, one could imagine different researchers that are studying the same problem to collect a common set of test results and final diagnostic categories (possible endpoints) in a similar way and to share their data for analysis.

Recommendations

Multiple logistic regression is currently the most popular technique for the analysis of diagnostic studies including multiple tests, especially in the case of dichotomous test results and disease outcomes. The most rewarding approach is to start with a simple one-test model and progressively adding other tests together with the relevant interactions. Both efficiency and clinical relevance may increase if tests are entered in the model as clusters, starting with "easy" or less costly tests or following the normal progression of a clinical approach (see option 4). The main alternative in current research practice is the use of CART-type tree-building methods (see option 2). Comparisons have not provided clear indications that one or the other approach would be more valid. We suggest that researchers should concentrate on one of these methods, try to master it in detail and consequently use it, always keeping in mind that alternatives are available, each with their own advantages and disadvantages.

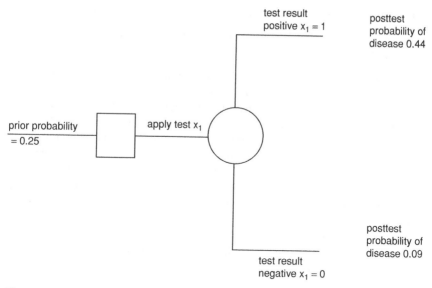

Figure 8.2 Decision/probability tree for the application of test x_1 (see data in Table 8.2).

Acknowledgments

We are grateful for the very helpful comments of Petra Macaskill on a previous version of this text.

Appendix: Deriving test characteristics from a logistic regression analysis

To show how test characteristics can be derived from logistic regression analysis we use a single test example based on a simple 2×2 table.[1] Table 8.2 summarizes data for a study population of 900 subjects investigated with a dichotomous test x to diagnose or exclude disease D. We would speak about x_1 if data on more test variables ($x_2, x_3, \ldots, x_i$) would be available. The prior probability of D, P(D), is $225/900 = .25$. Values of other relevant diagnostic measures such as sensitivity, specificity, likelihood ratios, odds ratio and posterior probabilities are presented in the table. A simple one test *prediction rule* for disease D, based on these data for this study population with prior disease probability .25, can be formulated as follows:

Apply test x:

- if x is positive ($x = 1$), then the posterior probability of D, $P(D|x = 1)$, is $180/405 = .44$;
- if x is negative ($x = 0$), then the posterior probability of D, $P(D|x = 0)$, is $45/495 = .09$.

Figure 8.2 summarizes this in a simple decision and probability tree.

The data in Table 8.1 can be expressed in a basic *logistic regression function*:

Ln (posterior odds), which is equivalent to Ln $(P(D|x)/(1 - P(D|x)))$,
$$= -2.30 + 2.08* x$$

where, as is known for logistic regression, the left term is the logit of D: the natural logarithm of the posterior disease odds given the test result for x_1.

Furthermore, -2.30 is the intercept, equivalent to the natural logarithm of the posterior disease odds for a negative test result ($= $ Ln $(.09/(1 - .09))$).

In addition, 2.08 is the logistic regression coefficient for independent variable x (that is, the test), and represents the natural logarithm of the odds ratio for the relationship between x and D in Table 8.1 ($= $ Ln 8.0). This quantity contains full information on the discrimination of the test since—as can be easily shown in a 2×2 table—the odds ratio is the ratio of the likelihood ratio of the positive test result (LR+) and the likelihood ratio of the negative test result (LR−): OR $=$ LR+/ LR−, so Ln OR $=$ Ln (LR+/ LR−) $= 2.08$.

If one wants to include directly the information of the prior disease odds, one can, again, use an equivalent expression (1):

$$Ln\ (P(D|x)/(1 - P(D|x))) = -1.10 + 2.08 \times (x - 0.58)$$

The intercept value -1.10 is equivalent to the natural logarithm of the prior disease odds ($= $ Ln$(.25/(1 - .25))$). The value .58 is representing the (virtual) indifferent value of x, (designated as x_0) for which posterior odds $=$ prior odds. The general formulation of the regression equation is then: Ln (posterior odds) $=$ Ln (prior odds) $+ B(x - x_0)$, with for x $= x_0$, Ln(prior odds)$=$ Ln(posterior odds).

It can be shown (1) that:

$$x_0 = \frac{Ln(\text{prior odds}) - Ln(\text{posterior odds}|x = 0)}{B},$$

in which B is the logistic regression coefficient representing Ln OR.

The advantage of this representation, in fact being a logistic expression of Bayes's formula, is that the relationship with the prior odds of the study population has clearly been retained and that the test information is added to it. In addition, in contrast to the usual representation of logistic regression, all *test characteristics can be directly derived from this* function:

$$LR+ = e^{B(1-x_0)} = 2.718^{2.08 \times (1-0.58)} = 2.4$$

$$B(-x_0)LR- = e = 2.718^{2.08 \times (-0.58)} = 0.30$$

$$\text{Sensitivity} = \frac{e^{-Bx_0} - 1}{e^{-B} - 1} = \frac{2.718^{-2.08 \times 0.58} - 1}{2.718^{-2.08} - 1} = 0.80$$

$$\text{Specificity} = \frac{e^{-B(1-x_0)} - 1}{e^{-B} - 1} = \frac{2.718^{-2.08 \times (1-0.58)} - 1}{2.718^{-2.08} - 1} = 0.66$$

Table 8.1 Which diagnostic indicators can be derived from the software output?*

	Simple tree building	CART	Standard logistic regression	Manipulated logistic regression	Neural network	Latent class analysis
Prevalence	Calculated	Outprint	Outprint	Outprint	Calculated	Outprint
PPV	Calculated	Calculated	Calculated	Calculated	Calculated	Outprint
NPV	Calculated	Calculated	Calculated	Calculated	Calculated	Outprint
Sensitivity	Calculated	Calculated	calculated†	Calculated†	Calculated	Outprint
Specificity	Calculated	Calculated	calculated†	calculated†	Calculated	Outprint
LR+	Calculated	Calculated	calculated†	calculated†	Calculated	Outprint
LR−	Calculated	Calculated	calculated†	calculated†	Calculated	Outprint
Odds ratio	Calculated	Calculated	Outprint	Outprint	Calculated	Outprint
AUC	Not	Not	Outprint	Outprint	Not	Not

Calculated: to be derived using simple calculations by the user. Standard error or 95% confidence interval not easily available.

Outprint: indicator and standard error or 95% confidence interval presented in standard outprint.

AUC, area under the curve; CART, classification and regression tree; LR, likelihood ratio, NPV = negative predictive value, PPV = positive predictive value.

*This may be slightly different in different software packages.

† Calculated according to reference 1.

Table 8.2 Example: relation between the result of test and the presence or absence of disease D

Test Result	Disease D+	Status D−	Total
positive: x = 1	180	225	405
negative: x = 0	45	450	495
Total	225	675	900

prior probability = 225/900 = .25
posterior probability of a positive test result (positive predictive value) = 180/405 = 0.44
posterior probability of a negative test result (1 − negative predictive value) = 45/495 = 0.09
sensitivity = 180/225 = .80
specificity = 450/675 = .67

$$\text{likelihood ratio positive (LR+)} = \frac{\text{sensitivity}}{1 - \text{specificity}} = 2.4$$

$$\text{likelihood ratio negative (LR−)} = \frac{1 - \text{sensitivity}}{\text{specificity}} = .30$$

$$\text{odds ratio (= cross product)} = \frac{180 \times 450}{225 \times 45} = 8.0$$

Also confidence intervals can be computed.[1] A practical problem is that at this moment no software is available in the standard statistical packages to routinely perform these calculations.

In applying a logistic regression function for diagnostic prediction to an individual subject with certain characteristics (that is, specific values for x variables), we can substitute the individual values for the x variables. This yields the natural logarithm of the estimated posterior disease odds for this subject. Then, using some elementary algebra we can calculate the *posterior probability* P(D|x). For the single test situation of Table 8.2, this will give the following results for subjects with positive and negative test outcomes, respectively:

$$P(D|x = 1) = \frac{1}{1 + e^{-(-1.10 + 2.08*(1 - .58))}} = .44$$

and

$$P(D|x = 0) = \frac{1}{1 + e^{-(-1.10 + 2.08*(-.58))}} = .09$$

These latter two outcomes are equivalent to the predictive value of a positive test and 1− the predictive value of the negative test respectively.

Of course, the same results would have been found by substitution into the usual logistic regression function. In Table 8.3, computer output for the logistic regression analysis for the Table 8.2 data is given, also including standard errors of the coefficients.

Table 8.3 Results of logistic regression analysis for a single test situation, including standard errors of the coefficients, for the usual approach and the approach using $(x - x_0)$ instead of x (Basic data in Table 8.2)

Variable	Ordinary		Proposed	
	coefficient	(SE)	coefficient	(SE)
Intercept X	−2.30	(.16)	−1.10	(.09)
(X − .58)	2.08	(.19)	2.08	(.19)

Analogous to the one test example, also multiple test situations can be worked out using multiple logistic regression analysis with $x_1, x_2, x_3, \ldots,$ x_i representing test 1, test 2, test 3, and test i, respectively, and with $x_{10}, x_{20},$ $x_{30}, \ldots, x_{i0}$ representing the respective indifferent x-values for these tests. The general elaboration for the regression function for a two-test situation, taking also possible interactions between the test results into consideration, is as follows:

Ln(posterior odds), equivalent to $\text{Ln}(P(D|x_1, x_2)/(1 - P(D|x_1, x_2))$

$$= \text{Ln(prior odds)} + B_1(x_1 - x_{10}) + B_{21}x_1(x_2 - x_{210}) + B_{20}(1 - x_1)(x_2 - x_{200})$$

in which B_1 is the regression coefficient for x_1, and B_{21} and B_{20} are the regression coefficients for x_2 if $x_1 = 1$ and $x_1 = 0$, respectively; x_{10}, x_{210}, and x_{200} are the indifferent values of x_1 and of x_2 in case of $x_1 = 1$, and of x_2 in case of $x_1 = 0$, respectively.

This implies that in the two-test situation the impact of x_2 may be different depending on whether the first test is positive (with $x_1 = 1$) or negative (with $1 - x_1 = 1$).

In Figure 8.3, the two-test situation with interaction between tests is represented in a diagnostic probability tree. When there are more than two test variables, the preferred sequence of the test can vary between the various "branches" of the diagnostic tree. 1

The relationship between Bayes's rule and logistic regression has also been pointed out by Spiegelhalter en Knill-Jones:[13,14] the natural logarithm of the likelihood ratio, Ln LR, can be used as *"weight of evidence"* in a additive logistic model starting from the Ln (prior disease odds). For a positively discriminating test this weight of evidence has a positive value, and for a negatively discriminating test the weight is negative.

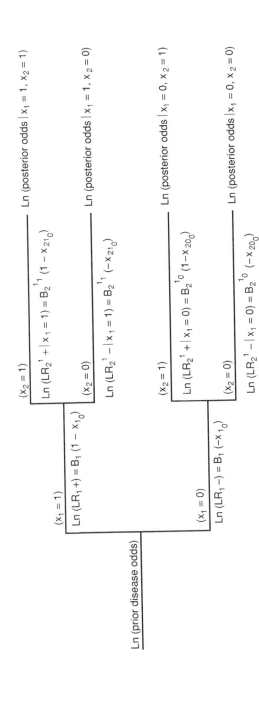

Figure 8.3 Logistic regression equation for a two-test situation represented in diagnostic probability tree, with x_1 and x_2 being the results for these (dichotomous) tests. In case of interaction (OR being different over the outcome categories of x_1), not only the posterior odds but also the test characteristics (e.g., likelihood ratios) are branch-specific.

References

1. Knottnerus JA. Application of logistic regression to the analysis of diagnostic data: exact modeling of a probability tree of multiple binary variables. *Med Decis Making.* 1992;**12**:93–108.
2. Bruyninckx R, Buntinx F, Aertgeerts B, et al. The diagnostic value of macroscopic haematuria for the diagnosis of urological cancer in general practice. *Br J Gen Pract.* 2003;**53**:31–35.
3. Pepe MS. *The statistical evaluation of medical tests for classification and prediction.* Oxford: Oxford University Press; 2003.
4. Connell FA, Koepsell TD. Measures of gain in certainty from a diagnostic test. *Am J Epidemiol.* 1985;**121**:744–53.
5. Aertgeerts B, Buntinx F, Ansoms S, et al. Screening properties of questionnaires and laboratory tests for the detection of alcohol abuse or dependence in a general practice population. *Br J Gen Pract.* 2001;**51**:206–17.
6. Harper PR. A review and comparison of classification algorithms for medical decision making. *Health Policy.* 2005;**71**:315–31.
7. Marshall RJ. The use of classification and regression trees in clinical epidemiology. *J Clin Epidemiol.* 2001;**54**:603–9.
8. Tsien CL, Fraser HSF, Long WL, et al. Using classification tree and logistic regression methods to diagnose myocardial infarction. Medinfo 1998. Proceedings of the 9th World Congress on Medical Informatics; 1998. pp. 493–97.
9. Hastie T, Tibshirani R, Friedman, J. *The elements of statistical learning: data mining, inference and prediction.* Springer-Verlag: New York; 2001.
10. Van den Bruel A, Aertgeerts B, Bruyninckx R, et al. Signs and symptoms for the diagnosis of serious infections in children: a prospective study in primary care. *Brit J Gen Pract .*2007;**57**:538–46.
11. Biesheuvel CJ, Vergouwe Y, Steyerberg EW, et al. Polytomous logistic regression analysis could be applied more often in diagnostic research. *J Clin Epidemiol.* 2008;**61**(2):125–34. Epub 2007 Jun 29.
12. Albert A. On the use and computation of likelihood ratios in clinical chemistry. *Clin Chem.* 1982;**28**:1113–19.
13. Spiegelhalter DJ, Knill-Jones RP. Statistical and knowledge-based approaches to clinical decision-support systems, with an application in gastroenterology. *J R Stat Soc [Ser A].* 1984;**147**:35–77.
14. Spiegelhalter DJ, Crean GP, Holden R, et al. Taking a calculated risk: predictive scoring systems in dyspepsia. *Scand J Gastroenterol.* 1987;**22**(Suppl 128):152–60.
15. Chan SF, Deeks JJ, Macaskill P, et al. Three methods to construct predictive models using logistic regression and likelihood ratios to facilitate adjustment for pretest probability give similar results. *J Clin Epidemiol.* 2008;**61**(1):52–63. Epub 2007 Jul 16.
16. Hopstaken RM, Muris JWM, Knottnerus JA, et al. Contributions of symptoms, signs, erythrocyte sedimentation rate, and C-reactive protein to a diagnosis of pneumonia in acute lower respiratory tract infection. *Br J Gen Pract.* 2003;**53**:358–64.
17. De Lepeleire J, Heyrman J, Baro F, et al. A combination of tests for the diagnosis of dementia had a significant diagnostic value. *J Clin Epidemiol.* 2005;**58**:217–25.
18. Baxt WG, Skora J. Prospective validation of an artificial neural network trained to identify acute myocardial infarction. *Lancet.*1996;**347**:12–15.
19. Ripley BD. *Pattern recognition and neural networks.* Cambridge University Press; 1996.

20. Olsson SE, Ohlsson M, Öhlin H, et al. Neural networks – a diagnostic tool in acute myocardial infarction with concomitant left bundle branch block. *Clin Physiol*. 2002;**22**:295–99.
21. Rindskopf D, Rindskopf W. The value of latent class analysis in medical diagnosis. *Stat Med*. 1986;**5**:21–27.
22. Lucas PJF, van der Gaag LC, Abu-Hanna A. Bayesian networks in biomedicine and health-care. *Artif Intell Med*. 2004;**30**:201–14.
23. Lipsky AM, Lewis RJ. Placing the Bayesian network approach to patient diagnosis in perspective. *Ann Emerg Med*. 2005;**45**:291–94.
24. Van den Bruel A, Aertgeerts B, Buntinx F. Results of diagnostic accuracy studies are not always validated. *J Clin Epidemiol*. 2006;**59**:559–66.
25. Buntinx F, Truyen J, Embrechts P, et al. Chest pain: an evaluation of the initial diagnosis made by 25 Flemish general practitioners. *Fam Pract*. 1991;**8**:121–24.
26. Hay AD, Gorst C, Montgomery A, et al. Validation of a clinical rule to predict complications of acute cough in preschool children. *Br J Gen Pract*. 2007;**57**:530–37.
27. Starmans R, Muris JW, Fijten GH, et al. The diagnostic value of scoring models for organic and nonorganic gastrointestinal disease, including the irritable-bowel syndrome. *Med Decis Making*. 1994;**14**:208–16.
28. Stoffers HE, Kester AD, Kaiser V, et al. Diagnostic value of signs and symptoms associated with peripheral arterial occlusive disease seen in general practice: a multivariable approach. *Med Decis Making*. 1997;**17**:61–70.
29. Knottnerus JA. Prediction rules: statistical reproducibility and clinical similarity. *Med Decis Making*. 1992;**12**:286–87.
30. Knottnerus JA. Diagnostic prediction rules: principles, requirements, and pitfalls. *Prim Care*. 1995;**22**:341–63.
31. Buntinx F, Truyen J, Embrechts P, et al. Evaluating patients with chest pain using CART. *Fam Pract*. 1992;**9**:149–53.
32. Khan KS, Bachmann LM, ter Riet G. Systematic reviews with individual patient data meta-analysis to evaluate diagnostic tests. *Eur J Obstetr Gynecol Reprod Biol*. 2003;**108**:121–25.

CHAPTER 9

Standards for reporting on diagnostic accuracy studies

Patrick M. M. Bossuyt and Nynke Smidt

Summary box

- In the evaluation of new and existing medical tests, establishing a test's diagnostic accuracy is an essential step.
- Accuracy studies with shortcomings in study design can produce biased results.
- Evidence accumulates that many published research articles fail to include key elements about study methods and findings.
- Standards for the Reporting of Diagnostic accuracy studies (STARD) were developed by an international group to improve the reporting of diagnostic accuracy studies.
- The STARD statement and the 25-item checklist have been published and adopted by major clinical and subspecialty journals.
- A similar initiative has been organized for prognostic tumor markers in oncology.

Introduction

In recent decades, the number of medical tests has been increasing at a rapid pace. New tests are developed at a fast rate and the technology of existing tests is continuously being improved.

As for all new medical technologies, new diagnostic tests should be thoroughly evaluated prior to their introduction into daily practice. A rigorous evaluation process of diagnostic tests before introduction into clinical practice could not only reduce the number of unwanted clinical consequences related to misleading estimates of test accuracy but also limit health care costs by preventing unnecessary testing.

The Evidence Base of Clinical Diagnosis: Theory and Methods of Diagnostic Research. 2nd edition. Edited by J. André Knottnerus and Frank Buntinx. © 2009 Blackwell Publishing, ISBN: 978-1-4051-5787-2.

Unfortunately, the evaluation of medical tests is less advanced than that of treatments.[1-3] Exaggerated and biased results from poorly designed and reported diagnostic studies could trigger their premature dissemination and lead physicians into making incorrect treatment decisions.

In the evaluation of new and existing medical tests, establishing a test's diagnostic accuracy is an essential step. Diagnostic accuracy studies evaluate a test's ability to identify patients with disease, or, more generally, the target condition, among those suspected for it. In studies of diagnostic accuracy, results from one or more tests are compared with the results obtained with the reference standard on the same subjects who are suspected of having a particular target condition.

The accurate and transparent reporting of research has become a matter of increasing concern as evidence accumulates that many published research articles fail to include key information about the study methods and findings. This concern has in turn led to efforts to try to identify which aspects of a study should be reported.

The STARD statement (Standards for the Reporting of Diagnostic accuracy studies) has been developed to improve the reporting of diagnostic accuracy studies. In this chapter we first summarize a series of sources of bias and variability in diagnostic accuracy studies, and the evidence about their effects. In the next section we describe the development of the STARD statement. The final section summarizes the uptake and effects of the STARD statement.

Sources of bias and variability in diagnostic accuracy studies

In studies of diagnostic accuracy, the results of one or more tests are compared with the results of the reference standard in the same patients. In such studies, the term test can refer to any method for obtaining additional information on a patient's health status. It includes information from history and physical examination, laboratory tests, imaging tests, function tests and histopathology.

Test accuracy applies to tests selected for other purposes than diagnosis. The target condition in testing can be a particular disease, a disease stage but also any other identifiable condition that may prompt clinical actions, such as further testing, or the initiation, modification or termination of treatment. While the term *disease* describes a state that is often tightly defined based on microbiological, pathological, or histological findings, a *target condition* is a more general term, that groups subjects similar in clinical history, examination and test results, and prognosis, and known to be better off with a particular course of medical management.

The reference standard is the best available method for establishing the presence or absence of the target condition in the tested patients. The reference standard can be a single method, or a combination of methods, to establish the presence of the target condition. It can include laboratory tests, imaging tests, pathology, but also dedicated clinical follow-up of subjects. In most cases, the test under evaluation, also called the index test, is a less invasive, quicker test than the reference standard.

The term diagnostic accuracy refers to expressions of the agreement between the index test and the reference standard, obtained from a comparison or cross-classification of the index test results and the results of the reference standard. Diagnostic accuracy can be expressed in many ways, including sensitivity and specificity, likelihood ratios, diagnostic odds ratio, and the area under a receiver operator characteristic (ROC) curve.

There are several potential threats to the internal and external validity of a study of diagnostic accuracy. Poor internal validity will produce bias: the estimates do not correspond to what one would have obtained using better methods. In other words, there is systematic error. Poor external validity limits the generalizability of the findings. The results of a study with poor generalizability, even if unbiased, do not correspond to the data needs for decision making.

As measures of diagnostic accuracy express the behavior of a test under particular circumstances, test behavior will differ depending on the group of patients that undergoes testing. Test evaluations should therefore include an appropriate spectrum of patients in whom the target condition is suspected in clinical practice. The ideal study takes a consecutive series of patients, inviting all patients suspected of the target condition within a specific period and specifying the amount of prior testing these patients have received. These patients then undergo the index test and all are subjected to the reference test. This resembles the cohort design, as it is known in epidemiology.

The word consecutive is heavily misused in the literature and has almost lost its meaning. It refers to total absence of any form of selection, beyond the a priori definition of the criteria for inclusion and exclusion, and explicit efforts to identify patients qualifying for inclusion. Not inviting consecutive patients can lead to spectrum or selection bias.[4]

Alternative designs are possible. Some studies first select patients known to have the target condition, and then contrast the results of these patients with those from a control group. These designs are similar to case-control designs in epidemiology, yet they differ from them in a number of ways. For that reason, the label 'two-gate designs' has been proposed. These "two-gate" accuracy studies use two sets of inclusion criteria, one for the diseased, and a second set for those without the target condition.[5] The selection of the control group in "two-gate" designs is critical. If the control group consists of healthy participants, diagnostic accuracy will be overestimated.[6,7] Patients suspected for the target condition who have negative test results on the reference standard usually have other signs, complaints, and conditions that prompted the ordering of the tests. These conditions are bound to give some false positive results. Healthy volunteers are usually without such complaints and are less likely to obtain false positive results.

In an accuracy study, the reference standard may not always be applied to all patients tested with the index test. This may happen if the reference standard is an invasive procedure, but it could also be due to negligence, or other factors. If not all patients are verified with the reference standard, verification bias may occur. We make a distinction between two forms of verification bias, partial verification bias and differential verification bias.

Partial verification applies when not all patients are tested. It will lead to bias if the selection is not purely random but is associated with the results of the index test and the strength of prior suspicion. Partial verification can result in workup bias, when patients with positive or negative diagnostic test results are preferentially referred to receive verification of diagnosis by the reference standard procedure.

Even if all patients are verified, a different form of verification bias can happen if more than one reference standard is used, and the two reference standards correspond to different manifestations of disease. This can lead to differential verification bias.

The timing of the reference standard can be critical. Larger intervals between test and verification by the reference standard may lead to disease progression bias. In that case, the disease is at a more advanced stage when the reference standard is performed and clear cases appear to have been missed by the index test. As the time interval grows larger, the actual condition of the patient may change, leading to more expressed forms of alternative conditions.

Review bias occurs when interpretation of the index test or reference standard is influenced by knowledge of the results of the other test. Diagnostic review bias occurs when the results of the index test are known while interpreting the reference standard. Analogously, test review bias can be present when results of the reference standard are known while interpreting the results of the index test.

In some cases, it may be inevitable or preferable to use a panel of experts to assign a final diagnosis, and to disclose the index test results to that panel, in addition to data on follow-up and other procedures. When the result of the index test is used in establishing the final diagnosis, incorporation bias may occur. Using the index test results as part of the reference standard is likely to increase the amount of agreement between index test results and the reference standard, leading to an overestimation of the various measures of diagnostic accuracy.[8]

These and other sources of bias and variability in diagnostic accuracy studies have been systematically reviewed by Whiting and collaegues, based on the available literature.[8] Lijmer and colleagues gained further empirical support for the baising effect of design deficiencies by collecting and re-analyzing a series of 18 meta-analyses of a wide range of medical tests.[6] Within each meta-analysis, they retrieved the original studies in the respective systematic review and scored their design features. Then, using multivariable meta-regression modeling, they evaluated whether studies with particular design deficiencies, such as partial verification, produced more optimistic estimates of the accuracy of studies than studies of the same test, for the same purpose, without such design deficiencies.

The results of the 218 test evaluations confirmed the prior suspicions. Tests with design deficiencies, in particular those using healthy controls and differential verification, found higher accuracy estimates.

The results of Lijmer *et al.* were replicated by the same research group. Rutjes and colleagues evaluated a larger set of different meta-analyses (n = 31), covering 487 primary accurracy studies, and evaluated more design feature (n = 15) with even more refined statistical methods.[7] Their results confirmed that shortcomings in study design can affect estimates of diagnostic accuracy, but Rutjes also observed that the magnitude of the effect may vary from one situation to another.

Developing the STARD statement

In this era of evidence-based medicine, clinicians and other decision makers turn to the scientific literature for high-quality evidence about the usefulness, precision, and accuracy of diagnostic tests. Such evidence is needed more than ever as the list of diagnostic tests grows exponentially, while even more biomarkers, proteomics and applications of gene expression profiling will be added in the years to come.

The reviews of Lijmer and Rutjes did not only show the biasing effects of design deficiencies, they also showed that essential information on key elements of design, conduct and analysis of diagnostic studies was often not reported. Rutjes and collaegues found that about half the studies failed to report the dates of the includion period, almost 20% did not report the sex and age of the study participants. Design features were also often not mentioned, or described in a confusing way.

These results confirmed previous findings. A survey of studies of diagnostic accuracy published in four major medical journals between 1978 and 1993 revealed that the methodological quality was mediocre at best.[9] Smidt and colleagues found that reporting of diagnostic accuracy in 124 papers in major clinical journals was less than optimal, even in journals with high impact factors.[10] The absence of critical information about the design and conduct of diagnostic studies has also been confirmed and lamented by many other authors of systematic reviews.

This is a reason for great concern, as complete and accurate reporting would allow the reader to detect the potential for biases in a study and to judge the generalisability and applicability of the results.

At the 1999 Cochrane Colloquium meeting in Rome, the Diagnostic and Screening Test Methods Working Group within the Cochrane Collaboration discussed the low methodological quality and substandard reporting of diagnostic test evaluations. The working group felt that the first step to correct these problems was to improve the quality of reporting of diagnostic studies. The objective of the then formed Standards for Reporting of Diagnostic Accuracy (STARD) initiative became the improvement of the quality of reporting of diagnostic accuracy studies. Following the successful CONSORT initiative, the STARD initiative aimed at the development of a checklist of items that should be included in the report of a study of diagnostic accuracy.

A STARD steering committee started with an extensive literature search and extracted a list of 75 potential items. This search included the Medline, EMBASE, BIOSIS, and the methodological database from the Cochrane Collaboration up to July 2000. In addition, the steering committee members examined reference lists of retrieved articles, searched personal files, and contacted other experts in the field of diagnostic research. They reviewed all relevant publications and extracted an extended list of potential checklist items.

Two general considerations help to shape the content and format of the checklist. First, the STARD group believes that one general checklist for studies of diagnostic accuracy, rather than different checklists for each field, was likely to be more widely disseminated and accepted by authors, peer reviewers, and journal editors. Although the evaluation of an imaging test differs from that of test in the laboratory, these differences may be more in degree than of kind. The second consideration was the development of a checklist specifically aimed at studies of diagnostic test accuracy. The STARD group did not include general issues in the reporting of research findings, like the recommendations contained in the Uniform Requirements for Manuscripts submitted to Biomedical Journals (see www.icmje.org).

Subsequently, the STARD steering committee convened a two-day consensus meeting on September 16 and 17, 2000, in Amsterdam for invited experts from the following interest groups: researchers, editors, methodologists, and professional organizations. During the consensus meeting, participants eliminated and consolidated items to form a final 25-item checklist (Table 9.1).

In addition, the STARD group put considerable effort in the development of a flow diagram prototype for test accuracy studies. The flow diagram provides information about the method of patient recruitment, the order of test execution, the number of patients undergoing the test under evaluation and the reference test, the number of patients with positive and negative test results and number of patients with indeterminate test results. Such a flow diagram has the potential to communicate vital information about the design of a study and the flow of participants in a transparent manner (Figure 9.1).

Potential users field-tested the first version of the checklist and flow diagram. The checklist was placed on the CONSORT website with a call for comments. The STARD group received valuable remarks during the various stages of evaluation and assembled the final, single-page checklist. Table 9.1 shows the STARD checklist and Figure 9.1 shows a prototypical flow diagram of a diagnostic accuracy study.

Uptake of STARD

The STARD statement was published in the first issues in 2003 of seven leading general and specialty journals, including *Annals of Internal Medicine*, *Radiology*, *BMJ*, and *Clinical Chemistry*, and, subsequently, in several other journals.[11–24].

Table 9.1 STARD checklist for reporting of studies of diagnostic accuracy

Section and topic	Item no.		On page no.
TITLE/ABSTRACT/ KEYWORDS	1	Identify the article as a study of diagnostic accuracy (recommend MeSH heading "sensitivity and specificity").	
INTRODUCTION	2	State the research questions or study aims, such as estimating diagnostic accuracy or comparing accuracy between tests or across participant groups.	
METHODS			
Participants	3	The study population: The inclusion and exclusion criteria, setting, and locations where data were collected.	
	4	Participant recruitment: Was recruitment based on presenting symptoms, results from previous tests, or the fact that the participants had received the index tests or the reference standard?	
	5	Participant sampling: Was the study population a consecutive series of participants defined by the selection criteria in item 3 and 4? If not, specify how participants were further selected.	
	6	Data collection: Was data collection planned before the index test and reference standard were performed (prospective study) or after (retrospective study)?	
Test methods	7	The reference standard and its rationale.	
	8	Technical specifications of material and methods involved including how and when measurements were taken, and/or cite references for index tests and reference standard.	
	9	Definition of and rationale for the units, cutoffs and/or categories of the results of the index tests and the reference standard.	
	10	The number, training, and expertise of the persons executing and reading the index tests and the reference standard.	
	11	Whether or not the readers of the index tests and reference standard were blind (masked) to the results of the other test and describe any other clinical information available to the readers.	

(continued)

Table 9.1 (*continued*)

Section and topic	Item no.		On page no.
Statistical methods	12	Methods for calculating or comparing measures of diagnostic accuracy, and the statistical methods used to quantify uncertainty (e.g., 95% confidence intervals).	
	13	Methods for calculating test reproducibility, if done.	
RESULTS			
Participants	14	When study was performed, including beginning and end dates of recruitment.	
	15	Clinical and demographic characteristics of the study population (at least information on age, gender, spectrum of presenting symptoms).	
	16	The number of participants satisfying the criteria for inclusion who did or did not undergo the index tests and/or the reference standard; describe why participants failed to undergo either test (a flow diagram is strongly recommended).	
Test results	17	Time-interval between the index tests and the reference standard, and any treatment administered in between.	
	18	Distribution of severity of disease (define criteria) in those with the target condition; other diagnoses in participants without the target condition.	
	19	A cross tabulation of the results of the index tests (including indeterminate and missing results) by the results of the reference standard; for continuous results, the distribution of the test results by the results of the reference standard.	
	20	Any adverse events from performing the index tests or the reference standard.	
Estimates	21	Estimates of diagnostic accuracy and measures of statistical uncertainty (e.g., 95% confidence intervals).	
	22	How indeterminate results, missing data and outliers of the index tests were handled.	
	23	Estimates of variability of diagnostic accuracy between subgroups of participants, readers or centers, if done.	
	24	Estimates of test reproducibility, if done.	
DISCUSSION	25	Discuss the clinical applicability of the study findings.	

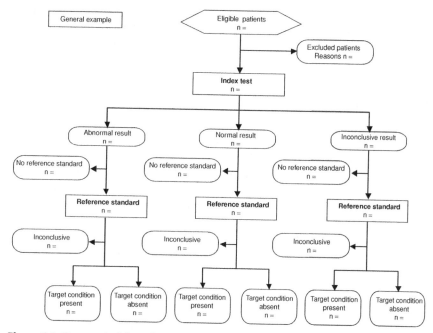

Figure 9.1 Prototypical flow diagram of a diagnostic accuracy study.

The STARD Statement was accompanied by a separate explanatory document, explaining the meaning and rationale of each item and briefly summarizing the available evidence.[25,26] The documents are also available on several websites, including that of *Clinical Chemistry*, CONSORT, and STARD (see www.stard-statement.org). Publication of the STARD documents was accompanied by several editorials, with statements of endorsement from editors and their boards.[27–42]

An early evaluation of 265 diagnostic accuracy studies published in 2000 (pre-STARD) and in 2004 (post-STARD) in high-impact journals revealed that the quality of reporting in articles on diagnostic accuracy has improved after the publication of the STARD statement, but there is still room for improvement.[43] Papers published in 2004 reported on average 14 of the 25 essential STARD items.

A possible reason for the slow uptake could be the way the STARD statement is used within the editorial process. Smidt and colleagues identified the top 50 journals that frequently publish studies on diagnostic accuracy, and examined the instructions for authors on each journal's website, extracting all text mentioning STARD or other text regarding the reporting of diagnostic accuracy studies. They found variable language in journals that had adopted the STARD statement. Most adopting journals refer to the STARD statement, without describing their expectations regarding the use of the STARD statement.

The STARD group plans new initiatives to improve the quality of reporting of accuracy studies, and intends to release updates of STARD when new evidence on sources of bias or variability becomes available. So far, no such updates have been deemed necessary.

Other Initiatives

The STARD initiative was followed by other initiatives aimed at strengthening the reporting of clinical and biomedical research.

Over many years, thousands of reports on tumor markers in oncology have yielded very few markers that have emerged as clinically useful. A major recommendation of the NCI-EORTC First International Meeting on Cancer Diagnostics (From Discovery to Clinical Practice: Diagnostic Innovation, Implementation, and Evaluation) held in Nyberg, Denmark, in July 2000, was the development of guidelines for the reporting of tumor marker studies. That meeting identified poor study design and analysis, assay variability, and inadequate reporting of studies as some of the major barriers to progress in the field. The Statistics Subcommittee was then charged with addressing statistical issues of poor design and analysis, and the reporting of tumor marker prognostic studies. Reporting guidelines were agreed to be the first priority.

The resulting REMARK recommendations were published simultaneously in September 2005 in five cancer journals: *British Journal of Cancer*, *European Journal of Cancer*, *Journal of Clinical Oncology*, *Journal of the National Cancer Institute*, and *Nature Clinical Practice Oncology*.[44-50]

Based on the evidence collected in the development of STARD, Whiting and colleague developed a quality appraisal instrument, to be used by authors of systematic reviews of test accuracy. The resulting QUADAS instrument contains 14 items, including patient spectrum, reference standard, disease progression bias, verification bias, review bias, clinical review bias, incorporation bias, test execution, study withdrawals, and indeterminate results.[51-53].

If medical journals, authors, editors, and reviewers more widely adopt the STARD checklist and the flow diagram, the quality of reporting of studies of diagnostic accuracy should improve to the advantage of the clinicians, researchers, reviewers, journals, and the public.

Acknowledgments

STARD, REMARK, and QUADAS and the other initiatives could not have reached publication without major efforts from many people, in particular those listed as authors on or acknowledged as contributors in the publications.

References

1. Knottnerus JA, van Weel C, Muris JW. Evaluation of diagnostic procedures. *BMJ*. 2002;**324**:477-80.

2. Straus SE. Bridging the gaps in evidence based diagnosis. *BMJ.* 2006;**333**:405–6.
3. Buntinx F, Knottnerus JA. Are we at the start of a new era in diagnostic research? *J Clin Epidemiol.* 2006;**59**:325–26.
4. Lachs MS, Nachamkin I, Edelstein PH, et al. Spectrum bias in the evaluation of diagnostic tests: lessons from the rapid dipstick test for urinary tract infection. *Ann Intern Med.* 1992;**117**:135–40.
5. Rutjes AW, Reitsma JB, Vandenbroucke JP, et al. Case-control and two-gate designs in diagnostic accuracy studies. *Clin Chem.* 2005;**51**:1335–41.
6. Lijmer JG, Mol BW, Heisterkamp S, et al. Empirical evidence of design-related bias in studies of diagnostic tests. *JAMA.* 1999;**282**:1061–66.
7. Rutjes AW, Reitsma JB, Di Nisio M, et al. Evidence of bias and variation in diagnostic accuracy studies. *CMAJ.* 2006;**174**:469–76.
8. Whiting P, Rutjes AWS, Reitsma JB, et al. Sources of variation and bias in studies of diagnostic accuracy. *Ann Intern Med.* 2004;**140**:189–202.
9. Reid MC, Lachs MS, Feinstein AR. Use of methodological standards in diagnostic test research. Getting better but still not good. *JAMA.* 1995;**274**:645–51.
10. Smidt N, Rutjes AWS, Van der Windt AWM, et al. Quality of reporting of diagnostic accuracy studies. *Radiology.* 2005;**235**:347–53.
11. Bossuyt PM, Reitsma JB. Standards for reporting of diagnostic accuracy group. The STARD initiative. *Lancet.* 2003; **361**:71.
12. Bossuyt PM, Reitsma JB, Bruns DE, et al. Towards complete and accurate reporting of studies of diagnostic accuracy; the STARD initiative. *Clin Chem.* 2003;**49**:1–6.
13. Bossuyt PM, Reitsma JB, Bruns DE, et al. Towards complete and accurate reporting of studies of diagnostic accuracy: the STARD initiative. *Radiology.* 2003;**226**: 24–28.
14. Bossuyt PM, Reitsma JB, Bruns DE, et al. Standards for Reporting of Diagnostic Accuracy: toward complete and accurate reporting of studies of diagnostic accuracy: the STARD initiative. *Ann Intern Med.* 2003;**138**:40–44.
15. Bossuyt PM, Reitsma JB, Bruns DE, et al. Standards for Reporting of Diagnostic Accuracy: toward complete and accurate reporting of studies of diagnostic accuracy: the STARD initiative. *BMJ.* 2003;**326**:41–44.
16. Bossuyt PM, Reitsma JB, Bruns DE, et al. Standards for Reporting of Diagnostic Accuracy: toward complete and accurate reporting of studies of diagnostic accuracy: the STARD initiative. *Am J Clin Pathol.* 2003;**119**:18–22.
17. Bossuyt PM, Reitsma JB, Bruns DE, et al. Standards for Reporting of Diagnostic Accuracy: Toward complete and accurate reporting of studies of diagnostic accuracy: the STARD initiative. *Clin Biochem.* 2003;**36**:2–7.
18. Bossuyt PM, Reitsma JB, Bruns DE, et al. Standards for Reporting of Diagnostic Accuracy: toward complete and accurate reporting of studies of diagnostic accuracy: the STARD initiative. *Clin Chem Lab Med.* 2003;**41**:68–73.
19. Bossuyt PM, Reitsma JB, Bruns DE, et al. Standards for Reporting of Diagnostic Accuracy: toward complete and accurate reporting of studies of diagnostic accuracy: the STARD initiative. *Acad Radiol.* 2003;**10**:664–69.
20. Bossuyt PM, Reitsma JB, Bruns, et al. Toward complete and accurate reporting of studies of diagnostic accuracy: the STARD initiative. *AJR Am J Roentgenol.* 2003;**181**:51–55.
21. Bossuyt PM, Reitsma JB, Bruns DE, et al. Standards for Reporting of Diagnostic Accuracy. Toward complete and accurate reporting of studies of diagnostic accuracy: the STARD initiative. *Ann Clin Biochem.* 2003;**40**:357–63.

22. Bossuyt PM, Reitsma JB, Bruns DE Gatsonis PP, Glasziou PP, Irwig LM, Lijmer JG, Moher D, Rennie D, De Vet HC; Standards for Reporting of Diagnostic Accuracy. Toward complete and accurate reporting of studies of diagnostic accuracy: the STARD initiative. *Clin Radiol.* 2003;**58**:575–80.

23. Bossuyt PM, Reitsma JB, Bruns DE, et al. Standards for Reporting of Diagnostic Accuracy: toward complete and accurate reporting of studies of diagnostic accuracy: the STARD initiative. *Fam Pract.* 2004;**21**:4–10.

24. Khan KS, Bakour SH, Bossuyt PM. Evidence-based ostetric and gynaecologic diagnosis: The STARD checklist for authors, peer-reviewing, and readers of test accuracy studies. *BJOG* 2004; **111**:638–640.

25. Bossuyt PM, Reitsma JB, Bruns. Standards for Reporting of Diagnostic Accuracy: the STARD statement for reporting of diagnostic accuracy: explanation and elaboration. *Clin Chem* 2003;**49**:7–18.

26. Bossuyt PM, Reitsma JB, Bruns DE. Standards for Reporting of Diagnostic Accuracy: the STARD statement for reporting of diagnostic accuracy: explanation and elaboration. *Ann Intern Med.* 2003;**138**:W1–12.

27. Rennie D. Improving reports of studies of diagnostic tests: the STARD initiative. *JAMA.* 2003;**289**:89–90.

28. Bruns DE. The STARD initiative and the reporting of studies of diagnostic accuracy. *Clin Chem.* 2003;**49**:19–20.

29. McQueen M. Evidence-based laboratory medicine: addressing bias, generalisability and applicability in studies on diagnostic accuracy: the STARD initiative. *Clin Biochem.* 2003;**36**:1–2.

30. McQueen M. Evidence-based laboratory medicine: addressing bias, generalisability and applicability in studies on diagnostic accuracy: the STARD initiative. *Clin Chem Lab Med.* 2003;**41**:1.

31. Holloway RG. Improving the flow of diagnostic information. The importance of STARD for authors and readers. *Neurology.* 2003;**61**:600–601.

32. Gatsonis C. Do we need a checklist for reporting the results of diagnostic test evaluations? The STARD proposal. *Acad Radiol.* 2003;**10**:599–600.

33. Trenti T. Evidence-based laboratory medicine as a tool for continuous professional improvement. *Clin Chim Acta.* 2003;**333**:155–67.

34. Ell PJ. STARD and CONSORT: time for reflection. *Eur J Nucl Med Mol Imaging.* 2003;**30**:803–4.

35. Price CP. Improving the quality of peer reviewed literature on diagnostic tests: the STARD initiative. *Clin Chim Acta.* 2003;**334**:1–3.

36. McQueen MJ. The STARD initiative: a possible link to diagnostic accuracy and reduction in medical error. *Ann Clin Biochem.* 2003;**40**:307–8.

37. Hansell DM, Wells AU. Towards complete and accurate reporting of studies of diagnostic accuracy: the STARD initiative. *Clin Radiol.* 2003;**58**:573–74.

38. Meyer GJ. Guidelines for reporting information in studies of diagnostic test accuracy: The STARD initiative. *J Pers Assess.* 2003;**81**:191–3.

39. Jones R. Reporting studies of diagnostic accuracy: the STARD initiative. *Fam Pract.* 2004;**21**:3.

40. Khan KS, Bakour SH, Bossuyt PM. Evidence-based obstetric and gynaecologic diagnosis: the STARD checklist for authors, peer-reviewers and readers of test accuracy studies. *BJOG.* 2004;**111**:638–40.

41. Selman TJ, Khan KS, Mann Ch. An evidence-based approach to test accuracy studies in gynecologic oncology: the "STARD" checklist. *Gyn Oncol.* 2005;**96**:575–78.

42. Johnston KC, Holloway RG. There is nothing staid about STARD: progress in the reporting of diagnostic accuracy studies. *Neurology.* 2006;**67**:740–41.
43. Smidt N, Rutjes AWS, Van der Windt DAWM, et al. The quality of diagnostic accuracy studies since the STARD statement: has it improved? *Neurology.* 2006;**67**:792–97.
44. McShane LM, Altman DG, Sauerbrei W, et al. Reporting recommendations for tumor MARKer prognostic studies (REMARK). *Breast Cancer Res Treat.* 2006;**100**:229–35.
45. McShane LM, Altman DG, Sauerbrei W, et al. REporting recommendations for tumor MARKer prognostic studies (REMARK). *Exp Oncol.* 2006;**28**:99–105.
46. McShane LM, Altman DG, Sauerbrei W, et al. REporting recommendations for tumor MARKer prognostic studies (REMARK). *Nat Clin Pract Urol.* 2005;**2**:416–22.
47. McShane LM, Altman DG, Sauerbrei W, et al. REporting recommendations for tumor MARKer prognostic studies (REMARK). *Nat Clin Pract Oncol.* 2005;**2**:416–22.
48. McShane LM, Altman DG, Sauerbrei W, et al. REporting recommendations for tumour MARKer prognostic studies (REMARK). *Br J Cancer.* 2005;**93**:387–91.
49. McShane LM, Altman DG, Sauerbrei W, et al. REporting recommendations for tumor marker prognostic studies (REMARK). *J Natl Cancer Inst.* 2005;**97**:1180–84.
50. McShane LM, Altman DG, Sauerbrei W, et al. REporting recommendations for tumour MARKer prognostic studies (REMARK). *Eur J Cancer.* 2005;**41**:1690–96.
51. Whiting P, Rutjes AW, Reitsma JB, et al. The development of QUADAS: a tool for the quality assessment of studies of diagnostic accuracy included in systematic reviews. *BMC Med Res Methodol.* 2003;**3**:25.
52. Whiting PF, Weswood ME, Rutjes AW, et al. Evaluation of QUADAS, a tool for the quality assessment of diagnostic accuracy studies. *BMC Med Res Methodol.* 2006;**6**:9.
53. Hollingworth W, Medina LS, Lenkinski RE, et al. Interrater reliability in assessing quality of diagnostic accuracy studies using the QUADAS tool: a preliminary assessment. *Acad Radiol.* 2006;**13**:803–10.

CHAPTER 10

Guidelines for conducting systematic reviews of studies evaluating the accuracy of diagnostic tests

Frank Buntinx, Bert Aertgeerts, and Petra Macaskill

Summary box

- A systematic review should include all available evidence from computerized databases and other sources.
- The search strategy must be based on an explicit description of the subjects receiving the reference test, the diagnostic test of interest, its accuracy estimates, and the study design. Titles and abstracts of the identified citations should be screened using prespecified inclusion criteria.
- Two reviewers should independently assess the methodological quality of each selected paper and extract the required information.
- Sources of heterogeneity should be examined. If this is based on a priori existing hypotheses, subgroup analyses can be performed.
- Whether meta-analysis with statistical pooling can be conducted depends on the number and methodological quality of the primary studies. The use of random effect models for obtaining summary estimates of diagnostic test performance is recommended, even if there is no apparent heterogeneity.
- Statistical methods for the meta-analysis of diagnostic test performance include recently developed hierarchical models such as the hierarchical SROC model and the bivariate model.

The Evidence Base of Clinical Diagnosis: Theory and Methods of Diagnostic Research. 2nd edition.
Edited by J. André Knottnerus and Frank Buntinx. © 2009 Blackwell Publishing.
ISBN: 978-1-4051-5787-2.

Introduction

Systematic reviews and meta-analyses of studies evaluating the accuracy of diagnostic and screening tests (in this chapter, we will refer to them generically as diagnostic systematic reviews) are appearing more often in the medical literature.[1,2] The decision of the Cochrane Collaboration to include diagnostic systematic reviews has boosted methods development in this field, which has its own difficulties in addition to the more general problems associated with reviews of trials. Diagnostic accuracy studies generally report two outcome measures (e.g., sensitivity and specificity) instead of one (e.g., relative risk) as is usual in trials. Additionally, these two measures are negatively correlated. The common occurrence of between study heterogeneity in diagnostic reviews and the likely presence of a threshold effect add to the list of issues to address. This largely complicates the quantitative approach to diagnostic reviews and dictates the need for hierarchical (also referred to as multilevel) methods.

We present a set of practical guidelines based on evidence and recent work within the Cochrane Collaboration to facilitate the understanding of and appropriate adherence to methodological principles when conducting diagnostic systematic reviews. We reviewed reports of systematic searches of the literature for diagnostic research,[3-8] methodological criteria to evaluate diagnostic research,[1,9-12] and explore heterogeneity,[13-18] and added recent methods for statistical pooling of data on diagnostic accuracy.[19-23]

Guidelines for conducting diagnostic systematic reviews are presented in a stepwise fashion and are followed by comments providing further information.

How to search the literature for studies evaluating the accuracy of diagnostic tests

Introduction

Conducting a comprehensive, objective, and reproducible search looking for all the available evidence is one of the cornerstones of a systematic review. Identifying all relevant studies and documenting the search for studies with sufficient detail so that it can be reproduced is largely what distinguishes a systematic review from a traditional narrative review. The reviewer has to design a search strategy based on a clear and explicit description of terms for the target condition and the index test. These elements are usually specified in the criteria for inclusion of primary studies in the review. The aim of the search strategy is to find all relevant primary studies from the literature. The literature encompasses several types of published material, including articles, dissertations, editorials, conference proceedings, and reports. Sources of and methods by which these publications can be found vary from the efficient electronic databases to time-consuming procedures of hand searching and contacting experts. A search strategy will focus on sensitivity rather than on precision. Sensitivities of more than 90% are feasible, whereas precisions of less than 10% have to be accepted.[24]

Developing a search strategy is an elaborative process in which terms that are used could be changed and other terms could be added. Additionally, searches with these terms have to be performed in different databases, and these databases have different search boxes. Sometimes MeSH terms can be used (MEDLINE, EMBASE), but sometimes they cannot (CENTRAL). Because of the specificity of different databases, close collaboration with an information specialist is an advantage to gather all the relevant information.

Search strategy

The *search terms* should at least include the index test and the clinical condition of interest. If the sensitivity of the search is too large, one can restrict the search by using additional terms (e.g., terms for the reference test, year of publication), using title words, excluding case reports, or using methodology filters. Search strategies have been developed through PubMed for MEDLINE.[6,24–25] Nevertheless, these "quick and dirty" strategies appear to be useful in clinical situations to obtain the most relevant information but are not sensitive enough to obtain all relevant information needed for a systematic review. The search terms could be used solely or in combination using either OR, AND, or NOT Booleans. Once a search strategy has been established, the formulation of the search can be stored and repeated later. Not only primary diagnostic studies have to be searched but also previous narrative reviews or systematic reviews and meta-analyses on the topic.

Afterward researchers should check the *reference list* of all relevant articles obtained. The reference list should be checked even from included and excluded papers, editorials, conference proceedings, and reviews (narrative or systematic reviews). This is what we call backward tracking of citations. The next step is *forward tracking* via citation indices and related articles. Examples are the ISI Citation Indices list paper and Google Scholar. PubMed now also offers a "related articles" option based on comparison of text words. *Unpublished or ongoing studies* also need to be detected. As a producer of a systematic review, you should look for authors of important reviews about that topic or contact experts in the field. In contrast to the register of ongoing trials, there is not yet such a database of ongoing diagnostic studies. In some cases, conference proceedings and grey literature must also be checked to avoid publication bias.

Databases

A search for relevant studies generally begins with health-related electronic bibliographic databases. Searches of electronic databases are generally the easiest and least time-consuming way to identify an initial set of relevant papers. When working with databases, it is crucial that the relevant databases are identified and that adequate combinations of search terms are used. Of the large number of electronic databases, authors should choose at least MEDLINE and EMBASE, combined with Medion and DARE. Authors should also search within other relevant databases specific for the subject of the review.

Hundreds of electronic bibliographic databases exist. A comprehensive on-line guide *Gale Directory of Online Portable and Internet Databases* is accessible through Dialog file 230 (www.dialog.com). Some databases, such as MED-LINE and EMBASE, cover all areas of health care and index journals published from around the world, mostly in English. Pascal covers several French journals. Other databases, such as the Australasian Medical Index, the Chinese Biomedical Literature Database, the Latin American Caribbean Health Sciences Literature (LILACS), and the Japan Information Centre of Science and Technology File on Science, Technology and Medicine (JICST-E) index journals, are published in specific regions of the world. Others, such as the Cumulative Index of Nursing and Allied Health (CINAHL), focus on specific areas of health, or on special document types (MEDICONF focus on medical conferences).

A few databases are specific for review articles focused on diagnostic accuracy studies: The MEDION database of the university of Maastricht (www.mediondatabase.nl) contains more than 1,000 references of published diagnostic reviews and methodological papers; the Database of Abstracts of Reviews of Effects (DARE), a database produced by the NHS Centre for Reviews and Dissemination in York, United Kingdom, contains a considerable number of abstracts of systematic reviews, including diagnostic reviews (www.nhscrd.york.ac.) and the database of the International Federation of Clinical Chemistry (IFCC) that consists of diagnostic reviews in clinical chemistry (www.ifcc.org).

An overview of the most important databases is indexed in Box 10.1.

Documenting the search strategy

The search strategy for each electronic database should be described in sufficient detail so that the process can be duplicated. The title of the databases searched (e.g., MEDLINE, EMBASE), name of the provider (OVID, Silverplatter), date the search was run, years covered by the search, the complete search strategy used in that particular database, and a one or two sentence summary of the search strategy, indicating which lines of the search strategy were used to identify the records related to the health condition and test should be provided. A flowchart (see Appendix 1) should be provided to give an overview of the obtained articles from the different databases or search methods (hand searching, citation tracking, etc.).

Retrieving the articles and inclusion criteria

Once the search is completed, two independent reviewers should screen the titles and abstracts of the identified citations using specific prespecified inclusion criteria. These can be pilot tested on a sample of articles. If disagreements cannot be resolved by consensus, or if insufficient information is available, a third reviewer and/or the full papers should be consulted.

- *Reference test:* The accuracy of a diagnostic or screening test should be evaluated by comparing its results with a "gold standard," criterion standard, or reference test accepted as the best available by content experts. The reference test may be a single test, a combination of different tests, or the clinical follow-up of patients.[26] The publication should describe the reference test, as it is an essential prerequisite for the evaluation of a diagnostic test.
- *Population:* Detailed information about the participants in diagnostic research is often lacking. Participants should be defined explicitly in terms of age, gender, complaints, signs, and symptoms, and their duration. At least a definition of participants with and without the disease, as determined by the reference test, should be available.
- *Outcome data:* Information should be available to allow the construction of the diagnostic 2×2 table with its four cells: true positives, false negatives, false positives, and true negatives.
- *Language:* If a review is limited to publications in certain languages, this should be reported.

Comments

As the patient mix (spectrum of disease severity) is different at different levels of care, a diagnostic review may focus on a specific setting (primary care, etc.) or include all levels. This information may be important for subgroup analyses in case of heterogeneity. All evidence available should be reviewed, regardless of the language of publication. However, it is not easy to identify non-English publications, as they are often not indexed in computerized databases. In the field of intervention research, there is some evidence of bias when excluding non-English publications.[27–28] Although large samples are no guarantee against selection bias, small samples seldom result from a consecutive series of patients or a random sample. Small studies are very vulnerable to selection bias. Minima of 20 and 50 participants have been used but may even be too low, depending on the type of study, the estimates of diagnostic accuracy, the resulting precision,[29] and the prevalence of the disease.

Methodological quality

The methodological quality of each selected paper should be assessed independently by at least two reviewers having sufficient knowledge of both methodological and content-specific issues. Chance-adjusted agreement should be reported, and disagreements solved by consensus or arbitration. To improve agreement, reviewers should pilot their quality assessment tools in a subset of included studies or studies evaluating a different diagnostic test. External validity criteria provide insight into the generalizability of the study and judge whether the test under evaluation was performed according to accepted standards. Internal and external validity criteria, describing participants, diagnostic test, and target disease of interest, and study methods may be used in

Box 10.1 Most important databases for diagnostic accuracy studies: according to the *Cochrane Manual*, chapter 5.

Name	**DARE**
	Database of Abstracts of Reviews of Effects
Producer	NHS Centre of Reviews and Dissemination, York, UK
	http://nhscrd.york.ac.uk/welcome.htm
Years of coverage	1994–present (incl. some records having an earlier publication date)
Journals covered	
Document types	Journal articles, reports, conference papers
Producer's information on scope	Reviews of potentially high methodological quality on effects of therapeutic interventions and diagnostic tests.
Update frequency	Quarterly
Growth rate	350 annually
Controlled terms	MeSH
Special fields	Systematic reviews
Special features	Free access (through NHS CRD, DIMDI)
	Quality assessment and summary is added to most references.
Compared to MEDLINE	Only systematic reviews
Available	Most complete version: directly from NHS CRD
	http://nhscrd.york.ac.uk/welcome.htm
	Cochrane Library, Datastar, DIMDI, OVID Online
Name	**CINAHL**
	Cumulative Index of Nursing and Allied Health Literature
Producer	Cinahl Information Systems, Glendale USA
	www.cinahl.com
Years covered	1982–present
Journals covered	>1,200 (nursing, allied health)
Document types	Journal articles, books, dissertations, conference proceedings, standards of professional practice, educational software, audiovisual materials
Scope	"Authoritative coverage of the literature related to nursing and allied health. Virtually all English-language publications are indexed..."
Update frequency	Online weekly; Local monthly

(*continued*)

Box 10.1 (*continued*)

Controlled terms	>10,000 subject headings. Approximately 70% of these headings also appear in MEDLINE. CINAHL supplements these headings with more than 2.000 terms designed specifically for nursing and allied health.
Special fields	Instrumentation; example: Nursing Home Behavior Problem Scale (NHBPS Special Interest Category; examples: Critical Care, Gerontologic Care
Special features	Cited References (added to selected publications in 1994); contain the bibliographic details of publications cited by the author. Backward and forward citation tracking.
Compared to MEDLINE	Additional publications on nursing and allied health subjects More document types as sources More controlled terms (index terms) for nursing and allied health subjects Cited publications searchable as of 1994.
Available	Directly through database producer: CinahlDirect www.cinahl.com/cdirect/cdirect.htm Online: OCLC FirstSearch (1982–), Datastar (1982–), ProQuest (1982–, incl. linking to 250 e-journals full text), EBSCO Publishing (1982–), OVID Online (1982–) Cdrom/local: OVID, SilverPlatter.
Name	**EMBASE and EMBASE ALERT** **Excerpta Medica Database**
Producer	Elsevier Science bv, Amsterdam, the Netherlands www.elsevier.com
Years covered	1974–present EMBASE most recent 8 weeks EMBASE ALERT
Journals covered	+3,750–+4,000 (biomedical)
Document types	Journal articles, conference papers published in journals
Scope	"The most current database today on (bio)medical, pharmacological and drug-related subjects. Indexing terms added within 10 working days (on average) upon the receipt of the original journal."
Update frequency	Online weekly (embase.com more often?), tapes monthly
Growth rate	400–450,000 annually

Box 10.1

Controlled terms	Controlled vocabulary EMTREE (polyhierarchically structured thesaurus) 38–39,000 terms + 150–170,000 synonyms Classification codes EMCLASS CAS Registry Numbers No indexing terms in EMBASE ALERT
Special fields	Pharmacology, drug research, health economics, hospital management, public health, occupational health, environmental medicine and pollution control, toxicology and drug dependence, forensic sciences.
Special features	Qualification of controlled terms by "links" (subheadings): 14 disease links to modify (qualify) EMTREE disease terms, 17 drug links, plus 47 special links on routes of drug administration since 2000, to qualify EMTREE drug terms. Embase.com integrates EMBASE and MEDLINE databases
Compared to MEDLINE	Additional non-U.S.A. and non-U.K. publications. Less focus on English-language sources. Faster assignment of indexing terms. Better coverage of drug research and pharmacology, more indexing terms for drug related subjects. More preclinical research. Original titles searchable (not possible in PubMed)
Available	Directly from Elsevier (http:/embase.com). Datastar (1974–), Dialog (1993–), DIMDI (1974–), OVID Online (1980–) Tapes for local use: OVID Technologies (incl. SilverPlatter) (1980)
Name	**JICST-Eplus** **Japan Science**
Producer	Japan Science and Technology Corporation (JST) www.jst.go.jp/en
Years covered	1985–present
Journals covered	+6,000 (science, technology, medicine)
Document types	Journals, serials, conference proceedings, technical reports, governmental publications.
Scope	"JICST-EPLUS covers Japanese literature on chemistry and the chemical industry, engineering, pharmacology, the life sciences, and medical science. Additionally, it contains a 'previews' section of unindexed records that appear approximately four months earlier than the fully indexed records."

(continued)

Box 10.1 (*continued*)

Update frequency	Weekly
Growth rate	12,300 weekly
Controlled terms	Thesaurus (controlled terms) and Classification Codes
Special fields	Multidisciplinary
Special features	35% English
Compared to MEDLINE	Additional publications of Japanese origin
Available	Datastar (1985–), Dialog (1985–), STN International (1985–)
Name	**MedionDatabase**
Producer	Maastricht University and Leuven University, Departments of General Practice www.mediondatabase.nl
Years of coverage	? –present
Journals covered	– (depending of databases and other sources searched)
Document types	Systematic reviews, methodological studies
Producer's information on scope	Overview of published systematic reviews on diagnostic studies. Methodological studies on systematic reviews of diagnostic studies, systematic reviews of diagnostic studies, systematic reviews of genetic diagnostic tests. No real quality requirements have been used.
Update frequency	"as much as possible," generally around 5 times a year
Growth rate	?
Controlled terms	List of keywords; ICPC codes
Special fields	Diagnostic tests, diagnosis.
Special features	
Compared to MEDLINE	Preselection of interesting category of systematic reviews
Available	Directly through database producer: www.mediondatabase.nl
Name	**MEDLINE and OLDMEDLINE**
Producer	U.S. National Library of Medicine (NLM), Bethesda, U.S.A. www.nlm.nih.gov
Years covered	1950–1965 OLDMEDLINE 1966-present MEDLINE
Journals covered	+4,600 (basic biomedical and clinical sciences)
Document types	Journal articles, conference papers published in journals

Box 10.1

Scope	NLM's premier bibliographic database containing references to journal articles covering basic biomedical research and the clinical sciences.
Update frequency	Daily (PubMed, OCLC), weekly (other online vendors, DVD SilverPlatter), monthly (CD SilverPlatter)
Growth rate	500,000 annually
Controlled terms	Controlled vocabulary MeSH (Medical Subject Headings) (polyhierarchically structured thesaurus) 22,500 terms + 130.000 "additional entries" (synonyms etc) No MeSH indexing in OLDMEDLINE, MEDLINE records in process ('PREMEDLINE'), and (in PubMed only) records with status qualification "PubMed".
Special fields	Nursing, dentistry, veterinary medicine, history of science, bioethics, complementary medicine
Special features	Qualification of controlled terms by 83 subheadings, organized in 19 searchable groups. Subject and Journal subsets. Clinical Queries and Related Articles search (through PubMed only) Free access (through NLM—PubMed and NLM Gateway, and through DIMDI).
Compared to other databases	Extensive coverage of dentistry.
Available	Directly from NLM (OLDMEDLINE, MEDLINE plus additional PubMed content) via PubMed (http://pubmed.gov) or the NLM Gateway (http://gateway.nlm.nih.gov/gw/Cmd) Datastar (1966–), Dialog (1966–), DIMDI (OLDMEDLINE, MEDLINE 1966–), OCLC FirstSearch (1966–), OVID Online (1966–) CD-ROM: DialogOnDisk (1966–), SilverPlatter (1966–), OVID (1966–)
Name	**PASCAL**
Producer	Institut de l'Information Scientifique et Technique du Centre National de la Recherche Scientifique (INIST-CNRS), France www.inist.fr
Years covered	1973–present
Journals covered	+6,000 (science, technology, medicine)
Document types	Journal articles, books, dissertations, conference proceedings, reports, patents

(continued)

Box 10.1 (*continued*)

Scope	Multilingual, multidisciplinary database that covers the core scientific literature science, technology, and medicine (31% medicine).
Update frequency	Online weekly (except Dialog: monthly), CD-ROM monthly (OVID) or quarterly (DialogOnDisc)
Growth rate	14,600 references/week
Controlled terms	Controlled vocabulary and classification codes (ex. 002B08J002B08J; Life sciences; Medical sciences; Dermatology) In English, French, and Spanish
Special fields	Interdisciplinary topics
Special features	Titles in original language and translated to French and/or English Priority given to French and European literature
Compared to MEDLINE	Additional European publications More document types as sources Controlled terms (index terms) not only in English but also in French and Spanish
Available	Directly through INIST ConnectSciences Portal (last 3 months free http://connectsciences.inist.fr) Datastar (1984–), Dialog (1973–), OCLC/PICA (1984–), Questel.Orbit (1973–). CD-ROM: OVID Technologies (1987–), DialogOnDisc (1990–)
Name	**PsycINFO (previously PsycLIT)**
Producer	American Psychological Association, Arlington U.S.A. www.apa.org
Years covered	1887– (non-English 1978–)
Journals covered	+1,900
Document types	Journal articles, conference papers, books, book chapters, dissertations, reports
Scope	An abstract database of the international literature in psychology and related behavioral and social sciences, including psychiatry, sociology, anthropology, education, pharmacology, and linguistics. Clinical, nonclinical and experimental psychology.
Update frequency	Weekly (monthly on DIMDI and SilverPlatter CD)
Growth rate	75,000 annually

Box 10.1

Controlled terms	Controlled vocabulary in records from 1967: Thesaurus of Psychological Index Terms. More than 7,000 controlled terms and cross-references. Also a classification system comprising 22 major categories and 135 subcategories.
Special fields	
Special features	99–100% of records have abstracts. From 2,000 cited references added to records of journal articles and books.
Compared to MEDLINE	More on psychology, psychiatry. Older literature. More records have abstract.
Available	Directly through APA during a 24-hour period at a time (payable by credit card only) www.psycinfo.com Datastar (1887–), Dialog (1887–), DIMDI (1887–), OCLC FirstSearch (1887–), OVID Online (1887–) CD-Rom/local: SilverPlatter (1887–), OVID (1887–)
Name	**SCIENCE CITATION INDEX (SCI)** **SOCIAL SCIENCES CITATION INDEX (SSCI)**
Producer	Institute of Scientific Information (ISI), Philadelphia U.S.A., London U.K. www.thomsonisi.com
Years covered	1945–
Journals covered	SCI 5,900 SSCI 1,700 (plus selected, relevant items from 5,800)
Document types	Journal articles
Scope	SSI: covers worldwide literature in the fields of science, technology, and biomedicine SSCI: covers worldwide literature from all areas of social sciences, including social medicine, psychology, and psychiatry.
Update frequency	Weekly
Growth rate	SCI: 650,000 annually SSCI: 120,000 annually
Controlled terms	None
Special fields	Multidisciplinary
Special features	Forward citation tracking. Related Records search.
Compared to MEDLINE	Older literature. Citation tracking.
Available	Directly from ISI as part of Web of Science (1945–) through Web of Knowledge (www.isiwebofknowledge.com). Datastar (SCI/SSCI 1972–), Dialog (SCI/SSCI 1972–), DIMDI (SCI 1974–/SSCI 1973–)

meta-analysis to assess the overall "level of evidence" and in sensitivity and subgroup analyses (see "Data extraction" and "Data analysis" sections).

It is important to remember that studies may appear to be of poor methodological quality because they were either poorly conducted or poorly reported. Methodological appraisal of the primary studies is frequently hindered by lack of information. In these instances, reviewers may choose to contact the studies' authors or to score items as "don't know" or "unclear."

The assessment of the methodological quality is the last step before collecting data and analyzing the results from the selected studies. Recently, the QUADAS tool was published to assess the methodological quality of diagnostic accuracy studies[30] (see Box 10.2). Reviewers should assess all recommended QUADAS items and consider whether there are additional items that should be included in their assessment. Reviewers should produce a document with clear details on how to score each item. At least two reviewers should perform the quality assessment and an explicit procedure to solve disagreement (discussion or arbitrage or both) should be described. The results of the quality assessment should also be presented in a table, on an item-by-item basis.

A modified version of the QUADAS that contains 11 items is proposed as the starting point for quality assessment of primary diagnostic accuracy studies.

Each item is scored as "yes," "no," or "unclear" based on all the information that is retrieved from the original paper or information from the authors. If there is insufficient information to judge a particular item, this item should be scored as "unclear."

The first item of the modified QUADAS tool refers to the generalizability or applicability of results (spectrum bias) based on the health care setting where the study was conducted, the study design and the inclusion/exclusion criteria applied in the study.

The second item concerns the use of an appropriate reference test, that is, could the reference test correctly identify the target condition? Because the apparent accuracy of a test depends upon the reliability of the reference test, this is an important step in the quality appraisal of a diagnostic accuracy study.

The time frame between the reference test and the index test is the third QUADAS item. This is important because of possible progression or regression of the disease. Ideally, both tests should be performed on the same patients at the same time. Nevertheless, the importance of this item will depend on the target disease (e.g., chronic conditions, infectious diseases).

(Partial) verification or workup bias (item 4) occurs when not all of the subjects are verified by the reference test. This occurs sometimes if an expensive or invasive reference test is indicated. Although researchers could avoid bias by testing a random selection of patients with the reference test, the selection is not usually random. Item 5 investigates differential verification bias, that is, did patients receive the same reference standard regardless of the index test result? This usually occurs when patients testing positive on the index test receive a more accurate, often invasive, reference standard than those with a negative test result. Information about the numbers of participants receiving different tests needs to be provided by the authors of the original studies.

Box 10.2 The original QUADAS tool (14 items).

BMC Medical Research Methodology 2003, 3: http://www.biomedicentral.com/1471-2288/3/25

Table 10.2 The QUADAS tool

Item		Yes	No	Unclear
1.	Was the spectrum of patients representative of the patients who will receive the test in practice?	()	()	()
2.	Were selection criteria described?	()	()	()
3.	Is the reference standard likely to correctly classify the target condition.	()	()	()
4.	Is the time period between reference standard and index test short enough to be reasonably sure that the target condition did not change between the two tests?	()	()	()
5.	Did the whole sample or a random selection of the sample, receive verification using a reference standard of diagnosis.	()	()	()
6.	Did patients receive the same reference standard regardless of the index test result?	()	()	()
7.	Was the reference standard independent of the index test (i.e., the index test did not form part of the reference standard)?	()	()	()
8.	Was the execution of the index test described in sufficient detail to permit replication of the test?	()	()	()
9.	Was the execution of the reference standard described in sufficient detail to permit its replication?	()	()	()
10.	Were the index test results interpreted without knowledge of the results of the reference standard?	()	()	()
11.	Were the reference standard results interpreted without knowledge of the results of the index test?	()	()	()
12.	Were the same clinical data available when test results were interpreted as would be available when the test is used in practice?	()	()	()
13.	Were uninterpretable/intermediate test results reported?	()	()	()
14.	Were withdrawals from the study explained?	()	()	()

Item 6 assesses the independence of the reference and the index tests. If the index test was part of the reference standard, the resulting incorporation bias will tend to increase the amount of agreement and hence overestimate the measures of diagnostic accuracy of the index test.

Items 7 and 8 are similar to the blinded outcome assessment in random controlled trials. This review bias will be avoided if the interpretation of the index test is blinded from the interpretation of the reference test and vice versa.

Studies have shown that the availability of clinical information could affect the accuracy of the index test in a positive way. Item 9 assesses the availability of clinical data during the interpretation of results within the study compared to the same clinical situation in real life.

Item 10 checks whether uninterpretable or intermediate test results were reported. This item is difficult to assess because the required information is not always reported. Finally, item 11 evaluates the withdrawals from the study. This is comparable with loss to follow-up within random controlled trials, and the approach to handling losses has great potential for biasing the results.

Data extraction

Two reviewers should independently extract the required information from the primary studies. Detailed information must be extracted about the participants included in the study and about the testing procedures. The cutoff point used in dichotomous testing, reasons for the choice of cut-point, and the number of participants excluded because of indeterminate results or infeasibility, are required.

Accuracy may be presented in different ways. For the meta-analysis of dichotomous tests (see statistical pooling) it is necessary to construct the diagnostic 2 × 2 table: absolute numbers in the four cells are needed. Totals of "diseased" and "nondiseased" participants are needed to estimate prior probability (pretest probability) and to reconstruct the 2 × 2 table. These data are used to compute sensitivity, specificity, likelihood ratios, predictive values and/or receiver operator characteristic (ROC) curves. If possible, the 2 × 2 table should be generated for all relevant subgroups. Further information to extract includes year of publication, setting, and country or region of the world where the study was performed.

Comments

A standardized data extraction form may be used simultaneously with, but separately from, the quality assessment form. This approach facilitates data extraction and comparison between reviewers. The form should be piloted to ensure that all reviewers interpret data in the same way. As in other steps of the review where judgments are made, disagreements should be recorded and resolved by consensus or arbitration.

Lack of details about test results or cutoff points, inconsequential rounding of percentages, and data errors require common sense and careful data handling when reconstructing 2 × 2 tables. Details can be requested from the authors of the studies, but these attempts are often unsuccessful, as the raw data may no longer be available.

Example

In a review of the accuracy of the CAGE questionnaire for the diagnosis of alcohol abuse, sufficient data were made available in only nine of the 22 studies selected, although the authors of the review tried to contact the original authors by all possible means.[31]

Data analysis

Whether a meta-analysis—statistical analysis and calculation of summary estimates of diagnostic test performance—can be conducted depends on the number and methodological quality of primary studies included and the degree of heterogeneity between them. Because diagnostic accuracy studies are often heterogeneous and present limited information it is typically difficult to complete a meta-analysis. If heterogeneity is identified, important information is obtained from attempts to explain it. For instance, the effect that each validity criterion has on the estimates of diagnostic accuracy and the influence of previously defined study characteristics should be explored as potential explanations of the observed study to study variation.[13–17] If meta-analysis is not possible or advisable, the review can be limited to a qualitative descriptive analysis of the diagnostic research available (best evidence synthesis).[32]

For the analysis, we recommend the following steps: (1) presentation of the results of individual studies; (2) searching for the presence of heterogeneity in accuracy and/or threshold effect; (3) dealing with heterogeneity; (4) deciding if statistical pooling is appropriate; and (5) statistical pooling. Appropriate methods to be used in each of these steps are described and discussed below.

Describing the results of individual studies

Reporting the main results of all included studies is an essential part of each review. It provides the reader with the outcome measures and gives an insight into their heterogeneity. In one or two tables, each study is presented with some background information (year of publication, geographical region, number of diseased and nondiseased patients, setting and selection of the patients, methodological characteristics) and a summary of the results. In view of the asymmetrical nature of most diagnostic tests (some tests are good to exclude a disease, others to confirm it), it is important to report pairs of complementary outcome measures, that is, both sensitivity and specificity, or likelihood ratio of a positive and of a negative test, or a combination of these. Predictive values are less generally reported as they are influenced by the prior probability, which differ markedly between populations. The diagnostic odds ratio (DOR) can be added as an overall measure of discrimination of the test. However, on its own, the DOR is less informative for the readers as the same odds ratio can relate to different combinations of sensitivity and specificity.

$$DOR = \frac{sensitivity/(1 - sensitivity)}{(1 - specificity)/specificity}$$

Main outcome measures should all be reported with their 95% confidence intervals (95% CI).

Searching for heterogeneity

The degree of heterogeneity (as against homogeneity) between studies is a measure of the differences between the studies. A set of diagnostic studies are perfectly homogeneous if they are similar with respect to their design, disease prevalence, disease spectrum, setting, and characteristics of the populations. They should also report similar inclusion, selection and referral patterns and previous testing that influenced the presence of the patients in the study population, and all details of the measurements of both the test to be studied and the reference test, analysis, and reporting. Sometimes such differences are not apparent from the methods sections of the individual papers, thereby limiting your ability to detect the *presence of heterogeneity* from the available information. The information may not be reported in the methods section of the paper because of limitation of space and readability requirements, or because the authors of the original studies have not reported the operationalization in sufficient detail. In such situations, differences in the accuracy measures between individual study results may indicate the presence of heterogeneity without information on its possible causes. Some people call this statistical heterogeneity, although it is of course only one way to detect the presence of heterogeneity as such. Identifying the presence of such statistical signs of heterogeneity can be straightforward.

In some cases, just looking at the data—the "eyeball test"—will enable the meta-analyst to judge whether a relation between an accuracy parameter and a study characteristic is both present and clinically relevant. Summarizing the study results in a forest plot (separately for each accuracy parameter) will make the overview easier. Ideally, the forest plot will comprise two parts showing both sensitivity and specificity side-by-side for each study. The data should also be displayed as a scatter plot of sensitivity plotted against 1-specificity for each study to assess whether the heterogeneity mainly relates to sensitivity, specificity, or both. However, from such displays, it is difficult to determine visually whether the variation between studies is due predominantly to random (sampling) error, or whether there is also true heterogeneity. Rigorous analysis of these data must take proper account of the within and between study variability, as described later in this chapter.

Another graphical approach that may be useful in assessing heterogeneity is a Galbraith plot[33] of the log odds ratio (or another measure of accuracy) of each study divided by its standard error (z statistic) plotted against the reciprocal of the standard error. A regression line through zero represents the overall log odds ratio. Parallel lines starting two units above and below this line define the region in which approximately 95% of studies should lie if there is no heterogeneity, hence outliers should closely be examined. However, as noted earlier, variation between studies can result from random error, heterogeneity, or both. Although a χ^2 test for homogeneity of diagnostic accuracy measures[34] is sometimes used, the power of such tests tends to be low. Consequently, these tests have limited value for diagnostic studies where heterogeneity is very likely to be present in sensitivity and/or specificity. It is generally advisable to assume that heterogeneity is present when conducting a meta-analysis of diagnostic studies.

Threshold (cut-point) effect

Clearly, the choice of the cut-point in a test with an outcome on a continuous scale will influence the diagnostic characteristics of the test. If a higher test result indicates a higher likelihood of the disease (indicated by a positive reference test result), increasing the cut-point will result in an increased specificity and a decreased sensitivity. Review-based estimates of diagnostic accuracy such as sensitivity, specificity and likelihood ratios will differ if not all studies use the same cut-point for a positive test result (or for the reference standard).

In many tests with a dichotomous test result, however, the decision whether the result is positive or negative partly results from interpretation by the test observer. Some observers will find it easier than others, for example, to detect a color change in a dipstick test, a cellular nucleus that is too large under microscopy, or a tumor to be present on a chest radiography. This situation is similar to differences in cut-point used for test results on a continuous scale and should be taken into consideration in a similar way when analyzing study results. It is sometimes called an implicit (because it is not measurable) cut-point effect. Aspects other than inter-observer variation such as between-study differences in testing operationalization, disease spectrum, and background characteristics such as age or co-morbidity patterns may also have the same effect.

A threshold (cut-point) effect will generally result in heterogeneity in both sensitivity and specificity, and a negative correlation between them across studies. However, a strong correlation between both parameters will often result in a homogeneous diagnostic $\log_e$ odds ratio (lnDOR).

Example

Box 10.3 shows a scatter plot of (1-specificity, sensitivity) pairs for 14 studies that evaluated peak systolic velocity (PSV) (Doppler ultrasound) to detect renal artery stenosis. Each study is denoted by an ellipse centered on the (1-specificity, sensitivity) pair for that study. The horizontal and vertical dimensions of each ellipse are proportional to the number of nondiseased and diseased respectively for that study. The display serves to highlight variation in both test positivity (threshold) and accuracy between studies. Variation resulting from an explicit or implicit cut-point effect, will result in the points appearing to be scattered about an underlying ROC curve.[19,35] Studies using a lower cut-point for test positivity (showing high sensitivity and low specificity) will be shown in the right upper quadrant of the figure.

Box 10.3 Variation in test performance of 14 studies that evaluated peak systolic velocity (PSV) to detect renal artery stenosis.

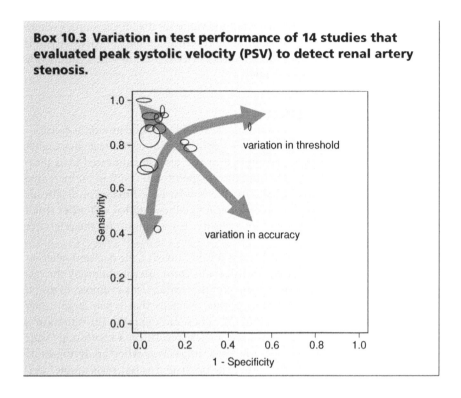

Dealing with heterogeneity

Interpretation of heterogeneity is often the most fascinating and productive part of a meta-analysis. In the presence of heterogeneity, the meta-analyst should start with assessing its clinical relevance. This is essentially a matter of clinical judgment. If the degree of heterogeneity is considered to be relevant, the reviewer can proceed in different ways.

One option is to restrict the review to a (homogeneous) subset of studies using strict inclusion and exclusion criteria. Of course, such a decision should be taken as soon as the (probable) presence of heterogeneity and its reasons become clear, that is, after studying the methodological characteristics of the individual studies or even before.

Example

In a review of the diagnostic value of macroscopic hematuria for the diagnosis of urological cancers in primary care, the positive predictive values (PPV) indicated a homogeneous series of five studies with a pooled PPV of 0.19 (95% CI 0.17–0.23) and one other with a PPV of 0.40.[36] The reason for this high PPV was mentioned in the original study: "GPs' services in the region are extremely good and cases of less serious conditions are probably adequately shifted out and treated without referral,"[36a] leading to a highly selected study population with a high prior probability. In this situation, the outlier can be excluded and the analysis continued with the homogeneous group of remaining studies.

Another option is to conduct subgroup analyses, ideally using subgroups defined in the protocol. The reviewer should search for causes of heterogeneity, stratify the studies according to categories for such causes, and pool results of homogeneous subgroups. For instance, in the same review on the diagnostic value of macroscopic hematuria for the diagnosis of urological malignancies,[36] sensitivity results were very heterogeneous. As could be expected, the degree of heterogeneity could largely be reduced after examining bladder, ureter, and kidney tumors separately (see Box 10.4). Of course, this is only possible if sufficient subgroup analyses are reported in the original publications or can be retrieved from the authors.

Box 10.4 Subgroup analysis resulting in homogeneous subgroups.

Pooled sensitivity of macroscopic hematuria
for the diagnosis of urological cancer
subgroup analysis

Localization	No. of studies	x^2 homogeneity (P)	Pooled sensitivity (95% CI)
BLADDER			
All	7	0.62	0.83 (0.80–0.85)
<40 years only	4	0.77	0.82 (0.74–0.88)
URETER			
All	4	0.01	0.66 (0.53–0.77)
Painless	2	0.39	0.55 (0.45–0.65)
With pain	1		0.20 (0.07–0.34)
Kidney			
All	3	0.03	0.48 (0.36–0.60)

When feasible, this is a rewarding way of dealing with heterogeneity as it provides you with the opportunity to find new things that are clinically relevant, that is, differences in the diagnostic accuracy of a test according to patient subsets. For example, you may detect that a test is helpful in younger people, but not in the elderly or vice versa. This is the case for screening mammography that has a far higher sensitivity in women above age 50 compared with younger women.[37]

If subgroup characteristics are detected during the analysis stage of the review (and not prestated in the protocol), there is a net risk of data dredging. If a sufficient number of subgroups are examined you will most likely find homogeneous ones, possibly with clinically irrelevant results. When heterogeneity can be expected on the basis of the individual studies' methods description, the decision about which subgroups are to be analyzed separately should be made before looking at the study results. In the case of unexplained (statistical) heterogeneity, this is of course impossible. The post hoc nature of such choice should be mentioned in the report of the review. Such subgroup results should be considered with caution and subsequent studies should try to confirm or refute the findings.

If sufficient studies are available, statistical modeling can be used to explore heterogeneity by including study and patient characteristics as possible covariates in the model. Multivariate models are used to assess the independent effect of study characteristics, adjusted for the influence of other variables.

Deciding on the statistical model to be used

Fixed effect versus random effects models

A *fixed effect model* assumes that all studies represent a random sample of one large (hypothetical) common study, and that differences between study outcomes only result from random (sampling) error. Pooling is relatively simple as it only requires calculation of a weighted average of the individual study results. Studies are weighted by the inverse of the variance of the parameter of test accuracy, or by the number of participants.

A *random effects model* assumes that in addition to the presence of random error, differences between studies can also result from real differences between study populations and procedures. Both sources of variability are taken into account when computing the weighting factor for each study. The method of Der Simonian and Laird, initially published for the meta-analysis of trials, is a simple example of a random effects model.[38]

Homogeneous studies

If parameters are homogeneous, and they show no threshold effect, their results can be pooled and a fixed effect model used.[39] However, if there is evidence of a threshold effect, Summary ROC (SROC) analysis is appropriate.

Heterogeneous studies

If heterogeneity is present, the reviewer has the following options:
1 Refrain from pooling and restrict the analysis to a qualitative overview.
2 Conduct subgroup analysis based on prior factors and pool within homogeneous subgroups.
3 Analyze the data using a random effects model. (Note: such an analysis should be preceded by descriptive subgroup analyses.)

In view of the poor methodological quality of most of the diagnostic studies that have been carried out, heterogeneity in test performance is to be expected in systematic reviews of diagnostic studies.[18] Hence, it is advisable to use random effects models for the meta-analysis of diagnostic studies, even if there is no apparent heterogeneity. Distinguishing between sources of variability also serves to ensure the validity of statistical testing and confidence intervals.

Statistical pooling

Pooling of proportions assuming homogeneous sensitivity and/or specificity

Separate pooling of sensitivity and specificity is not generally recommended as these two measures are usually correlated and so should be analyzed jointly.[40,41] However, in the absence of a threshold effect, and clear evidence of homogeneity in sensitivity and/or specificity across studies, it may be acceptable to use *fixed effect* pooling.[42]

Threshold effect: SROC curve

At present, SROC analysis provides the most general approach for the meta-analysis of diagnostic studies as it allows for a threshold effect between studies, and takes account of both sensitivity and specificity for each study. The most commonly used method is that of Littenberg and Moses[19,35] (see Appendix 3), which uses linear regression to model the natural logarithm of the DOR (D = lnDOR) of each study as a function of a proxy for the test threshold for that study. This proxy for test threshold (denoted by S) is based on the proportion of diseased and nondiseased subjects who test positive (see Appendix 3) The model is given by D = $a + b$S where a represents the intercept (interpreted as the mean lnDOR when S = 0) and b represents the slope. A nonzero slope indicates that test accuracy increases (or decreases) systematically as the threshold varies. The model is usually fitted by unweighted or weighted (using the inverse of the variance of D as the weighting factor) least squares, and both a and b are assumed to be fixed effects. Inverse transformation is required to generate the estimated SROC curve, and the curve is usually restricted to lie within the range of the observed data.

This method is very useful for descriptive analyses to obtain an SROC curve based on all studies and within subgroups. However, the method does not take separate account of the within and between study variability in test accuracy. In addition, the explanatory variable (S) is subject to sampling error thereby violating an important assumption of the least squares method.[22] Because of these limitations, the use of covariates in this model to test for differences in test accuracy across subgroups of studies could be unreliable and is not recommended. This is also the case when comparing the accuracy of two or more tests, which is a frequent reason to perform a diagnostic meta-analysis. The more recent development of hierarchical models that do not suffer from these limitations provides a more appropriate approach for statistical inference.

Hierarchical models

Two hierarchical models have been adopted for the meta-analysis of diagnostic studies: the hierarchical SROC (HSROC) model[22,43] and the bivariate model.[20,21,44] Although the models have been shown to be mathematically equivalent,[45] they nevertheless approach the analysis somewhat differently.

HSROC model

The HSROC model can be conceptualized as a two-level (multilevel) model that focuses on the estimation of a summary ROC curve. At the first level, the within-study sampling error is taken into account by assuming a binomial error distribution for the sensitivity and 1-specificity for each study. Each study provides an estimate of test accuracy (lnDOR) and a proxy for threshold which are both taken to be random effects that follow a normal distribution at level 2 (see Appendix 3). Test accuracy, threshold, and the dependence between them (shape of the SROC) can be modeled as a function of study-level covariates. Hence, the model can be used to assess whether the expected accuracy, threshold, and/or shape of the summary ROC curve vary across subgroups. An expected operating point (expected sensitivity and specificity) and corresponding 95% confidence region can be obtained for each fitted curve. The estimated likelihood ratios for a positive and negative test, and their 95% confidence intervals, can then be obtained at this expected operating point. The model may be fitted in SAS[46] using PROC NLMIXED to obtain the required estimates.[47] A more complex, fully Bayesian analysis can also be conducted.[22]

Bivariate model

The bivariate method directly models the logit(sensitivity) and logit(specificity), while accounting for the correlation between them (see Appendix 3). It can also be conceptualized as a two-level model that assumes a binomial error distribution for the sensitivity and specificity for each study at level one. At level two, the logit(sensitivity) and logit(specificity) are assumed to be normally distributed, correlated random effects. For this model, the focus is on using study level covariates to model systematic variation in sensitivity or specificity. Although the main output from this method is the expected operating point and corresponding 95% confidence region, the estimated likelihood ratios at the expected operating point(s) and the summary ROC curve(s) can also be derived.[45] It is best to fit the model taking account of the binomial error distribution by using PROC NLMIXED in SAS,[46] or GLLAMM in STATA.[48]

The choice between the HSROC and bivariate models is largely governed by whether the meta-analyst is more concerned with how the position and shape of the SROC curve varies with study and patient characteristics, or how the expected sensitivity and specificity vary with these factors. Software availability may also influence the choice of method.

Pooling of ROC curves

The results of diagnostic studies with a dichotomous gold standard outcome, and a test result that is reported on a continuous scale, are generally presented as an ROC curve with or without the related area under the curve (AUC) and its 95% CI. To pool such results, the reviewer has three options: to pool sensitivities and specificities for all relevant cutoff points using the methods described above assuming that sufficient raw data are available to construct the 2 × 2 tables; to pool the AUCs; or to model and pool the ROC curves themselves.

Comments

Although methods have been developed for pooling AUCs,[49] the AUC like all one-dimensional measures provides no information about the asymmetrical nature of a diagnostic test. It cannot distinguish between curves with a high sensitivity at moderate values of the specificity and those with a high specificity at moderate values of the sensitivity.

Where data are available at multiple test thresholds for each study, an ROC curve can be obtained for each study. Ideally, we would want to perform a meta-analysis that utilizes all available information from the ROC curves across studies to obtain a summary ROC curve. A Bayesian model has been developed to implement this approach.[23] However, a high level of statistical expertise is required to fit the model because of its complexity.

A method has also been developed to enable direct pooling of ROC curves that requires only the published curves and the number of positive and negative participants on the gold standard test as input.[50] Once again, the approach is complex to implement requiring often complex data extraction, estimation of parameters and corresponding standard errors for the study of specific ROC curves, and the use of random effects modeling to obtain summary estimates for these parameters. These summary estimates are then used to obtain the summary ROC.

In addition to causing calculation problems in specific situations, pooling published ROC curves[50] also hides the test values from the picture. Although this is not a problem when evaluating a test method, or when comparing different methods, it limits the possible use of the pooled curve for evaluating the diagnostic value of each specific test result. Moreover, a published curve can be a fitted estimate of the real curve based on the initial values, and any bias or imprecision resulting from this estimation will be included in the pooled estimates.

Data presentation

All results should include a scatter plot of (1–specificity, sensitivity) pairs for each study plotted in ROC space. Subgroups may be denoted by different colors or symbols to highlight important patterns in the data. If SROC curves have been estimated, these can be superimposed on the scatter plot and the expected ("average") operating point for a test can be marked on the SROC with a 95% confidence region displayed for that point. Predicted sensitivity at a given specificity (or vice versa) can also be estimated from the SROC.

Example

Box 10.5 shows the same 14 studies depicted in Box 10.3 that evaluated PSV for the detection of renal artery stenosis. Different symbols have been used to denote the 10 studies that excluded occluded arteries from their evaluation, and the 4 studies that did not. HSROC analysis was used to assess whether test performance differed between these subgroups of studies. The results showed no evidence that accuracy (lnDOR) depended on threshold, but despite the small number of studies, there was evidence that the expected accuracy of studies that excluded occluded arteries was higher than those that did not (relative DOR 4.4, 95% CI 1.1 − 17.1, P = 0.034). The expected operating point and corresponding confidence region was computed for each subgroup as shown in Box 10.5. For studies that excluded occluded arteries, the expected sensitivity and specificity were 0.87 (95% CI 0.81, 0.93) and 0.95 (95% CI 0.92, 0.98), respectively. The corresponding estimates for the remaining four studies were 0.76 (95% CI 0.63, 0.89) and 0.89 (95% CI 0.83, 0.96). These estimates can also be obtained from the bivariate model.

Box 10.5 Estimated SROC and expected operating point with corresponding 95% confidence region for subgroups of studies that did, and did not, exclude occluded arteries.

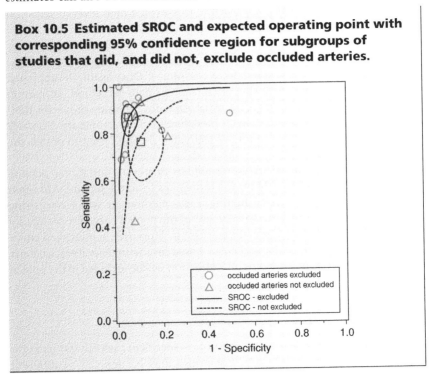

The expected sensitivity and specificity can be used to obtain the predicted positive and negative likelihood ratios at that point on the SROC, and both the HSROC and bivariate models can provide confidence intervals for these To make the results more accessible to clinicians, these likelihood ratios can be used to obtain the predictive values by using the mean or median prior (pretest) probabilities of each subgroup. Alternatively, likelihood ratios could be reported so that users can calculate posttest probabilities based on the pretest probabilities applicable to their patients. However, the generalizability of the results to populations with pre-test probabilities outside the range of the studies used to generate the SROC may be questionable.

Discussion

Although the methodology to conduct a systematic review and meta-analysis of diagnostic research is developed to a certain extent, at least for dichotomized tests, the exercise itself remains quite a challenge. Systematic reviews have to meet high methodological standards and the results should always be interpreted with caution. Several complicating issues need careful consideration: (1) it is difficult to discover all published evidence, as diagnostic research is often inadequately indexed in electronic databases; (2) the studies are often poorly reported and a set of minimal reporting standards for diagnostic research has only recently been discussed; (3) the methodological quality and validity of diagnostic research reports is often limited (i.e., no clear definition of "diseased" participants, no blinding, no independent interpretation of test results, insufficient description of participants); (4) accuracy estimates are often very heterogeneous, yet examining heterogeneity is cumbersome and the process is full of pitfalls; (5) quantitative analysis of diagnostic reviews has become complex, requiring expert statistical input and sophisticated software that is not found in the current "simple" meta-analysis packages; (6) nevertheless, results have to be translated into information that is clinically relevant, taking into account the clinical reality at different levels of health care (prevalence of disease, spectrum of disease, available clinical and other diagnostic information). Even in a state of the art systematic review, the reviewers have to make many subjective decisions when deciding on the inclusion or exclusion of studies, on quality assessment and the interpretation of limited information, on the exclusion of outliers, and on choosing and conducting subgroup analyses. Subjective aspects have to be assessed independently by more than one reviewer, with tracking of disagreements and resolution by consensus or arbitration. These subjective decisions should be explicitly acknowledged in the report to allow the readers some insight into the possible consequences of these decisions on the outcomes of the review and the strength of inference derived from it.

Whereas some researchers question the usefulness of pooling the results of poorly designed research or meta-analyses based on limited information,[51,52] we think that examining the effects of validity criteria on the diagnostic accuracy measures and the analysis of subgroups adds valuable evidence to the field of diagnostic accuracy studies. The generation of a pooled estimate and/or SROC provides clinicians with useful information until better-conducted studies are published. The reader should remember that evidence about the influence of validity of studies on diagnostic accuracy is still limited.[2,11,53] Consequently, it is difficult to recommend a strict set of methodological criteria, recognizing that any minimum set of methodological criteria is largely arbitrary. The development of guidelines for systematic reviews of tests with continuous or ordinal outcomes, reviews of the (incremental) value of series of subsequent tests and reviews of comparisons between more than one test, remains another challenge, as the methodology is still limited or even nonexistent. It is possible that only individual patient meta-analyses will be able to fully address all these issues.

Appendix 1:   A flowchart of the searching and selection process.

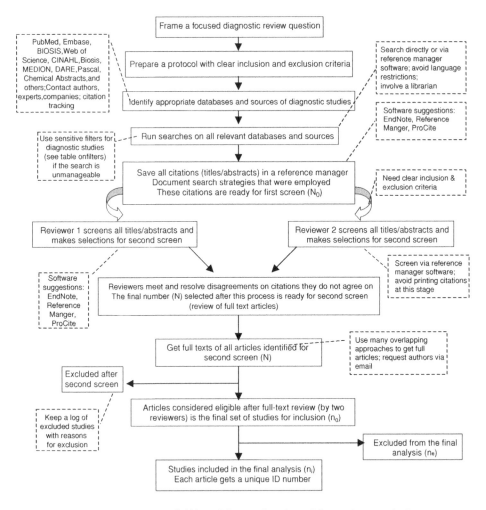

This flowchart has been adapted from: Pai M, *et al*. Systematic reviews of diagnostic test evaluations: what is behind the scenes? *Evid Based Med*. 2004—reproduced with permission from the BMJ Publishing Group.

Appendix 2: Other databases of significance to reviewers

Database	Why interesting?	Available
Allied and Complementary Health (AMED)	Additional content	Datastar, DIMDI, Ovid
Australasian Medical Index (AMI) producer Nat. Library of Australia www.nla.gov.au/ami	Geographic focus Australia 1968– 100 journals not in MEDLINE	Subscribing institutions/libraries For subscriptions contact www.RMITPublishing.com.au
BIOSIS, BIOSIS/RRM (Biological Abstracts)	Conference proceedings, reports Biomedicine 1969–, total >15 billion records	Datastar, Dialog, DIMDI, Ovid
Chemical Abstracts (CA) producer Chemical Abstracts Service, Am.Chem.Soc.	Conference proceedings, reports Search with CAS Registry numbers Pharmacology, clinical chemistry 1907–, total >22 billion records	STN, Datastar, Dialog, Scifinder
Conference Papers Index (CONFSCI) producer Cambridge Scientific Abstracts	Conference proceedings Life sciences 1973–, total >2 billion records	STN
Computer Retrieval of Information on Scientific Projects (CRISP)	Ongoing research projects U.S.A. Unpublished research	(free) http://crisp.cit.nih.gov
Digital Dissertations (Dissertation Abstracts)—producer ProQuest Information & Learning	Doctoral dissertations and master's theses. 1860–. Mainly U.S.A.	http://www.lib.umi.com/ dissertations (2 most current years free). OCLC FirstSearch, ProQuest
German Medical Science Meetings	Conference proceedings, medical	DIMDI
Health Services Research Projects in Progress (HSRPROJ)—producer U.S. Academy Science	Ongoing research USA—data from leading federal and private funders	(free) NLM Gateway http://gateway.nlm.nih.gov

(*continued*)

Appendix 2   (*continued*)

Database	Why interesting?	Available
ISI Proceedings (ISTPB, as of 1998 ISTP/ISSHP)	Conference proceedings 1978–. 80% with abstract. >60,000 meetings since 1990	DIMDI, Web of Knowledge www.webofknowledge.com
Literatura Latinoamericana y del Caribe en Ciencias de la Salud (LILACS; Latin American Health Sciences Literature.	Geographic focus Latin America and Caribbean.	Bibliotheca Virtual en Salud www.bvs.org.ar www.bireme.br/bvs/E/ebd.htm
MEDICONF—producer Fairbase Database Ltd Germany	Conference data. Directory, 1993–2007. Medical, pharmaceutical	Dialog, STN, (partly free at) producer's site www.mediconf.com
National Research Register U.K.	Ongoing research projects 2000– U.K. Unpublished research	(free) Update Software Ltd http://www.update-software.com/National/
SIGLE—producer Eur. Assoc. for Gray Lit. Exploitation, in cooperation with FIZ Karlsruhe	Grey literature 1976– mainly dissertations, reports. FTN (Germany) database included.	Ovid, STN

Appendix 3

Notation
TP = true positives, FP = false positives, TN = true negatives, FN = false negatives, i = study number, k = total number of studies, *logit* represents the log odds, *exp* represents the exponential function.

SROC method of Littenberg and Moses:
For each study compute:

$$\log \text{ diagnostic odds ratio D} = \ln\left[\frac{sensitivity}{1-sensitivity}\right] - \ln\left[\frac{1-specificity}{specificity}\right], \text{ and}$$

$$\text{proxy for test threshold S} = \ln\left[\frac{sensitivity}{1-sensitivity}\right] + \ln\left[\frac{1-specificity}{specificity}\right].$$

The fit the model D = $a + b$S using either unweighted least squares regression, or weight each study by the inverse variance of the lnDOR (i.e., D), where $\text{var(D)} = \frac{1}{\text{TP}} + \frac{1}{\text{FP}} + \frac{1}{\text{TN}} + \frac{1}{\text{FN}}$ (Note: 0.5 may be added to all counts in each

2 × 2 table to avoid division by zero.) After fitting the model, the SROC curve can be generated using the estimated values of a and b.[35]

HSROC model

Level 1

For each study $(i, i = 1, \ldots, k)$, the number testing positive (y_{ij}) for both the diseased $(j = 1)$ and nondiseased $(j = 2)$ groups is assumed to follow a binomial distribution $(B(\pi_{ij}, n_{ij})$, where π_{ij} represents the probability of a positive test result in group j, and n_{ij} represents the number of subjects in group j). The model takes the form $logit(\pi_{ij}) = (\theta_i + \alpha_i \, dis_{ij}) \exp(-\beta dis_{ij})$ where dis_{ij} is coded as -0.5 for the nondiseased and 0.5 for the diseased; θ_i are random effects for test threshold; α_i are random effects for accuracy for each study; and β is a fixed effect for dependence between accuracy and threshold.

Level 2

The θ_i are assumed to be normally distributed with mean Θ and variance τ_θ^2, and the α_i are assumed to be normally distributed with mean Λ and variance τ_α^2. The two distributions of random effects are assumed to be uncorrelated.

After fitting the model, the SROC curve can be generated from the estimated values of β, Θ, and Λ.[47]

Bivariate model

Level 1

For each study $(i, i = 1, \ldots, k)$, the number correctly diagnosed (y_{ij}) for both the diseased $(j = 1)$ and nondiseased $(j = 2)$ groups is assumed to follow a binomial distribution $(B(\pi_{ij}, n_{ij})$, where π_{ij} represents the probability of a correct diagnosis in group j, and n_{ij} represents the number of subjects in group j). Hence, the observed sensitivity in study i is y_{i1}/n_{i1} and specificity is y_{i2}/n_{i2}. Both sensitivity and specificity are taken to be random effects.

Level 2

The distribution of logit(sensitivity$_i$) is assumed to follow a normal distribution with mean μ_A and variance σ_A^2. Similarly, the distribution of logit(specificity$_i$) is assumed to follow a normal distribution with mean μ_B and variance σ_B^2. The two distributions are assumed to be correlated. After fitting the model, the expected sensitivity and specificity are computed using the estimates of μ_A and μ_B.[44]

References

1. Irwig L, Tosteson ANA, Gatsonis C, et al. Guidelines for meta-analyses evaluating diagnostic tests. *Ann Intern Med.* 1994;**120**:667–76.

2. Lijmer JG, Mol BW, Heisterkamp S, et al. Empirical evidence of design-related bias in studies of diagnostic tests. *JAMA*. 1999;**282**:1061–66.

3. Haynes RB, Wilczynski N, McKibbon KA, et al. Developing optimal search strategies for detecting clinically sound studies in Medline. *J Am Med Inform Assoc*. 1994;**1**:447–58.

4. Dickersin K, Scherer R, Lefebvre C. Identifying relevant studies for systematic reviews. *BMJ*. 1994;**309**:1286–91.

5. van der Weijden T, IJzermans CJ, Dinant GJ, et al. Identifying relevant diagnostic studies in MEDLINE: the diagnostic value of the erythrocyte sedimentation rate (ESR) and dipstick as an example. *Fam Pract*. 1997;**14**:204–8.

6. Devillé WLJM, Bezemer PD, Bouter LM. Publications on diagnostic test evaluation in family medicine journals: an optimal search strategy. *J Clin Epidemiol*. 2000;**53**:65–69.

7. Devillé WL, Buntinx F, Bouter LM, et al. Conducting systematic reviews of diagnostic studies: didactic guidelines. *BMC Med Res Methodol*. 2002;**2**(9):1–13.

8. Pai M, McCulloch M, Enanoria W, et al. Systematic reviews of diagnostic test evaluations: What's behind the scenes? *ACP J Club*. 2004;**141**(1):A11–13.

9. Jeaschke R, Guyatt GH, Sackett DL. User's guidelines to the medical literature: III. How to use an article about a diagnostic test, A: are the results of the study valid? *JAMA*. 1994;**271**:389–91.

10. Jeaschke R, Guyatt GH, Sackett DL. User's guidelines to the medical literature: III. How to use an article about a diagnostic test, B: what are the results and will they help me in caring for my patients? *JAMA*. 1994;**271**:703–7.

11. Greenhalgh T. How to read a paper: papers that report diagnostic or screening tests. *BMJ*. 1997;**315**:540–43.

12. Reid MC, Lachs MS, Feinstein AR. Use of methodological standards in diagnostic test research: getting better but still not good. *JAMA*. 1995;**274**:645–51.

13. Yusuf S, Wittes J, Probsfield J, et al. Analysis and interpretation of treatment effects in subgroups of patients in randomised clinical trials. *JAMA*. 1991;**266**:93–98.

14. Oxman A, Guyatt G. A consumer's guide to subgroup analysis. *Ann Intern Med*. 1992;**116**:78–84.

15. Thompson SG. Why sources of heterogeneity in meta-analysis should be investigated. *BMJ*. 1994;**309**:1351–55.

16. Colditz GA, Burdick E, Mosteller F. Heterogeneity in meta-analysis of data from epidemiologic studies: a commentary. *Am J Epidemiol*. 1995;**142**:371–82.

17. Mulrow C, Langhorne P, Grimshaw J. Integrating heterogeneous pieces of evidence in systematic reviews. *Ann Intern Med*. 1997;**127**:989–95.

18. Lijmer JG, Bossuyt PM, Heisterkamp SH. Exploring sources of heterogeneity in systematic reviews of diagnostic tests. *Stat Med*. 2002;**21**(11):1525–37.

19. Littenberg B, Moses LE. Estimating diagnostic accuracy from multiple conflicting reports: a new meta-analytic method. *Med Decis Making*. 1993;**13**:313–21.

20. van Houwelingen HC, Zwinderman KH, Stijnen T. A bivariate approach to meta-analysis. *Stat Med*. 1993;**12**:2273–84.

21. van Houwelingen HC, Arends LR, Stijnen T. Advanced methods in meta-analysis: multivariate approach and meta-regression. *Stat Med*. 2002;**21**:589–624.

22. Rutter C, Gatsonis C. A hierarchical regression approach to meta-analysis of diagnostic test accuracy evaluations. *Stat Med*. 2001;**20**:2865–84.

23. Dukic V, Gatsonis C. Meta-analysis of diagnostic test accuracy assessment studies with varying number of thresholds. *Biometrics*. 2003;**59**:936–46.

24. Bachmann LM, Coray R, Estermann P, Ter Riet G. Identifying diagnostic studies in MEDLINE: reducing the number needed to read. *Am Med Inform Assoc.* 2002;**9**(6):653–58.

25. Haynes 2004 Haynes RB, Wilczynski NL. Optimal search strategies for retrieving scientifically strong studies of diagnosis from Medline: analytical survey. *BMJ.* 2004;**328**(7447):1040.

26. Walter SD, Irwig L, Glasziou PP. Meta-analysis of diagnostic tests with imperfect reference standards. *J Clin Epidemiol.* 1999;**52**:943–51.

27. Grégoire G, Derderian F, Le Lorier J. Selecting the language of the publications included in a meta-analysis: is there a Tower of Babel bias? *J Clin Epidemiol.* 1995;**48**:159–63.

28. Egger M, Zellweger-Zahner T, Schneider M, et al. Language bias in randomised controlled trials published in English and German. *Lancet.* 1997;**350**(9074):326–29.

29. Obuchowski NA. Sample size calculations in studies of test accuracy. *Stat Meth Med Res.* 1998;**7**:371–92.

30. Whiting PF, Weswood ME, Rutjes AW, et al. Evaluation of QUADAS, a tool for the quality assessment of diagnostic accuracy studies. *BMC Med Res Methodol.* 2006; **6**:9.

31. Aertgeerts B, Buntinx F, Kester A. The value of the CAGE in screening for alcohol abuse and alcohol dependence in general clinical populations: a meta-analysis. *J Clin Epidemiol.* 2004;**57**:30–39.

32. Centre for Evidence Based Medicine. Levels of evidence and grades of recommendations. http://cebm.jr2.ox.ac.uk/docs/levels.html

33. Galbraith R. A note on graphical presentation of estimated odds ratios from several clinical trials. *Stat Med.* 1988;**7**:889–94.

34. Fleiss JL. The statistical basis of meta-analysis. *Stat Meth Med Res.* 1993;**2**:121–45.

35. Moses LE, Shapiro D, Littenberg B. Combining independent studies of a diagnostic test into a summary ROC curve: data-analytic approaches and some additional considerations. *Stat Med.* 1993;**12**:1293–316.

36. Buntinx F, Wauters H. The diagnostic value of macroscopic haematuria in diagnosing urological cancers: a meta-analysis. *Fam Pract.* 1997;**14**:63–68.

36a. Gillatt DA, O'Reilly PM. Haematuria analysed – a prospective study. *J. R. Soc. Med.* 187; **87**:115–117.

37. Vainio H, Bianchini F, eds. *Breast cancer screening (IARC handbooks of cancer prevention).* Vol. 7. Lyon: IARC Press; 2002.

38. DerSimonian R, Laird N. Meta-analysis in clinical trials. *Controlled Clin Trials.* 1986;**7**:177–88.

39. Deeks J. Systematic reviews of evaluations of diagnostic and screening tests. In: Egger M, Davey-Smith G, Altman D, eds. *Systematic reviews in health care: meta-analysis in context.* 2nd ed. London: BMJ Publishing Group; 2001.

40. Irwig L, Tosteson AN, Gatsonis CA, et al. Guidelines for meta-analyses evaluating diagnostic tests. *Ann Int Med.* 1994;**120**:667–76.

41. Irwig L, Macaskill P, Glasziou P, et al. Meta-analytic methods for diagnostic test accuracy. *J Clin Epidemiol.* 1995;**48**:119–30.

42. Midgette AS, Stukel TA, Littenberg B. A meta-analytic method for summarizing diagnostic test performances: receiver-operating-characteristic-summary point estimates. *Med Decis Making.* 1993;**13**:253–57.

43. Rutter C, and Gatsonis C. Regression methods for meta-analysis of diagnostic test data. *Acad Radiol*. 1995;**2**:S48–56.
44. Reitsma JB, Glas AS, Rutjes AWS, et al. Bivariate analysis of sensitivity and specificity produces informative summary measures in diagnostic reviews. *J Clin Epidemiol*. 2005;**58**:982–90.
45. Harbord RM, Egger M, Sterne JA. A modified test for small-study effects in meta-analyses of controlled trials with binary endpoints. *Stat Med*. 2006;**25**(20):3443–57.
46. SAS Institute. *The SAS system for Windows*. Version 9.1. Cary (NC): SAS Institute, 2003.
47. Macaskill P. Empirical Bayes estimates generated in a hierarchical summary ROC analysis agreed closely with those of a full Bayesian analysis. *J Clin Epidemiol*. 2004;**57**(9):925–32.
48. Rabe-Hesketh S, Pickles A, Skrondal A. GLLAMM Manual. University of California, Berkeley Division of Biostatistics Working Paper Series. Working Paper 160; 2004 Berkeley: University of California; http://www.bepress.com/ucbbiostat/paper160
49. McClish DK. Combining and comparing area estimates across studies or strata. *Med Decis Making*. 1992;**12**:274–79.
50. Kester A, Buntinx F. Meta-analysis of ROC-curves. *Med Decis Making*. 2000;**20**:430–39.
51. Greenland S. A critical look at some popular meta-analytic methods. *Am J Epidemiol*. 1994;**140**:290–301.
52. Shapiro S. Meta-analysis/Shmeta-analysis. *Am J Epidemiol*. 1994;**140**:771–77.
53. Oosterhuis WP, Niessen RWLM, Bossuyt PMM. The science of systematic reviewing studies of diagnostic tests. *Clin Chem Lab Med*. 2000;**38**:577–88.

CHAPTER 11

Producing and using clinical prediction rules

Tom Fahey and Johan van der Lei

Summary box

- Clinical prediction rules (CPRs) are tools that quantify the contribution of symptoms, clinical signs and available diagnostic tests, and in doing so stratify patients according to the probability of having a target disorder.
- CPRs can be used across the range of clinical decision-making diagnosis, prognosis, or therapy.
- A further distinction relates to "prediction" versus "decision" rules. Prediction rules stratify patients according to the probability of a target disorder either in terms of diagnosis or prognosis; decision rules additionally recommend a clinical course of action.
- Application of CPRs is based on Bayesian reasoning and the threshold diagnostic approach.
- Three phases of development of a CPR are necessary before it can be used in clinical practice: development, validation, and clinical impact analysis of the rule.
- There are recognized methodological standards that should be adhered to when developing and validating CPRs.
- At present, most CPRs are at the stage of initial development, fewer have been validated in different populations of patients and fewer still have been subject to impact analysis in broad clinical settings.
- Increasingly decision rules are being linked to computer-based clinical decision support systems (CDSSs) and other Information and Communication Technology (ICT) tools.
- When considering implementation a CPR, clinicians should consider system, physician and patient-related barriers.

The Evidence Base of Clinical Diagnosis: Theory and Methods of Diagnostic Research. 2nd edition.
Edited by J. André Knottnerus and Frank Buntinx. © 2009 Blackwell Publishing,
ISBN: 978-1-4051-5787-2.

Introduction

Clinical prediction rules (CPRs) are tools that quantify the contribution of symptoms, clinical signs and available diagnostic tests, and in doing so stratify patients according to the probability of having a target disorder.[1] The outcome of interest can be diverse and range across the diagnostic, prognostic, and therapeutic spectrum. Furthermore, CPRs have been developed, validated, and used across the primary, secondary, and tertiary care settings. Their value in helping clinicians to "rule in" or "rule out" a target disorder may well depend on the clinical setting in which the CPR is being used. In primary care, ruling out a disorder, providing reassurance, or adopting a "watchful waiting" strategy is more common than in a hospital setting where the emphasis is usually on establishing a firm diagnosis and commencing appropriate treatment. Developing and validating a CPR is a particular form of observational epidemiological research that requires reference to specific methodological standards.[2,3] Conventionally CPRs go through three distinct stages prior to full implementation in a clinical setting: (1) development of the CPR—establishing the independent and combined effect of explanatory variables that can include symptoms, signs or diagnostic tests; (2) narrow and broad validation—where the explanatory variables or clinical predictors in the derivation CPR set are assessed in separate populations; and lastly (3) impact analysis of the CPR—assessed by means of a randomized controlled trial (RCT) where the impact of applying the CPR in a clinical setting is measured either in terms of patient outcome, health professional behavior, resource use or any combination of these outcomes.[1,3] In this chapter, we will discuss CPRs in relation to the clinical context in which they are being used; we will provide a brief clinical overview of selected CPRs summarizing their method of presentation and implementation; we will review the general analytical approach when developing a CPR alongside the methodological challenges of developing, validating and assessing the impact of CPRs; lastly, we will make some tentative suggestions about implementation of CPRs in relation to information and communication technology (ICT) by means of computerized clinical decision support systems (CDSSs) and decision aids (DAs) through the medium of the Electronic Patient Record (EPR). More specific reference to examples of CPRs developed, validated, and implemented in the clinical area of primary prevention of cardiovascular disease will also be made.

Clinical context

The diagnostic framework

Use and application of CPRs is firmly based on probabilistic or Bayesian diagnostic reasoning.[4,5] With this approach, a clinician identifies a plausible target disorder that could be responsible for causing a patient's illness, and then quantifies the uncertainty by going through three cognitive steps: first, estimating the probability of the target disorder being present before any other additional diagnostic information is elicited, an estimation of the pretest probability of the target disorder; secondly, as new clinical information is obtained (from the history and physical examination), it raises or lowers the probability of the target disorder depending on the discriminatory power of each element of the finding from the history and physical examination, quantified in conditional probability terms, usually as a likelihood ratio; thirdly, the revised probability or posttest probability is interpreted in relation to diagnostic probability thresholds. By explicitly quantifying the contribution of an element of the history, physical examination or diagnostic test, CPRs can be readily applied to this diagnostic process.[1,4]

Observational studies have established that by eliciting key findings from the history and physical examination a substantial impact on subsequent diagnosis and management of patients can be made.[6] A rational approach to the clinical examination encourages clinicians to view symptoms and signs as laboratory tests with measurable sensitivities, specificities and predictive powers.[7] CPRs are explicit extensions of this process. The Rational Clinical Examination series, running in *JAMA* since 1992, has produced nearly 60 articles that summarize the literature on various aspects of the clinical examination and draw attention to areas where there is a paucity of evidence. Many of these articles contain summaries of CPRs. Alongside this mapping and summary of the clinical examination literature, the Clinical Assessment of the Reliability of the Examination (CARE) interest group has formed to design and run large, simple studies of the accuracy and precision of the clinical examination (see recommended websites).[8]

Error in the heuristics of decision making and their influence on CPRs

Heuristics are strategies that people learn or adopt when making decisions, coming to judgments, or solving problems, typically when facing complex problems or incomplete information. Heuristics work well under most circumstances, but in certain cases lead to systematic cognitive biases. These biases have been studied in the context of diagnostic decision making, so also influence diagnostic decision making when CPRs are being used as part of the diagnostic process. These biases may affect the use and implementation of CPRs in the following ways:

- Pretest probability—Estimates of pretest probability are dependent on previous clinical experience and the setting of clinical care that a clinician has been working in. Patients in secondary or tertiary care have higher proportions of more serious disease or more uncommon disease than in primary care settings, and this clinical experience influences the pretest probability estimates of clinicians.[9] However, when asked, clinicians can have surprisingly divergent estimates of pretest probability for the same patient, for example estimates of pretest probability for pulmonary embolism in a single patient varied from 5% to 80% in a group of hospital clinicians.[10] Explanations for divergent estimates may relate to clinician experience or expertise though recent studies show that medical expertise was not associated with closer estimates of pretest probability.[11] It is more likely that divergence in pretest probability relates to known errors in estimation of probability. These errors include availability bias—overestimating the frequency of vivid or easily recalled events; representativeness bias—estimating the probability of disease by judging how similar it is to a diagnostic category thereby confusing test sensitivity with posttest probability. For instance the symptom of cough is often present with pneumonia but the probability of pneumonia with cough as the only symptom is not high; support bias—overestimating probability in case of more explicit and detailed descriptions of a patient.[12] In the context of clinical encounters in primary care, pretest probability estimates have been published for common presenting symptoms such as cough, shortness of breath, general weakness/tiredness based on "reasons for encounter" in a Dutch national study of 267,897 patient encounters.[13] Knowledge and usage of such pretest probability estimates would avoid some of the cognitive biases in pretest probability estimation.

- Integrations and estimation of posttest probability errors in revision of probability can occur in several ways: anchoring and adjustment—posttest probabilities being sensitive to the starting point and the shift in probability needed to reach diagnostic certainty; order—when diagnostic information given later is given more weight; as well as errors in data interpretation. CPRs have the potential to overcome these heuristic biases, particularly if integrated and implemented by means of computerized clinical decision support systems (CDSSs).[14]

Thresholds approach to diagnosis

As part of the clinical application of CPRs the probabilistic approach to diagnostic reasoning is combined with the threshold approach to diagnosis.[15] Further action in relation to the posttest probability estimates depends on whether or not the posttest probability is above two different thresholds- the test-treatment threshold or the test threshold (Figure 11.1).[15] If the posttest probability is above the test-treatment threshold, a diagnosis is made and a management plan, including an assessment of the risks and benefits of treatment, for the target condition can be started. If the posttest probability falls below the test threshold, the patient is either reassured, alternative diagnoses are pursued, or a "watchful waiting" practice adopted. If the posttest probability falls between these thresholds into an intermediate range, then further diagnostic testing is continued until the posttest probability is revised and is either above the test-treatment threshold or below the test threshold (Figure 1.11).[9,15,16] In the context of using clinical prediction rules, a key issue relates to the value placed on what is felt to be a clinically important and cost effective intermediate testing range.[17] This is not a statistical issue but a matter of clinical judgment that relates to the seriousness of the target condition, the treatment options available, as well as the cost, availability and side effects of diagnostic tests.[17] Once diagnostic thresholds have been quantified, it is then

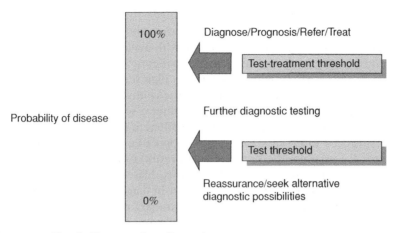

Figure 11.1 Threshold approach to diagnosis.

possible to recognize situations in terms of pre-test probability where testing is useful (intermediate range of probability) or less useful (very low or very high pre-test probability).[17] As a further reflection on the inherent nature of diagnostic uncertainty, it has been shown that overreliance on the value of applying tests that are highly sensitive (*Sen*sitive test that is *N*egative helps to rule *out* the diagnosis, or SnNout) or tests that are highly specific (*Sp*ecific test that is *P*ositive serves to rule in the diagnosis, or SpPin) symptoms, signs or diagnostic tests may not be as reliable as initially assumed.[5,18] Ideally, uncertainty when applying apparently highly sensitive or specific tests and converting to posttest probabilities should be conveyed by estimating post test probability with a 95% confidence interval around the estimate. The subsequent step of applying the estimated posttest probability and its 95% confidence interval is then judged against diagnostic thresholds (Figure 11.1).

When making clinical diagnoses it is likely that clinicians implement different but complementary approaches simultaneously: applying the probabilistic approach alongside consideration of all potential diagnoses on a differential diagnosis list (the possibilistic approach) as well as considering more serious conditions that if left untreated would have a major impact on a patient's prognosis (the severity approach).[9] Indeed the approach of matching probability with severity underpins the more formalized approach of decision analysis.[19] Furthermore, application of diagnostic tests depend on whether a clinician is attempting to definitively "rule in" a diagnosis—choosing a diagnostic test of high specificity / positive likelihood ratios much greater than one—often the case in secondary or tertiary care settings or whether the clinician is more concerned about "ruling out" a diagnosis—choosing a diagnostic test with high sensitivity / negative likelihood ratio much smaller than one—often the case in primary care settings.[9] Application of diagnostic tests is always context specific;[20] for instance, in low prevalence settings or in situations of screening,

ideal diagnostic tests would be highly sensitive—those patients testing negative could be confidently assured that they are without disease but would also
be highly specific—low false positive rate with avoidance of iatrogenic harm
from further diagnostic testing in healthy patients. Unfortunately, few single
diagnostic tests perform with simultaneous high sensitivity and specificity.[21]
A further word of caution is required in the context of applying the results
of diagnostic tests developed in different clinical settings to which they are
applied. Spectrum bias (population with a different clinical spectrum, usually
more advanced cases) or selection bias (population of patients included on
the basis of a prior positive or negative test result) can produce diagnostic test
estimates of higher sensitivity and specificity, biased measured of test accuracy. These biases are particularly apparent in diagnostic tests developed in
secondary care and applied to patients in primary care.[21,22] Last, aside from
diagnostic or prognostic considerations, other contextual issues in relation to
the application of CPRs will influence clinical behavior. Patient related factors, such as the acceptability and side effects of the diagnostic test; physician
related factors, such as fear of litigation; and organizational factors, such as
availability of diagnostic tests, will all influence clinical decision making and
may modify the use, application and interpretation of CPRs.[20]

Description and coverage of clinical prediction rules

Identification of CPRs is a challenge for several reasons Firstly, there are relatively few CPRs in quantity when compared to other types of study designs
posted in major online clinical literature databases, with only a fraction being
of high quality. Secondly, there is a plurality of terminology associated with
CPRs and there is a lack of standardized controlled indexing vocabulary assigned to CPR studies which makes extraction from large clinical literature
databases difficult.[23,24] Fortunately, search filters have been developed for the
retrieval of higher quality CPRs when searching the MEDLINE and EMBASE
clinical literature databases.[23-25]

CPRs have been developed across a broad range of health care areas. Three
reviews have summarized the CPRs published in four general medical journals
(*New England Journal of Medicine, Journal of the American Medical Association,
British Medical Journal*, and *Annals of Internal Medicine*) in three separate time
periods—1981–1984,[26] 1991–1994,[2] and 2000–2003.[27] During this time, the
absolute number of CPRs has not substantially increased, though there is a
greater number of studies reporting on validation rather than derivation of a
rule.[27] Table 11.1 provides some examples of CPRs, showing the stage of their
development and the clinical area covered.

Most CPRs function at the level of providing probabilistic information for
a target disorder usually in the form of a risk score or clinical algorithm that
stratifies individuals into different categories of risk.[27] As will be discussed,
implementation of CPRs involves transformation from prediction estimates
in the format of probability calculations, to decision rules in the format of

Table 11.1 Clinical prediction rules—some examples and format

Clinical area	Description of CPR	Recommendation and format	Stage of development of CPR
Red eye[52]	Population: adults presenting to their general practitioner with symptom of "red eye" Predictors: self reported medical history, symptoms, physical examination Reference standard: bacterial culture from each eye	Independent predictors of positive bacterial culture Clinical score converted into probability of positive bacterial culture	Development
Acute coronary syndrome[53]	Population: adults presenting to hospital admission with acute coronary syndrome (MI or unstable angina) Predictors: age, medical history, symptoms, physical examination, biomarkers, and ECG findings Reference standard: death and myocardial infarction at 6-month follow-up	Eight independent predictors of death or myocardial infarction Web-based nomogram calculating probability of in-hospital death or MI or at 6-month follow-up	Development and validation in a separate patient population
Vaginal birth after previous cesarean section[54]	Population: Pregnant women with one prior cesarean section who attempted vaginal birth at or after 40 weeks gestation Predictors: maternal age, height, previous vaginal birth, gestation at delivery, method of induction, fetal gender Reference standard: risk of emergency cesarean section and risk of intrapartum uterine rupture	Independent predictors of emergency cesarean section or intrapartum uterine rupture Adjusted log likelihood ratios converted into probability of cesarean section	Development and validation groups randomly split from the same national cohort

(continued)

Table 11.1 (*continued.*)

Clinical area	Description of CPR	Recommendation and format	Stage of development of CPR
4-year mortality in older adults[55]	Population: community-dwelling adults older than 50 years Predictors: demographic characteristics, specific comorbidities and functional measures Reference standard: death at 4-year follow-up	Independent predictors of 4-year mortality Clinical score converted into probability of 4-year mortality	Development in the east, west, and central population and validation in the southern population of a national cohort
Risk of stroke after transient ischemic attack (TIA)[56]	Population: patients diagnosed with TIA and reviewed in emergency departments and outpatient clinics in the U.K. or U.S. within one week of TIA Predictors: ABCD^2 score-age, blood pressure, clinical features, duration, diabetes Reference standard: assessment by neurologist of stroke (including medical record and imaging report)	Independent predictors of 2, 7, or 90 days stroke risk Clinical score converted into probability of stroke risk	Two separate development cohorts in U.K. and U.S.; four validation cohorts; overall ABCD^2 was derived from both derivation groups for 2-day stroke risk
Hip fracture[57]	Population: women aged $\geq$70 years in three rural populations in Sweden Predictors: FRAMO index(age $\geq$80 years, weight <60 kg, previous fragility fracture, need to use arms when rising from sitting position) Reference standard: hip-fracture, other fragility fracture (radiography reports), all cause mortality (national Swedish Population Register)	Independent predictors of 2-year hip fracture, fragility fracture and mortality Clinical score converted into probability of 2-year hip or fragility fracture, or all cause mortality	Derivation and applied to same total population

categorized clinical recommendations.[27] Table 11.1 shows that CPRs at the stage of development or validation usually frame their recommendations in probabilistic terms.

Methodological challenges

Analytical approach

A multivariable approach, usually in the form of logistic regression analysis assessing the presence of absence of the target disorder, enables the development of CPRs that take into account different sources of diagnostic or prognostic information: general patient characteristics (age, gender, social class), past medical history, presenting symptoms, physical examination findings, laboratory or other diagnostic data and in some clinical situations medication data.[17] The independent "weights" of these sources of data—in the form of logistic regression coefficients as the natural logarithms of the odds ratios for the presence of each predictor in the CPR—allow the calculation of post-probabilities for a target disorder when applied to individual patients.[3,17] Predicted posttest probabilities on the scale of 0% to 100% are generated. In terms of assessment of the performance of the CPR, these predicted posttest probabilities (equivalent to the test–treatment threshold in Figure 11.1) are compared against the observed classification according to the diagnostic or gold standard applied to the study population. This allows the CPR to be assessed like a conventional diagnostic test, generating the sensitivity, specificity, likelihood ratios and odds ratios at a particular disease threshold. By varying the disease threshold a receiver operating characteristic (ROC) curve for a CPR can be generated, allowing comparison between different combinations of symptoms, signs and diagnostic tests, using the area under the curve (AUC) as a summary measure for the overall predictive power of each CPR.[17] The cut-point chosen for a disease threshold is condition and context-specific and depends on the consequence of possible classification errors.

Methodological standards and levels of evidence

There is a recognized hierarchy of evidence when developing, validating, and evaluating the clinical impact of clinical prediction rules. Figure 11.2 shows these three stages and links these stages to four levels of evidence to the application of a CPR in clinical care.[1,3] A recent reviews suggest that impact analysis should be divided into narrow and broad impact, making five levels of evidence before a clinical prediction rule can be used with confidence in diverse clinical settings (Figure 11.2).[27] Currently, there is a dichotomy between the recommended level of evidence and the actual number of CPRs that have reached the highest level of evidence. Three review papers have mapped out the number of CPRs published in the same four general medical journals over the last 21 years,[2,26,27] the absolute number of CPRs has not changed substantially, 36 in 1985 up to 41 in 2006. In 1985, 55% of published CPRs were

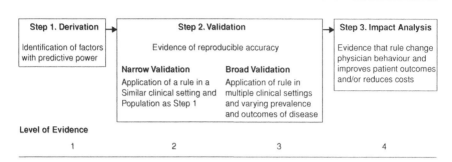

Figure 11.2 Stages in the development, validation and impact analysis of a Clinical Prediction Rule, with corresponding levels of evidence. Adapted from McGinn *et al.*[3]

still at Level 1 (derivation), while in 2006, 63% of published CPRs were concerned with narrow or broad validation (Levels 2 and 3).[27] Clinicians can still extract clinically relevant messages from developed CPRs, noting the most important predictors and consider giving less importance to variables that show less predictive power.[3] For example, in a CPR developed but not validated in children with acute cough, presence of fever and chest signs raised the probability of future reconsultation or complications. These predictors might play a role in differentiating those children who require more careful follow-up or who might benefit from antibiotic treatment to prevent complications,[28] but caution is required in uncritically applying these clinical predictors without broad validation of the CPR. External validation of a CPR for the presence of serious bacterial infection in children that initially showed good discrimination, area under the receiver-operating characteristic curve (AUROC) 0.83 fell on external validation to 0.57. In terms of calibration, prediction of low risk categories in the development model corresponded poorly with the observed level of risk in the validated model.[29]

Derivation

Diagnostic studies with methodological flaws tend to overestimate the accuracy of diagnostic tests.[30] Examples of biases associated with diagnostic accuracy studies include: spectrum bias, where the selection of patients is not representative of patients seen in usual clinical care, leading to exaggeration of sensitivity (test is developed in patients with serious or advanced disease) or specificity (test is developed in healthy subjects);[21] partial verification bias, where a reference test is not applied consistently to confirm the negative findings of the symptom, signs, or index test, leading to overestimation of sensitivity and underestimation of specificity or overestimation of both sensitivity and specificity; and incorporation bias, when the test under evaluation is also part of the reference standard, leading to overestimation of test accuracy as the experimental and reference test are no longer independent.[18,30]

Table 11.2 Methodological standards for Derivation and Validation of a Clinical Prediction Rule[3]

Derivation
1. Were all important predictors included in the derivation process?
2. Were all predictors present in a significant proportion of the study population?
3. Were all the outcome events and predictors clearly defined?
4. Were those assessing the outcome event blinded to the presence of the predictors and those assessing the presence of predictors blinded to the outcome event?
5. Was the sample size adequate (including adequate number of outcome events)?
6. Does the rule make clinical sense?

Validation
1. Were the patients chosen in an unbiased fashion and do they represent a wide spectrum of severity of disease?
2. Was there a blinded assessment of the criterion standard for all patients?
3. Was there an explicit and accurate interpretation of the predictor variables and the actual rule without knowledge of the outcome.
4. Was there 100% follow-up of those enrolled?

The methodological standards applied in the derivation of a CPR (Table 11.2), incorporate checks that address these and other biases. Like diagnostic test methodological standards,[30,31] failure to adhere to these criteria are likely to introduce biases that inflate the diagnostic accuracy of a developed CPR.[3]

Validation

Validation is the next key component when translating a CPR into clinical practice.[27] In the best circumstances, broad validation of a CPR (Level 3) involves application of the CPR to a new population with a different prevalence and spectrum of disease. However, in many instances because of constraints in time, opportunity and funding, narrow validation (Level 2) of applying the CPR in a similar clinical setting might be the best that can be achieved. Key issues include making sure that the CPR performs similarly in different populations when used by different clinicians who apply the CPR in routine clinical care in similar clinical settings.[3] Methodological standards for validation enable stronger inference concerning the robustness of the validation procedure to be made;[3] these standards are summarized in Table 11.2.

Reasons why validation is unsuccessful may be due to several underlying reasons. Chance effects can occur in smaller studies where a different set of predictor variables emerge in a different population of patients.[3] Several different forms of bias can occur. Selection in terms of the population may result in predictors being idiosyncratic to each selected population. More subtle biases occur in relation to CPRs that incorporate or involve prior diagnostic testing or referral procedures. Interaction bias occurs when CPRs developed in one setting, for instance secondary care are validated in another setting, such as primary care.[17] The methodological standards adopted for validation studies address these issues of chance, blinding of predictors and outcome as well adequate follow-up in the validation population.[3,17]

Predictive accuracy of a derived CPR can be assessed in two complementary ways: calibration and discrimination.[32] Calibration refers to whether the predicted probabilities agree with the observed probabilities. In terms of assessing calibration, if the predicted risk of an individual or a group of individuals is the same as the observed risk, then the model is perfectly calibrated or 100% reliable. Calibration is usually quantified by the ratio of predicted to observed outcome. Calibration can be graphically displayed with a calibration curve that plots predicted versus observed outcomes at pre-determined categories of risk and is assessed by the Hosmer–Lemeshow goodness-of-fit test.[32–34] Discrimination describes how well the CPR separates individuals who have or will get the disease outcome from with those that remain disease-free. Discrimination is typically measured by using the area under the AUROC. This area ranges from 1 (100%) representing perfect discrimination to 0.5 (50%) representing discrimination being no better than chance. For binary outcomes (which is how CPRs are usually represented as having or not having the target disorder), a validation model is evaluated by measuring the C statistic, which in this situation is identical to the AUROC (larger values indicate better discrimination).[32–34]

Clinical example-validation studies of primary prevention of cardiovascular disease

Assessment of cardiovascular disease (CVD) risk, based on the Framingham risk function was initially proposed in the early 1990s in response to the unreliability of preventing cardiovascular disease by means of single risk factor assessment.[35] In this instance, prognosis concerning future cardiovascular events (stroke or myocardial infarction) is quantified and estimated by means of multivariable risk assessment—a form of dia-prognostic research.[22] Multivariable risk assessment methods enables clinicians to combine risk factor information from their patients and calculate the risk that their patient will have a cardiovascular event within a specified time period.[36] This is important as the relative benefit of a risk-reducing treatment is generally equivalent across levels of risk, meaning the absolute benefit of the intervention is proportional to the absolute risk of the individual.[35] If the absolute risk of the patient is high, then the absolute benefits of risk reduction are also going to be high. If the absolute risk of disease is low, then any extra benefit from risk-reducing interventions will also be low and possible harms of the treatment may out-weight these small benefits. Consequently, effective targeting of resources is enhanced by identifying individuals at higher levels of absolute risk. The absolute risk charts developed from the multivariable risk functions are developed CPRs whereby each individual's predicted absolute risk can be calculated and treatment recommendation be made. Examples of three different cardiovascular risk functions are provided in the appendix, each being derived from different populations of patients.

In the context of levels of evidence, the Framingham risk is the currently recommended CPR used for the primary prevention of cardiovascular disease in the United Kingdom. Like any CPR, this derived rule requires narrow and broad validation.[3,27] The initial study assessed narrow validation by applying the Framingham risk function to a representative sample of 7735 men aged 40–59 years (at entry in 1978–1980) in 24 U.K. towns—the British Regional Heart Study (BRHS).[33] The risk of coronary heart disease (CHD) mortality over a 10-year period for each of the BRHS men free of cardiovascular disease and with complete risk factor information were calculated using the appropriate Framingham equations. The men were categorized into groups defined by quintiles of Framingham risk, systolic blood pressure, total to HDL cholesterol ratio and age. The average predicted event risk within each quintile for both endpoints was compared with the observed 10-year rates.[33]

Applying the CHD mortality equation to each of the men in the BRHS, the predicted number of CHD deaths within 10 years was 270 (4.1%) compared with an observed CHD death rate of 183 (2.8%) over the first 10 years of follow-up. Figure 11.3 shows predicted and observed CHD mortality rates across a range of risk factor levels (according to the quintiles of Framingham risk, systolic blood pressure, total to HDL cholesterol and age). The relative overprediction of CHD mortality risk by 47% (was similar for individuals at all baseline risk levels so that overprediction of absolute risk was greatest for individuals at highest risk. The relative overprediction was approximately constant at all levels of risk so it was possible to recalibrate and correct the predicted Framingham scores by dividing the calculated score for each individual by the amount of relative overprediction. Recalibrated probabilities of CHD death were obtained from the 10-year CHD predictions by dividing the final score by 1.47. After this correction the predicted risk became very close to the observed at all levels of risk with a substantial decrease in the chi-squared statistic for goodness-of-fit from 30.2 to 3.4.[33]

On the basis of this single, narrow validation study which represents Level 2 evidence, a systematic review of 27 other validation studies of the Framingham risk function in 71,727 patients was performed in order to assess the issue of broader validation.[37] Figure 11.4 summarizes the finding of predicted versus observed 10-year risk for CHD or CVD when the Framingham risk function is applied to different populations by means of an overall ratio of predicted to observed risk. Over or under-prediction is clearly related to the baseline or background risk of CHD or CVD in each population studied. CHD predicted to observed ratios ranged from an under-prediction of 0.43 (95% confidence interval 0.27 to 0.67) in a high risk population to an overprediction of 2.87 (95% confidence interval 1.91 to 4.31) in a lower risk population (Figure 11.4).[37]

These two examples of narrow (level 2 evidence) and broad (level 3 evidence) validation of the Framingham risk function shows that uncritical

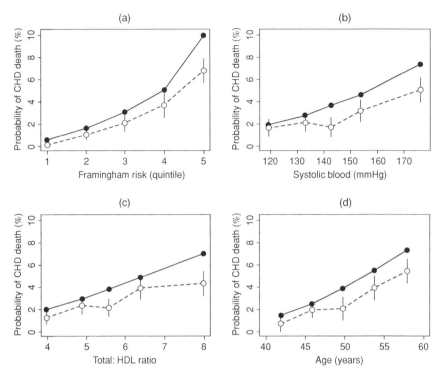

Figure 11.3 Narrow validation (Level 2 evidence) of the Framingham risk function in the British Regional Heart Study cohort. Adapted from Brindle *et al.*[33] Ten-year predicted (black) versus observed CHD death rates (white) by quintile of (a) Framingham risk, (b) systolic blood pressure, (c) total to HDL cholesterol ratio and (d) age.

application without reference to the background level of CHD or CVD risk is likely to produce over or under estimation of the true cardiovascular risk for an individual patient. Recalibration is worthwhile but requires knowledge of the background CVD/CHD risk in the population to which the CPR is to be applied. Background risk can also vary within a country as well as between countries.[33] More recent CPRs for the primary prevention of cardiovascular disease are based on larger, more representative populations,[38,39] or have focused on specific sub-groups of patients such as women.[34]

Impact analysis

Despite these efforts to summaries the literature on the value of the clinical examination, use, and application of CPRs in clinical practice is not well developed. Though the discriminatory power of symptoms and signs are identified as key components of effective clinical care, relatively little research has

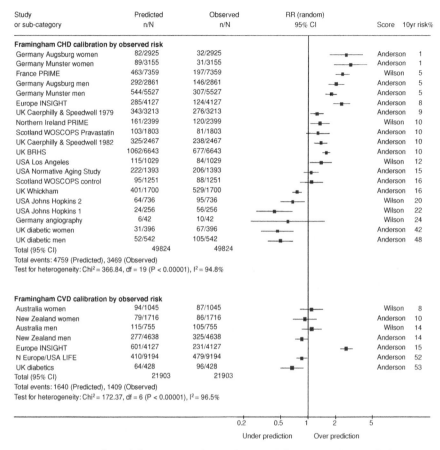

Study or sub-category	Predicted n/N	Observed n/N	RR (random) 95% CI	Score	10yr risk%
Framingham CHD calibration by observed risk					
Germany Augsburg women	82/2925	32/2925		Anderson	1
Germany Munster women	89/3155	31/3155		Anderson	1
France PRIME	463/7359	197/7359		Wilson	5
Germany Augsburg men	292/2861	146/2861		Anderson	5
Germany Munster men	544/5527	307/5527		Anderson	5
Europe INSIGHT	285/4127	124/4127		Anderson	8
UK Caerphilly & Speedwell 1979	343/3213	276/3213		Anderson	9
Northern Ireland PRIME	161/2399	120/2399		Wilson	10
Scotland WOSCOPS Pravastatin	103/1803	81/1803		Anderson	10
UK Caerphilly & Speedwell 1982	325/2467	238/2467		Anderson	10
UK BRHS	1062/6643	677/6643		Anderson	10
USA Los Angeles	115/1029	84/1029		Wilson	12
USA Normative Aging Study	222/1393	206/1393		Anderson	15
Scotland WOSCOPS control	95/1251	88/1251		Anderson	16
UK Whickham	401/1700	529/1700		Anderson	16
USA Johns Hopkins 2	64/736	95/736		Wilson	20
USA Johns Hopkins 1	24/256	56/256		Wilson	22
Germany angiography	6/42	10/42		Wilson	24
UK diabetic women	31/396	67/396		Anderson	42
UK diabetic men	52/542	105/542		Anderson	48
Total (95% CI)	49824	49824			
Total events: 4759 (Predicted), 3469 (Observed)					
Test for heterogeneity: Chi² = 366.84, df = 19 (P < 0.00001), I² = 94.8%					
Framingham CVD calibration by observed risk					
Australia women	94/1045	87/1045		Wilson	8
New Zealand women	79/1716	86/1716		Anderson	10
Australia men	115/755	105/755		Wilson	14
New Zealand men	277/4638	325/4638		Anderson	14
Europe INSIGHT	601/4127	231/4127		Anderson	15
N Europe/USA LIFE	410/9194	479/9194		Anderson	52
UK diabetics	64/428	96/428		Anderson	53
Total (95% CI)	21903	21903			
Total events: 1640 (Predicted), 1409 (Observed)					
Test for heterogeneity: Chi² = 172.37, df = 6 (P < 0.00001), I² = 96.5%					

```
              0.2      0.5    1      2      5
              Under prediction    Over prediction
```

Figure 11.4 Broader validation* (Level 3 evidence) of the Framingham risk function in cohort studies. Adapted from Brindle *et al.*[37]
Predicted to observed ratio of Framingham risk scores, ordered by increasing observed 10-year risk (%) in the validation populations.
   CHD, fatal and nonfatal coronary heart disease; CVD, cardiovascular disease; composite of fatal and nonfatal stroke or myocardial infarction.

reported on the use and application of CPRs in real-time clinical practice. For instance, several CPRs have been developed and validated using the presence of group A β-hemolytic streptococcal pharyngitis (sore throat) as the reference standard.[40] These CPRs include symptoms and signs such as history or measured fever, absence of cough, presence of tender cervical lymphadenopathy, tonsillar exudate and age of the patient.[40] Impact analysis of this rule in the context of a randomized controlled trial using chart stickers that prompted use and scoring of a sore throat CPR made no difference to the prescribing of unnecessary antibiotics or overall antibiotic use.[41]

The lack of impact analysis studies has been attributed to the fact that a transition is needed when assessing a CPR's impact on clinical care: changing a rule from estimates about the likely probability of a target disorder to recommendations about clinical care.[27] In addition, the methodological approach of impact analysis—experimental research requiring randomized comparison groups, differs from the methodological approach for derivation and validation of a prediction rule—observational research assessing and validating the independent predictive effects of clinical and diagnostic variables.[17,27] Lastly, clarity about the purpose of applying a CPR in clinical practice is required. Modifying practitioner performance is an intermediate step in relation to a change in patient outcome. Clear linkage is required between the probability estimates generated from a CPR and subsequent recommendations concerning management and therapy. Evidence from RCTs assessing the impact of the Framingham risk function illustrates the importance of linkage between probability estimates and clinical recommendations.

Current evidence from impact analysis studies of primary prevention of cardiovascular disease

A systematic review identified four randomized controlled trials that assessed the impact of the using the Framingham risk function in the primary prevention of cardiovascular disease.[37] In all RCTs, the intervention was formatted as paper-based cardiovascular risk charts categorizing individuals into 5-year cardiovascular risk categories. None of the RCTs translated this probabilistic information into clinical recommendations concerning treatment. One RCT compared two intervention arms—card-based and computer-based cardiovascular risk information—but only in terms of probabilistic information and not in terms of decision recommendations.[42] For all RCTs, the objective was to improve the intermediate outcomes of either lowering blood pressure or cholesterol, or increasing the intensity of drug therapy. All four RCTs did not show significant improvements in blood pressure or cholesterol, or in the intensification of drug treatment as a consequence of using the Framingham risk function in a chart format.[37]

For successful implementation of CPR, consideration should be given to several factors. First, framing of the rule requires transformation from prediction estimates framed as probability calculations, to a decision rule framed as categorized clinical recommendations.[27] The format in which the CPR is implemented—in an electronic format, ideally as part of a CDSS, requires integration with the electronic patient record (EPR). Lastly, several physician-related barriers have been identified that occur before, during and after the establishment of a CPR that require ongoing monitoring and performance assessment of the CPR in usual clinical practice.[27] Examples of these concerns include skepticism concerning recommendations of the CPR, medicolegal, and patient safety concerns, and lack of understanding and poor infrastructure to maintain the use of the CPR. What is clear is that simple provision of the CPR without adequate integration and ongoing support is likely to be insufficient

Table 11.3 Barriers and strategies to the effective implementation of clinical prediction rules (Adapted from Reilly *et al.* and Kawamoto *et al.*[27,43])

Barrier	Strategy
Physician related	
Introduction phase: skepticism, distrust, or disinterest	Enable discretionary use of CPR but involve physicians in development and validation, and collect data on how CPR could facilitate and aid physician's tasks
During use: failure to use CPR consistently and accurately	Track usage and provide feedback about impact on patient outcomes
After establishment of CPR: complaints not easy to use or poorly integrated	Develop as a CDSS, monitor usage and modify as appropriate involving users
System related	
Framing: probability estimates	Provide linkage to explicit clinical recommendation according to strata of risk based on CPR
Format: paper-based format	Integrate with electronic patient record; provide patient-specific advice as part of usual clinical activity
Usage	Provide as a CDSS or as a PDA, monitor usage and provide information on patient outcome
Patient related	
Concerns about lack of input from patient's	Modify CDSS to incorporate patient preferences in the form of a decision aid

to change clinical practice and alter patient outcome. Strategies to ensure ongoing implementation need to be considered and addressed (Table 11.3).[27]

Future implementation of CPRs—the electronic patient record and computerized clinical decision support systems (CDSSs)

CDSSs are information systems designed to improve clinical decision making. The underlying structure of a CDSS requires electronic, patient-specific data linked to a computerized knowledge base that provides patient-specific treatment recommendations via an algorithm.[14] Some CDSSs may require interaction between the system and the clinician. The clinician initiates a dialogue with the system and provides it with data by entering symptoms or answering questions. This has been the usual way in which the predictors for a CPR are entered into a CDSS to produce the probabilistic information on diagnosis or prognosis. Unfortunately, experience has shown that the acceptance of this type of CDSS by clinicians can be relatively low. Other systems are integrated with electronic medical records, and use the data in them as input.

In such settings, receiving decision support requires little or no additional data input on the part of the clinician. Some of the information generated for the Framingham risk equations operates at this level. Finally, some systems are directly connected to the devices that generate the data, for example, systems that interpret ECGs or laboratory data.

By applying the medical knowledge to the patient data, the CDSS generates patient-specific advice. Some CDSSs, especially those integrated with the electronic medical record; provide advice independent of a clinician's request for it—unsolicited advice. Examples are reminding systems that continuously screen patient data for conditions that should be brought to the clinician's attention (e.g., the patient's kidney function is decreasing, or the patient is eligible for preventive screening). Other systems, such as critiquing systems, may monitor the decisions of the clinician and report deviations from guidelines. The previously mentioned RCTs of CPRs using the Framingham risk function did generate patient-specific information concerning cardiovascular risk but did not translate this information into categorized clinical recommendations concerning drug treatment.[37]

Evidence from a systematic review of 64 RCTs of CDSSs shows improvements in practitioner performance compared to usual clinical care in terms of diagnostic systems, reminder systems, disease management systems and drug-dosing or monitoring systems. The effects on patient outcome are less well studied with current results being inconsistent.[14] A further review critiqued the elements of clinical decision support systems that were more likely to improve clinical practice.[43] They found several features that were closely linked to decision support systems' ability to improve patient care: automatic provision of decision support as part of clinical workload; provision of recommendations rather than just assessments; provision of decision support at the time and location of decision making; and computer based decision support.[43] CPRs are well suited to integration into a computer-based format with linkage to patient-specific advice using evidence-based clinical algorithms. Indeed, many of the Rational Clinical Examination Series guides summarize their recommendation as an algorithm with categorized clinical recommendations linked to risk categories. Figure 11.5 illustrates this approach in the management of urinary tract infection.

If a CDSS platform is used to implement a CPR, important methodological standards have been developed that relate to the validity of the CDSS in relation to integration and implementation of a CPR.[44] Particular attention is focused on the function of the CDSS with a range of possibilities that include prediction and diagnosis which may or may not be linked to assisting (tailoring recommendations) or suggesting (generating suggestions) roles. Also important is the application of a CDSS into the clinical setting it is to be used.[44]

Future developments
In the future, integration of CPRs into CDSSs or into personal digital assistants (PDAs) will require explicit linkage of probabilistic information into evidence-based clinical recommendations. Information and communication

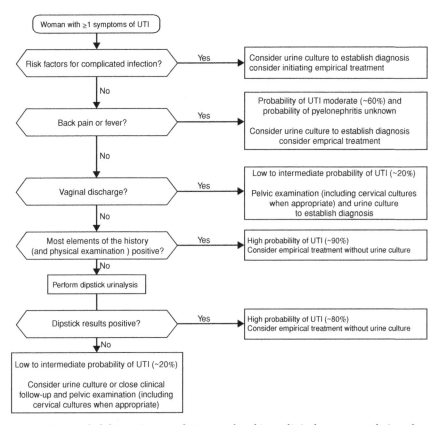

Figure 11.5 Probability estimates of UTI translated into clinical recommendations for the management of UTI. Adapted from Bent *et al.*[51]

technology (ICT) is increasingly popular amongst medical students and many medical schools deliver their curriculum through a virtual learning environment (VLEs). The next generation of doctors will be using ICT largely in daily clinical practice. Already PDAs program CPRs so as to estimate the probability of adverse events or complications for specific clinical conditions, for instance the risk of life-threatening complications or death in patients with acute pancreatitis.[45]

Alongside technological developments, an increase in morbidity coding will lead to a larger database of CPRs. For instance, a CPR could be triggered by entry of a specific morbidity code, prompting the health professional to input key elements of history, clinical examination finding and diagnostic test and producing recommendations concerning the prior probability and posttest probability for a target disorder. As previously discussed, probabilistic diagnostic information can be incorporated with patient-specific therapeutic recommendations in the form of a CDSS. Application of CPRs in clinical practice will require more flexible modeling for alternative differential diagnoses as well as for specific patient profiles or subgroups of patients.[17] Other analytical approaches such as "neural networks" will require evaluation, measured alongside conventional regression modeling and evaluation of usual clinical practice.[17] Lastly, patient's preferences concerning the optimal level of diagnostic certainty as well as the trade-offs between further diagnostic investigation versus iatrogenic harm, will require more sophisticated modelling of individual preferences using ICT. Decision analysis has the potential to model preferences alongside individualized probabilities derived from CPRs. For example a decision analysis decision aid (DA) was able to quantify cardiovascular risk and integrate patients' values so that individual treatment preferences about anti-hypertensive drug therapy could be made.[46] It is possible to produce patient-specific recommendations, incorporating each patient's individual preferences, into a format so that patients can become co-decision makers with health professionals. All these developments will require more powerful and sophisticated ICT tools embedded in each patient's EPR.

Conclusions

High-quality CPRs remain relatively uncommon in the medical literature.[27] However, we appear to be at the start of a new era in diagnostic research,[47] and progress in relation to the development, validation and impact analysis assessment of CPRs should be viewed within the broader context of this expanding field (Figure 11.2). The Cochrane Collaboration now includes systematic reviews of diagnostic accuracy studies in the Cochrane Library. This is likely to drive further methodology standards adopted in the conduct and reporting of individual diagnostic accuracy studies,[48] and in systematic reviews of diagnostic accuracy studies.[49]

Key issues to consider when putting a CPR to use in a clinical setting relate to the stage of development in its use and corresponding level of evidence (Figure 11.2). Knowledge of the required standards in terms of development and validation of a CPR is thus required (Table 11.2). Few CPRs have been broadly validated in relation to their impact on clinical care,[27] so wide dissemination and usage of CPRs is unlikely to occur in the near future. However, with developments in ICT, integration of CPRs into clinical databases is likely to be more commonplace and knowledge of the stages of CPR development alongside the level of evidence is becoming core clinical knowledge for health professionals. Implementation of CPRs is likely to take place alongside modification and refinements in CDSSs for health professionals and decision aids for patients. Unless practicing clinicians understand the methodological issues involved in the development, validation, and impact analysis of CPRs, they are likely to be misled by apparently simple but potentially biased CPRs, which have been integrated uncritically into ICT software programs. Last, if CPRs are to be used in clinical practice, developers of CPRs need to be aware of the barriers and solutions to the full implementation of CPRs in terms of clinicians, patients and the healthcare system involved (Table 11.3).

Recommended key references

Books
- Black ER, Bordley DR, Tape TG, *et al.*, eds. *Diagnostic strategies for common medical problems.* Philadelphia: American College of Physicians; 1999.
- Ebell MH. *Evidence-based diagnosis: a handbook of clinical prediction rules.* New York: Springer-Verlag; 2001.
- Guyatt GH, Rennie DR. *Users' guides to the medical literature: a manual for evidence-based clinical practice.* Chicago: American Medical Association Press; 2002.

Websites
- Clinical Assessment of the Reliability of the Examination (CARE): http://www.carestudy.com/CareStudy/Default.asp
- Centre for Evidence Based Medicine: http://www.cebm.net/
- Mount Sinai site for clinical prediction rules: http://www.mssm.edu/medicine/general-medicine/ebm/#cpr
- Rational Clinical Examination series—1998 to present: http://jama.ama-assn.org/cgi/collection/rational_clinical_exam

Examples of Cardiovascular risk functions

- Cardiovascular risk score based on the Framingham risk function: http://www.nhlbi.nih.gov/about/framingham/index.html
- Cardiovascular risk score based on the Framingham risk function and modified as the Joint British Societies Cardiovascular Disease Risk Prediction Chart:
  http://www.bhsoc.org/Cardiovascular_Risk_Charts_and_Calculators.stm
- Cardiovascular risk score based on eight randomized controlled trials of antihypertensive treatment in North American and Europe:[50] http://www.riskscore.org.uk/
- Cardiovascular risk score based on 12 European cohort studies: the SCORE risk charts:[38]
  http://www.escardio.org/initiatives/prevention/prevention-tools/SCORE-Risk-Charts.htm

A more recent review article suggests that Impact analysis should be further sub-divided into:[27]
- Narrow impact analysis: prospective demonstration in one setting that use of CPR improves physician behaviour, patient outcome and/or reduces costs (Level 4)
- Broad impact analysis: prospective demonstration in varied settings that use of CPR improves physician behaviour, patient outcome and/or reduces costs for a wide spectrum of patients (Level 5).

References

1. McGinn T, Guyatt G, Wyer P, et al. Diagnosis: clinical prediction rules. In: Guyatt G, Rennie D (eds.) *Users' guides to the medical literature*. Chicago: American Medical Association; 2004. pp. 471–83.
2. Laupacis A, Sekar N, Stiell I. Clinical prediction rules: a review and suggested modifications of methodological standards. *JAMA.* 1997;**277**:488–94.
3. McGinn TG, Guyatt GH, Wyer PC, et al. Users' guides to the medical literature XXII: How to use articles about clinical decision rules. *JAMA.* 2000;**284**:79–84.
4. Richardson WS. We should overcome the barriers to evidence-based clinical diagnosis! *J Clin Epidemiol.* 2007;**60**:217–27.
5. Sackett DL, Haynes RB, Guyatt GH, et al. *Clinical epidemiology: a basic science for clinical medicine.* Toronto: Little, Brown; 1991.
6. Reilly BM. Physical examination in the care of medical inpatients: an observational study. *Lancet.* 2004;**362**:1100–105.
7. Simel D, Rennie D. The clinical examination: an agenda to make it more rational. *JAMA.* 1997;**277**:572–74.
8. McAlister F, Straus SE, Sackett D. Why we need large, simple studies of the clinical examination: the problem and a proposed solution. *Lancet.* 1999;**354**:1721–24.
9. Richardson WS, Wilson MC, Guyatt GH, et al. Users' guides to the medical literature XV: how to use an article about disease probability for differential diagnosis. *JAMA.* 1999;**281**:1214–19.
10. McGinn T, Moore C, Ho W. Practice corner: using clinical prediction rules. *Evid Based Med.* 2002;7:132–34.
11. Cahan A, Gilon D, Manor O, et al. Clinical experience did not reduce the variance in physicians' estimates of pretest probability in a cross-sectional survey. *J Clin Epidemiol.* 2005;**58**:1211–16.
12. Elstein AS, Schwarz A. Evidence base of clinical diagnosis: clinical problem solving and diagnostic decision making: selective review of the cognitive literature. *BMJ.* 2002;**324**:729–32.
13. Okkes IM, Oskam SK, Lamberts H. The probability of specific diagnoses for patients presenting with common symptoms to Dutch family physicians. *J Fam Pract.* 2002;**51**:31–36.
14. Garg AX, Adhikari NKJ, McDonald H, et al. Effects of computerized clinical decision support systems on practitioner performance and patient outcomes: a systematic review. *JAMA.* 2005;**293**:1223–38.
15. Pauker SG, Kassirer JP. The threshold approach to clinical decision making. *New Engl J Med* 1980;**302**:1109–17.
16. Black ER, Bordley D, Tape TG, et al. *Diagnostic strategies for common medical problems.* Philadelphia: American College of Physicians; 1999.
17. Knottnerus JA. Diagnostic prediction rules: principles, requirements and pitfalls. *Prim Care.* 1995;**22**:341–63.
18. Pewsner D, Battaglia M, Minder C, et al. Ruling a diagnosis in or out with "SpPIn" and "SnNOut": a note of caution. *BMJ.* 2004;**329**:209–13.
19. Sox H, Blatt M, Higgins M, et al. *Medical decision making.* Boston: Butterworths; 1988.
20. Whiting P, Toerien M, de Salis I, et al. A review identifies and classifies reasons for ordering diagnostic tests. *J Clin Epidemiol.* 2007;**60**(10):981–89.

21. Knottnerus JA, van Weel C, Muris JWM. Evidence base of clinical diagnosis: Evaluation of diagnostic procedures. *BMJ.* 2002;**324**:477–80.
22. Knottnerus JA, Muris JW. Assessment of the accuracy of diagnostic tests: the cross-sectional study. *J Clin Epidemiol.* 2003;**56**:1118–28.
23. Holland J, Wilczynski N, Haynes RB. Optimal search strategies for identifying sound clinical prediction studies in EMBASE. *BMC Med Inform Decis Making.* 2005;**5**:11.
24. Ingui B, Rogers M. Searching for clinical prediction rules in Medline. *J Am Med Inform Assoc.* 2001;**8**:391–97.
25. Wong S, Wilczynski NL, Haynes RB, et al. Developing optimal search strategies for detecting sound clinical prediction studies in MEDLINE. *AMIA 2003 Symp Proc.* 2003;728–32.
26. Wasson JH, Sox HC, Neff R, et al. Clinical prediction rules: Applications and methodological standards. *New Engl J Med.* 1985;**313**:793–99.
27. Reilly BM, Evans AT. Translating clinical research into clinical practice: impact of using prediction rules to make decisions. *Ann Intern Med.* 2006;**144**:201–9.
28. Hay AD, Fahey T, Peters TJ, Wilson A. Predicting complications from acute cough in pre-school children in primary care: prospective cohort study. *Br J Gen Pract.* 2004;**54**:9–14.
29. Bleeker S, Moll H, Steyerberg E, et al. External validation is necessary in prediction research: a clinical example. *J Clin Epidemiol.* 2003;**56**:826–32.
30. Whiting P, Rutjes AWS, Reitsma JB, et al. Sources of variation and bias in studies of diagnostic accuracy. *Ann Intern Med* 2004;**140**:189–202.
31. Bossuyt PM, Reitsma JB, Bruns DE, et al. Towards complete and accurate reporting of studies of diagnostic accuracy: the STARD initiative. *BMJ.* 2003;**326**:41–44.
32. Diamond G. What price perfection? calibration and discrimination of clinical prediction models. *J Clin Epidemiol.* 1992;**45**:85–89.
33. Brindle P, Emberson J, Lampe F, et al. Predictive accuracy of the Framingham coronary risk score in British men: prospective cohort study. *BMJ.* 2003;**327**:1267–70.
34. Ridker PM, Buring JE, Rifai N, et al. Development and validation of improved algorithms for the assessment of global cardiovascular risk in women: the Reynolds risk score. *JAMA.* 2007;**297**:611–19.
35. Jackson R, Barham P, Bills J, et al. Management of raised blood pressure in New Zealand: a discussion document. *BMJ.* 1993;**307**:107–10.
36. Anderson KM, Odell PM, Wilson PWF, et al. Cardiovascular disease risk profiles. *Am Heart J.* 1991;**121**:293–98.
37. Brindle P, Beswick A, Fahey T, et al. The accuracy and impact of risk assessment in the primary prevention of cardiovascular disease: a systematic review. *Heart.* 2006;**92**:1752–59.
38. Conroy R, Pyorala K, Fitzgerald A, et al. Estimation of ten-year risk of fatal cardiovascular disease in Europe: the SCORE project. *Eur Heart J.* 2003;**24**:987–1003.
39. Sheffield JV, Larson EB. Update in general internal medicine. *Ann Intern Med.* 2003;**139**:285–93.
40. Ebell MH, Smith MA, Barry HC, et al. Does this patient have strep throat? *JAMA.* 2000;**284**:2912–18.
41. McIssac W, Goel V, To T, et al. Effect on antibiotic prescribing of repeated clinical prompts to use a sore throat score: lessons from a failed community intervention study. *J Fam Pract.* 2002;**51**:339–44.

42. Montgomery AA, Fahey T, Peters TJ, MacKintosh C, Sharp D. Evaluation of a computer-based clinical decision support system and chart guidelines in the management of hypertension in primary care: a randomised controlled trial. *BMJ*. 2000;**320**:686–90.

43. Kawamoto K, Houlihan CA, Balas EA, et al. Improving clinical practice using clinical decision support systems: a systematic review of trials to identify features critical to success. *BMJ*. 2005;**330**:765.

44. Randolph A, Haynes RB, Wyatt JC, et al. Users' guides to the Medical Literature XVIII. How to use an article evaluating the clinical impact of a computer-based clinical decision support system. *JAMA*. 1999;**282**:67–74.

45. Baumgart D. Personal digital assistants in health care: experienced clinicians in the palm of your hand. *Lancet*. 2005;**366**:1210–22.

46. Montgomery AA, Fahey T, Peters TJ. A factorial randomised controlled trial of decision analysis and an information video plus leaflet for newly diagnosed hypertensive patients. *Br J Gen Pract*. 2003;**53**:446–53.

47. Buntinx F, Knottnerus JA. Are we at the start of a new era in diagnostic research? *J Clin Epidemiol*. 2006;**59**:325–26.

48. Bossuyt PM, Reitsma JB, Bruns DE, et al. Towards complete and accurate reporting of studies of diagnostic accuracy: the STARD initiative. *BMJ*. 2003;**326**:41–44.

49. Whiting P, Rutjes A, Reitsma J, et al. The development of QUADAS: a tool for the quality assessment of studies of diagnostic accuracy included in systematic reviews. *BMC Med Res Method*. 2003;**3**:25.

50. Pocock SJ, McCormack V, Gueyffier F, et al. A score for predicting risk of death from cardiovascular disease in adults with raised blood pressure, based on individual patient data from randomised controlled trials. *BMJ*. 2001;**323**:75–81.

51. Bent S, Nallamothu B, Simel D. Does this woman have an acute uncomplicated urinary tract infection? *JAMA*. 2002;**287**:2701–10.

52. Rietveld RP, Riet GT, Bindels PJE. Predicting bacterial cause in infectious conjunctivitis: cohort study on informativeness of combinations of signs and symptoms. *BMJ*. 2004;**329**:206–10.

53. Fox KAA, Dabbous OH, Goldberg RJ, et al. Prediction of risk of death and myocardial infarction in the six months after presentation with acute coronary syndrome: prospective multinational observational study (GRACE). *BMJ*. 2006;**333**:1091.

54. Smith G, White I, Pell J, et al. Predicting cesarean section and uterine rupture among women attempting vaginal birth after prior cesarean section. *PLoS Med*. 2005;**2**:e252.

55. Lee SJ, Lindquist K, Segal MR, et al. Development and validation of a prognostic index for 4-year mortality in older adults. *JAMA*. 2006;**295**:801–8.

56. Claiborne Johnson S, Rothwell PM, Nguyen-Huynh M, et al. Validation and refinement of scores to predict very early stroke after transient ischeamic attack. *Lancet*. 2007;**369**:283–92.

57. Albertsson DM, Mellstrom D, Petersson C, et al. Validation of a 4-item score predicting hip fracture and mortality risk among elderly women. *Ann Fam Med*. 2007;**5**:48–56.

CHAPTER 12

Clinical problem solving and diagnostic decision making: a selective review of the cognitive research literature

Alan Schwartz and Arthur S. Elstein

Summary box

- Research on clinical diagnostic reasoning has been conducted chiefly within two research paradigms, problem solving and decision making.
- The key steps in the problem-solving paradigm are hypothesis generation, the interpretation of clinical data to test hypotheses, pattern recognition, and categorization.
- The decision-making paradigm views diagnosis as updating opinion with imperfect information; the normative rule for this process is Bayes's theorem. In practice, diagnosticians are susceptible to well-documented errors in probability estimation and revision.
- Problem based learning and ambulatory clinical experiences make sense from the viewpoint of cognitive theory because students generalize less from specific clinical experiences than educators have traditionally hoped.
- In residency training, both practice guidelines and evidence-based medicine are seen as responses to the psychological limitations of unaided clinical judgment.

Introduction

This chapter reviews the cognitive processes involved in diagnostic reasoning in clinical medicine and sketches our current understanding of these

The Evidence Base of Clinical Diagnosis: Theory and Methods of Diagnostic Research. 2nd edition.
Edited by J. André Knottnerus and Frank Buntinx. © 2009 Blackwell Publishing,
ISBN: 978-1-4051-5787-2.

principles. It describes and analyses the psychological processes and mental structures employed in identifying and solving diagnostic problems of varying degrees of complexity, and reviews common errors and pitfalls in diagnostic reasoning. It does not consider a parallel set of issues in selecting a treatment or developing a management plan. For theoretical background, we draw on two approaches that have been particularly influential in research in this field: problem solving[1,2,3,4,5,6] and decision making.[7,8,9,10,11]

Problem-solving research has usually focused on how an ill-structured problem situation is defined and structured (as by generating a set of diagnostic hypotheses). Psychological decision research has typically looked at factors affecting diagnosis or treatment choice in well-defined, tightly controlled problems. Despite a common theme of limited rationality, the problem-solving paradigm focuses on the wisdom of practice by concentrating on identifying the strategies of experts in a field to help learners acquire them more efficiently. Research in this tradition has aimed at providing students with some guidelines on how to develop their skills in clinical reasoning. Consequently, it has emphasized how experts generally function effectively despite limits on their rational capacities. Behavioral decision research, on the other hand, contrasts human performance with a normative statistical model of reasoning under uncertainty, Bayes's theorem. This research tradition emphasizes positive standards for reasoning about uncertainty, demonstrates that even experts in a domain do not always meet these standards, and thus raises the case for some type of decision support. Behavioral decision research implies that contrasting intuitive diagnostic conclusions with those that would be reached by the formal application of Bayes's theorem would give us greater insight into both clinical reasoning and the probable underlying state of the patient.

The psychological study of reasoning has been profoundly influenced by the "two-system" or "dual-process" theories of cognition.[12,13,14] Dual-process theories posit two distinct systems of judgment: one fast, automatic, and intuitive (System 1), and the other slow, effortful and analytic (System 2). A two-system viewpoint integrates research findings from the problem-solving and decision-making traditions and provides a useful set of educational implications that have received recent attention with promising results.

Problem solving: diagnosis as hypothesis selection

To solve a clinical diagnostic problem means, first, to recognize a malfunction and then to set about tracing or identifying its causes. The diagnosis is ideally an explanation of disordered function – where possible, a causal explanation. The level of causal explanation changes as fundamental scientific understanding of disease mechanisms evolves. In many instances, a diagnosis is a category for which no causal explanation has yet been found.

In most cases, not all of the information needed to identify and explain the situation is available early in the clinical encounter, and so the clinician must decide what information to collect, what aspects of the situation need attention, and what can be safely set aside. Thus, data collection is both sequential and selective. Experienced clinicians execute this task rapidly, almost automatically; novices struggle to develop a plan.

The hypothetico-deductive method

Early hypothesis generation and selective data collection

Difficult diagnostic problems are solved by a process of generating a limited number of hypotheses or problem formulations early in the workup and using them to guide subsequent data collection.[2] Each hypothesis can be used to predict what additional findings ought to be present, if it were true, and then the workup is a guided search for these findings; hence, the method is hypothetico-deductive. The process of problem structuring via hypothesis generation begins with a limited data set and occurs rapidly and automatically, even when clinicians are explicitly instructed not to generate hypotheses. Given the complexity of the clinical situation and the limited capacity of working memory, hypothesis generation is a psychological necessity. It structures the problem by generating a small set of possible solutions—a very efficient way to solve diagnostic problems. The content of experienced clinicians' hypotheses are of higher quality; some novices have difficulty in moving beyond data collection to considering possibilities.[3]

Data interpretation

To what extent do the data strengthen or weaken belief in the correctness of a particular diagnostic hypothesis? A Bayesian approach to answering these questions is strongly advocated in much recent writing[15,16] and is clearly a pillar of the decision making approach to interpreting clinical findings. Yet it is likely that only a minority of clinicians employ it in daily practice and that informal methods of opinion revision still predominate. In our experience, clinicians trained in methods of evidence-based medicine[17] are more likely to use a Bayesian approach to interpreting findings than are other clinicians.

Accuracy of data interpretation and thoroughness of data collection are separate issues. A clinician could collect data thoroughly but nevertheless ignore, misunderstand, or misinterpret some findings. In contrast, a clinician might be overly economical in data collection, but could interpret whatever is available accurately. Elstein *et al.*[2] found no significant association between thoroughness of data collection and accuracy of data interpretation. This finding led to an increased emphasis upon data interpretation in research and education, and argued for studying clinical judgment while controlling the database. This strategy is currently the most widely used in research on clinical reasoning. Sometimes clinical information is presented sequentially: the case unfolds in a simulation of real time, but the subject is given few or no options in data collection.[18,19,20] The analysis may focus on memory organization, knowledge utilization, data interpretation, or problem representation.[3,20,21] In other studies, clinicians are given all the data simultaneously and asked to make a diagnosis.[22,23]

Pattern recognition or categorization

Problem-solving expertise varies greatly across cases and is highly dependent on the clinician's knowledge of the particular domain. Clinicians differ more in their understanding of problems and their problem representations than in the reasoning strategies employed.[2] From this point of view, it makes more sense to consider reasons for success and failure in a particular case than generic traits or strategies of expert diagnosticians.

This has been called case or content specificity. It challenged the hypothetico-deductive model of clinical reasoning for several reasons: both successful and unsuccessful diagnosticians used hypothesis testing, and so it was argued that diagnostic accuracy did not depend as much on strategy as on mastery of domain content. The clinical reasoning of experts in familiar situations frequently does not display explicit hypothesis testing[5,24,25,26] but is instead rapid, automatic, and often nonverbal. The speed, efficiency, and accuracy of experienced clinicians suggest that they might not even use the same reasoning processes as novices, and that experience itself might make hypothesis testing unnecessary.[5] It is likely that experienced clinicians use a hypothetico-deductive strategy only with difficult cases.[27,28] Much of the daily practice of experienced clinicians consists of seeing new cases that strongly resemble those seen previously, and their reasoning in these situations looks more like pattern recognition or direct automatic retrieval. The question then becomes, what is retrieved? What are the patterns?

Pattern recognition implies that clinical reasoning is rapid, difficult to verbalize, and has a perceptual component. Thinking of diagnosis as fitting a case into a category brings some other issues into clearer view. How is a new case categorized? Two somewhat competing accounts have been offered, and research evidence supports both. Category assignment can be based on matching the case either to a specific instance—so-called instance-based or exemplar-based recognition—or to a more abstract prototype. In instance based recognition a new case is categorized by its resemblance to memories of instances previously seen.[5,25,29,30] For example, acute myocardial infarction (AMI) is rapidly hypothesized in a 50-year-old male heavy smoker with severe crushing, substernal chest pain because the clinician has seen previous instances of similar men with very similar symptoms who proved to have AMI. This model is supported by the fact that clinical diagnosis is strongly affected by context (e.g., the location of a skin rash on the body), even when this context is normatively irrelevant.[30] These context effects suggest that clinicians are matching a new case to a previous one, not to an abstraction from several cases, because an abstraction should not include irrelevant features.

The prototype model holds that clinical experience—augmented by teaching, discussion, and the entire round of training—facilitates the construction of abstractions or prototypes.[4, 31] Differences between stronger and weaker diagnosticians are explained by variations in the content and complexity of their prototypes. Better diagnosticians have constructed more diversified and abstract sets of semantic relations to represent the links between clinical features or aspects of the problem.[3, 32] Support for this view is found in the fact that experts in a domain are more able to relate findings to each other and to potential diagnoses, and to identify the additional findings needed to complete a picture.[27] These capabilities suggest that experts utilize abstract representations and do not merely match a new case to a previous instance.

One memory model that has received some attention in cognitive psychology and been successfully applied to clinical reasoning is fuzzy-trace theory.[33] According to fuzzy-trace theory, people simultaneously encode two kinds of representations in memory. The first, called the "verbatim" representation, is a precise encoding of the features of experience. The second, called the "gist" representation is a less precise (hence "fuzzy") trace that captures the essential meaning of the experience without the detailed features. Fuzzy-trace theory argues that while memory tasks assess the verbatim representation, most reasoning tasks in fact operate with the gist representation.[34] Better diagnosticians take more advantage of gist representations in their reasoning, and accordingly appear to gather and use less information than inexperienced diagnosticians.

The controversy about the methods used in diagnostic reasoning can be resolved by recognizing that clinicians, like people generally, are flexible in approaching problems: the method selected depends upon the perceived characteristics of the problem. There is an interaction between the clinician's level of skill and the perceived difficulty of the task.[35] Easy cases can be solved by pattern recognition or by going directly from data to diagnostic classification (forward reasoning).[24] Difficult cases need systematic hypothesis generation and testing. Whether a diagnostic problem is easy or difficult is a function of the knowledge and experience of the clinician who is trying to solve it. When we say that a diagnostic problem is difficult, we really mean that a significant fraction of the clinicians who encounter this problem will find it difficult, although for some it may be quite easy.

Errors in hypothesis generation and restructuring

Neither pattern recognition nor hypothesis testing is an error-proof strategy, nor are they always consistent with statistical rules of inference. Errors that can occur in difficult cases in internal medicine are illustrated and discussed by Kassirer and Kopelman.[20] Another classification of diagnostic errors is found in Bordage.[36] The frequency of errors in actual practice is unknown, and studies to better establish the prevalence of various errors are much needed.

Many diagnostic problems are so complex that the correct solution is not contained within the initial set of hypotheses. Restructuring and reformulating occur as data are obtained and the clinical picture evolves. However, as any problem solver works with a particular set of hypotheses, psychological commitment takes place and it becomes more difficult to restructure the problem.[37]

A related problem is that knowledge stored in long-term memory may not be activated unless triggered by a hypothesis or some other cognitive structure that provides an access channel to the contents of memory. This phenomenon has been demonstrated experimentally in a nonclinical context: recall of the details of the layout of a house varies depending on whether one takes the perspective of a burglar or a potential buyer.[38] We are unaware of an experimental demonstration of this effect in medical education, presumably because of the difficulty of ensuring that an experimental trigger has been effective. However, the complaint of many medical educators that students who can solve problems in the classroom setting appear to be unable to do so in the clinic with real patients, illustrates the role of social context in facilitating or hampering access to the memory store. On the other side of this equation, there are students who struggle academically but are competent clinicians, presumably because the clinical context facilitates their thinking. These observations are all consistent with Bartlett's[39] classic proposal that memory is organized schematically, not in the storage of unconnected bits. Stories help us to remember the details and provide guidance as to what details "must be there." This phenomenon has been demonstrated in medical students[6] and may contribute to continuing interest in medical case studies and narrative medicine.[40,41]

Decision making: diagnosis as opinion revision

Bayes's theorem

From the point of view of decision theory, reaching a diagnosis involves updating an opinion with imperfect information (the clinical evidence).[10,11,15,42] The normative mathematical rule for this task is Bayes's theorem. The pretest probability is either the known prevalence of the disease or the clinician's subjective probability of disease before new information is acquired. As new information is obtained, the probability of each diagnostic possibility is continuously revised. The posttest probability—the probability of each disease given the information—is a function of two variables, pretest probability and the strength of the evidence. The latter is measured by a "likelihood ratio," the ratio of the probabilities of observing a particular finding in patients with and without the disease of interest.

If the data are conditionally independent, each posttest probability becomes the pretest probability for the next stage of the inference process. Using Bayes's theorem becomes hopelessly complicated and impractical when this assumption is violated and more than two correlated cues are involved in a diagnostic judgment, as is often the case in clinical medicine. In these situations, linear and logistic regression techniques are commonly used to derive an equation or clinical prediction rule. A review of these methods is beyond the scope of this chapter. We simply point out that the coefficients (weights) in a regression equation depend on the composition of the derivation sample. Bayes's theorem distinguishes the effect of disease prevalence and the strength of the evidence on the diagnostic judgment, but ordinary regression analytical methods confound these variables in the regression coefficients. (For alternative regression approaches that address this problem, see[43]). If the index disease is overrepresented in the derivation sample, a prediction rule should be applied cautiously to populations where the prevalence of that disease is different. Despite this limitation, these rules are useful. Clinical applications of statistically derived prediction rules can outperform human judgment;[44] this is the rationale for a range of clinical prediction rules that have been developed during the past two decades. Reports of the accuracy of such rules and the reasons for their success have been available in the psychological literature on judgment for over 40 years,[45] but application in clinical practice has been slow because of continuing concerns about:

- whether a rule derived from a particular population generalizes accurately to another
- eroding the professional authority and responsibility of clinicians, and
- whether guidelines (at least in the United States) are intended more to ration care and contain costs than to improve quality.[46,47]

Both evidence-based medicine (EBM) and decision analysis are efforts to introduce quantification into the diagnostic process and still leave a substantial role for clinical judgment.[48,49] EBM leaves the application of research results, including a clinical guideline, up to the clinical judgment of the clinician, who should be guided by canons for interpreting the literature. Decision analysis proposes to offer the clinician insight into the crucial variables in a decision problem, together with a recommended strategy that maximizes expected utility (e.g., see Col *et al.*[50]). Both attempt to avoid quasi-mandatory prescriptive guidelines and to leave room for professional discretion.

Bayes's theorem is a normative rule for diagnostic reasoning: it tells us how we *should* reason, but it does not claim that we use it to revise opinion. It directs attention to two major classes of error in clinical reasoning: in the assessment of either pretest probability or the strength of the evidence. The psychological study of diagnostic reasoning from the Bayesian viewpoint has focused on errors in both components.[51]

Errors in probability estimation

Availability

People are prone to overestimate the frequency of vivid or easily recalled events and to underestimate the frequency of events that are either very ordinary or difficult to recall.[52,53] Diseases or injuries that receive considerable media attention (e.g., injuries due to shark attacks) are often considered more probable than their true prevalence. This psychological principle is exemplified clinically in *overemphasizing rare conditions*. Unusual cases are more memorable than routine problems. The clinical aphorism "When you hear hoof beats, think horses, not zebras" calls attention to this bias.

Representativeness

Earlier, clinical diagnosis was viewed as a categorization process. The strategy of estimating the probability of disease by judging how similar a case is to a diagnostic category or prototype can lead to an overestimation of the probability of a disease in two ways. First, posttest probability can be confused with test sensitivity.[54,55] For example, although fever is a typical finding in meningitis, the probability of meningitis given fever alone as a symptom is quite low. Second, representativeness neglects base rates and implicitly considers all hypotheses as equally likely. This is an error, because if a case resembles disease A and disease B equally well, and there are 10 times as many cases of A as of B, then the case is more likely an instance of A. This heuristic drives the "conjunction fallacy": incorrectly concluding that the probability of a joint event (such as the combination of multiple symptoms to form a typical clinical picture) is greater than the probability of any one of those events alone. The joint event may be more representative (typical) of the diagnostic category, but it cannot be more probable than a single component.

Probability distortions

Normative decision theory assumes that probabilities are mentally processed linearly; that is, they are not transformed from the ordinary probability scale. Because behavioral decision research has demonstrated several violations of this principle, it has been necessary to formulate descriptive theories of risky choice that will better account for choice behaviour in a wide range of situations involving uncertainty.

One of the earliest of these theories is prospect theory (PT),[56] which was formulated explicitly to account for choices involving two-outcome gambles (or one two-outcome gamble and a certain outcome). Cumulative prospect theory (CPT)[57] extends the theory to the multi-outcome case. Both PT and CPT propose that decision makers first edit the decision stimulus in some way, and then evaluate the edited stimulus. Options are evaluated by using an expected-utility-like rule, except that a transformation of the probabilities, called decision weights, are multiplied by subjective values and summed to yield the valuation of a lottery. Probabilities are transformed by a function that is sensitive to both the magnitude of each probability and its rank in the cumulative probability distribution. Hence, it is a *rank-dependent* utility theory.

In general, small probabilities are overweighted and large probabilities underweighted. This "compression error"[58] results in discontinuities at probabilities of 0 and 1, and permits this model to predict "certainty effect" violations of expected utility theory (in which the difference between 99% and 100% is psychologically much greater than the difference between, say, 60% and 61%). Cumulative prospect theory and similar rank-dependent utility theories provide formal descriptions of how probabilities are distorted in risky decision making. The distortions are exacerbated when the probabilities are not precisely known,[59] a situation that is common in clinical medicine.[60] It should be stressed that cumulative prospect theory does not assert that individuals are in fact carrying out mentally a set of calculations that are even more complex than those required to calculate expected utility. Rather, the theory claims that observed choices (that is, behaviour) can be better modeled by this complex function than by the simpler expected-utility rule.

Support theory
Several probability estimation biases are captured by support theory,[61,62] which posits that subjective estimates of the frequency or probability of an event are influenced by how detailed the description is. More explicit descriptions yield higher probability estimates than compact, condensed descriptions, even when the two refer to exactly the same events (such as "probability of death due to a car accident, train accident, plane accident, or other moving vehicle accident" versus "probability of death due to a moving vehicle accident"). This theory can explain availability (when memories of an available event include more detailed descriptions than those of less available events) and representativeness (when a typical case description includes a cluster of details that "fit," whereas a less typical case lacks some of these features). Clinically, support theory implies that a longer, more detailed case description will be assigned a higher subjective probability of the index disease than a brief abstract of the same case, even if they contain the same information about that disease. Thus, subjective assessments of events, although often necessary in clinical practice, can be affected by factors unrelated to true prevalence.[63]

Errors in probability revision

Errors in interpreting the diagnostic value of clinical information have been found by several research teams.[2,6,64,65]

Fixedness
Several different but related errors result in diagnosticians being overly resistant to change in their diagnoses. These include conservatism, pseudodiagnosticity, and biased interpretation.

In clinical case discussions, data are commonly presented sequentially, and diagnostic probabilities are not revised as much as is implied by Bayes's theorem. This phenomenon has been called "conservatism" and was one of the earliest cognitive biases identified.[66] One explanation of conservatism is that diagnostic opinions are revised up or down from an initial anchor, which is either given in the problem or formed subjectively. Final opinions are sensitive to the starting point (the "anchor"), the shift ("adjustment") from it is typically insufficient, so the final judgment is closer to the anchor than is implied by Bayes's theorem.[47] This bias in *processing* information leads to the collection of more information than is normatively necessary to reach a desired level of diagnostic certainty. The common complaint that clinicians overuse laboratory tests is indirect evidence that these biases operate in clinical practice.

"Pseudodiagnosticity"[67] or "confirmation bias"[58] is the tendency to seek information that confirms a hypothesis rather than the data that facilitate efficient testing of competing hypotheses. For example, in one study, residents in internal medicine preferred about 25% of the time to order findings that would give a more detailed clinical picture of one disease, rather than findings that would allow them to test between two potential diagnoses.[58] Here, the problem is knowing what information would be useful, rather than overestimating the value (likelihood ratio) of the information, or failing to combine it optimally with other data.[59]

A third related error is *interpreting* information as consistent with hypotheses already under consideration.[2,6,68] Where findings are distorted in recall, it is generally in the direction of making the facts more consistent with typical clinical pictures.[2] Positive findings are overemphasized and negative findings tend to be discounted.[2,69] From a Bayesian standpoint these are all errors in assessing the diagnostic value of information, that is, errors in subjectively assessing the likelihood ratio. Even when clinicians agree on the presence of certain clinical findings, wide variations have been found in the weights assigned in interpreting cues,[23] and this variation may be due partly to the effect of the hypotheses being considered.[64]

As a result of these biases, new information that might disconfirm a hypothesis is less often sought, less often recognized, and less often given enough weight in revising a diagnosis than is normatively appropriate.

Confounding the probability and value of an outcome

It is difficult for everyday judgment to keep separate accounts of the probability of a particular disease and the benefits that accrue from detecting it. Probability revision errors that are systematically linked to the perceived cost of mistakes demonstrate the difficulties experienced in separating assessments of probability from values.[70,71] For example, there is a tendency to overestimate the probability of more serious but treatable diseases because a clinician would hate to miss one.[61]

Order effects

Bayes's theorem implies that clinicians given identical information should reach the same diagnostic opinion, regardless of the order in which the information is presented. However, final opinions are also affected by the order of presentation: information presented later in a case is given more weight than that presented earlier.[18,72] This may partly explain why it is difficult to get medical students to pay as much attention to history and the physical examination as their teachers would wish. High-tech laboratory tests tend to have very high likelihood ratios, and they are obtained late in the diagnostic work up.

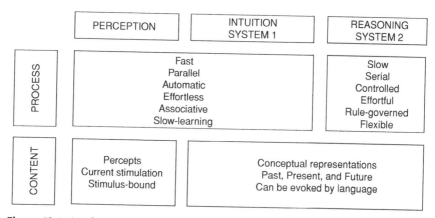

Figure 12.1 Attributes of the two judgmental systems as well as the perceptual system. Reproduced from Kahneman's Nobel prize lecture (2003), with permission of The Nobel Foundation.

Two-system theories of cognition

The psychological study of reasoning has been profoundly influenced by the "two-system" or "dual-process" theories of cognition.[12,13,14] Dual-process theories posit two distinct systems of judgment, both of which operate in parallel.

The first, designated System 1, is an intuitive judgment system that shares many features with perception. System 1 is fast and automatic, and underlies pattern recognition, prototypicality, and heuristic processing. It is also influenced by the emotional state of the judge and the emotional content of the judgment. In contrast, System 2 is a slow, effortful, and analytic mode of judgment that applies rules in an emotionally neutral manner. When appropriate data are available, System 2 yields the most normatively rational reasoning but is easily disrupted by high cognitive load. Figure 12.1, reproduced from Kahneman's Nobel Prize lecture, illustrates the attributes of the two judgmental systems as well as the perceptual system.[13] Indeed, it has been suggested that our perceptual system tacitly and automatically encodes such information as the frequency of events and associations between co-occurring events.[14]

Kahneman (2003) points out that in making judgments, the two systems interact in one of four ways. If no intuitive response is evoked from System 1, the judgment is produced by System 2. On the other hand, if an intuitive response is evoked, System 2 operates on the intuitive response, and may endorse it as evoked, use it as an anchor and adjust the judgment based on other features of the situation, or identify it as incompatible with a subjectively valid rule and block it from overt expression.[13] A key feature of this description is the notion that both systems operate together; System 1 processing cannot be suppressed, although the intuitive responses it generates may be. Gigerenzer and colleagues have argued extensively for the adaptive nature of "fast and frugal" System 1 heuristics.[73] Fuzzy-trace theory, discussed earlier, specifically argues that gist processing (a System 1 function) represents the apex of the development of reasoning.[34]

A two-system viewpoint integrates research findings from the problem-solving and decision-making traditions and explains several of the findings about individual and contextual differences in reasoning reviewed above. Moreover, it provides a useful set of educational implications that have received recent attention with promising results and are discussed below.

Educational implications

Two recent innovations in undergraduate medical education and residency training, problem-based learning and evidence-based medicine, are consistent with the educational implications of this research.

Problem-based learning (PBL)[74,75,76] can be understood as an effort to introduce formulating and testing clinical hypotheses into a preclinical curriculum dominated by biological sciences. The cognitive–instructional theory behind this reform was that, because experienced clinicians use this strategy with difficult problems, and as practically any clinical situation selected for instructional purposes will be difficult for students, it makes sense to call this strategy to their attention and to provide opportunities to practice it, first using case simulations and then with real patients.

The finding of case specificity showed the limits of a focus on teaching a general problem solving strategy. Problem solving expertise can be separated from content analytically, but not in practice. This realization shifted the emphasis toward helping students acquire a functional organization of content with clinically usable schemata. This became the new rationale for problem-based learning.[77,78,79]

Because transfer from one context to another is limited, clinical experience is needed in contexts closely related to future practice. The instance-based model of problem solving supports providing more experience in outpatient care because it implies that students do not generalize as much from one training setting to another as has traditionally been thought. But a clinician overly dependent on context sees every case as unique, as all of the circumstances are never exactly replicated. The unwanted intrusion of irrelevant context effects implies that an important educational goal is to reduce inappropriate dependence on context. In our opinion, there are two ways to do this:

1 Emphasize that students should strive to develop prototypes and abstractions from their clinical experience. Clinical experience that is not subject to reflection and review is not enough. It must be reviewed and analyzed so that the correct general models and principles are abstracted. Most students do this, but some struggle, and medical educators ought not to count upon its spontaneous occurrence. Well-designed educational experiences to facilitate the development of the desired cognitive structures should include extensive focused practice and feedback with a variety of problems.[5,80] The current climate, with its emphasis on seeing more patients to compensate for declining patient care revenues, threatens medical education at this

level because it makes it more difficult for clinical preceptors to provide the needed critique and feedback, and for students to have time for the necessary reflection.[73]

2 A practical Bayesian approach to diagnosis can be introduced. EBM[17,81] may be viewed as the most recent—and, by most standards, the most successful— effort to date to apply these methods to clinical diagnosis. EBM uses likelihood ratios to quantify the strength of the clinical evidence, and shows how this measure should be combined with disease prevalence (or prior probability) to yield a post-test probability. This is Bayes's theorem offered to clinicians in a practical, useful format! Its strengths are in stressing the role of data in clinical reasoning, and in encouraging clinicians to rely on their judgment to apply the results of a particular study to their patients. Its weaknesses, in our view, are that it does not deal systematically with the role of patient preferences in these decisions, or with methods for quantifying preferences, and that it blurs the distinction between probability-driven and utility-driven decisions.

In our experience teaching EBM, residents soon learn how to interpret studies of diagnostic tests and how to use a nomogram[82,83] to compute posttest probabilities. The nomogram, or a 2×2 table, combines their prior index of suspicion (a subjective probability) and the test characteristics reported in the clinical literature. It has been more difficult to introduce concepts of decision thresholds (at what probability should management change?) and the expected value of information (should a test that cannot result in a change in action be performed at all?). Lloyd and Reyna, however, have recently discussed a fuzzy-trace theory approach for designing EBM educational interventions that may simplify instruction around these concepts.[84]

Recently, Norman and Eva have championed the view that clinicians apply multiple reasoning strategies as necessary to approach diagnostic problems.[85,86] Their research suggests that training physicians in multiple knowledge representations and reasoning modes, including both "analytic" (System 2) and "nonanalytic" (System 1) approaches, may yield the best overall performance. They emphasize flexibility as a key feature of expertise, and argue for teaching around examples that mimic the way problems would actually be encountered.

Methodological guidelines

1 Psychological research on clinical reasoning began in a thinking-aloud tradition, which remains attractive to many investigators. It seems quite natural to ask a clinician to articulate and discuss the reasoning involved in a particular case, and to record these verbalizations for later analysis. Whatever its shortcomings, this research strategy has high face validity. Because the clinicians involved in these studies frequently discuss real cases,[2,20] content validity on the clinical side is assured.

The problems of this approach are easily summarized: first, it is labor intensive, and therefore most studies have used small samples of both clinicians and cases. Therefore, they lack statistical power and are best suited for exploratory analysis. But to demonstrate statistically significant differences between experts (senior attending clinicians) and novices (medical students or junior house officers), researchers must take into account two facts: (1) within any group of clinicians at any level of clinical experience, or within any speciality, there is a great amount of variation, both in reasoning and in practice. With small samples, within-group variance will make it difficult to demonstrate significant between-group differences; and (2) the performance of clinicians varies considerably across cases. These two features imply that research on diagnostic reasoning must use adequate samples of both clinicians and cases if there is to be any hope of reaching generalisable conclusions. Most research to date has not paid adequate attention to issues of sample size (of both cases and research participants) and statistical power.

2 Many important cognitive processes are not available to consciousness and are not verbalized. Indeed, the more automatic and overlearned a mental process is (the more it relies on System 1), the less likely is it that one can verbalize how the process works. Once a person has lived for some time at a given address, it becomes impossible to tell how one knows that address: it is simply "known." Closer to our concerns, participants do not report that a subjective probability is overestimated because of the availability bias: the existence of the bias is inferred by comparing estimates with known frequencies. For these reasons, much recent work has shifted toward a research paradigm modeled on experimental cognitive psychology: research participants are presented with a task and their responses are recorded. Their verbalizations are one more source of data, but are not treated as a true account of internal mental processes. Instead, the "true account" (at an appropriate level of abstraction) is inferred from the relationship between task and subject variables and responses, which is often characterized by a mathematical model that provides falsifiable predictions. This research has yielded many of the findings summarized in this chapter, but it is at times criticized for using artificial tasks (lack of face validity) and, consequently, not motivating the participants adequately. The generalizability of the results to real clinical settings is then questioned.

3 More attention should be given, in general, to the operation and interaction of dual cognitive processes (i.e., System 1 and System 2) in the study of diagnostic reasoning. The two-system account offers an intriguing set of predictions about how expertise might be manifest (e.g., that experts may develop both stronger System 1 intuitions and have a more powerful set of System 2 analytical tools at their disposal). At the same time, it provides a methodological caution against conducting research that ignores the parallel operation of the two systems.

4 Selection bias is a potential threat to the validity of both types of studies of clinical reasoning. Senior clinicians in any clinical domain can decline to participate in research far more easily than can medical students or house

officers in the same domain. Therefore, the more experienced participants in a study are usually volunteers. Attention should be paid to issues of selection bias and response rate as potential limitations; thought should be given to their possible effects on the validity and generalizability of the results of the study.

5 Behavioral decision research conducted to date has been concerned primarily with demonstrating that a particular phenomenon exists, for example demonstrating biases in probability estimation, such as availability and representativeness. Statistical tests of significance are used to demonstrate the phenomena. From an educational standpoint, we ought to be more interested in identifying how prevalent these biases are and which are most likely to affect treatment and management. Thus, more research is needed to assess the prevalence of these errors and to determine how often treatment choices are affected by diagnostic errors caused by these biases. If these facts were known, a more rational, systematic curriculum could be developed that could focus on preventing or managing the most prevalent errors.

Conclusion

This chapter has selectively reviewed 30 years of psychological research on clinical diagnostic reasoning, focusing on problem solving and decision making as the dominant paradigms of the field. This research demonstrates the limitations of human judgment, although the research designs employed make it difficult to estimate their prevalence. Work in cognitive psychology suggests that both a fast, automatic judgmental system and a slow, deliberative judgment system operate simultaneously, and the interaction of these systems explains a considerable number of limitations in judgments as well as predicting successful performance in many tasks. Problem based learning and evidence-based medicine are both justified by the psychological research about judgment limitations, violations of Bayesian principles in everyday clinical reasoning, and the finding of limited transfer across clinical situations, although we do not believe that these innovations were initially directed by an awareness of cognitive limitations. Within graduate medical education (residency training), the introduction of practice guidelines based on evidence has been controversial because guidelines may be perceived as efforts to restrict the authority of clinicians and to ration care. The psychological research helps to explain why formal statistical decision supports are both needed and likely to evoke controversy.

Acknowledgments

Preparation of this review was supported in part by grant RO1 LM5630 from the National Library of Medicine.

References

1. Newell A, Simon HA. *Human problem solving.* Englewood Cliffs (NJ): Prentice-Hall; 1972.
2. Elstein AS, Shulman LS, Sprafka SA. *Medical problem solving: an analysis of clinical reasoning.* Cambridge (MA): Harvard University Press; 1978.
3. Bordage G, Lemieux M. Semantic structures and diagnostic thinking of experts and novices. *Acad Med.* 1991;**66**(9 Suppl):S70–S72.
4. Bordage G, Zacks R. The structure of medical knowledge in the memories of medical students and general practitioners: categories and prototypes. *Med Educ.* 1984;**18**:406–16.
5. Schmidt HG, Norman GR, Boshuizen HPA. A cognitive perspective on medical expertise: theory and implications. *Acad Med.* 1990;**65**:611–21.
6. Friedman MH, Connell KJ, Olthoff AJ. Medical student errors in making a diagnosis. *Acad Med.* 1998;**73**(10 Suppl):S19–S21.
7. Kahneman D, Slovic P, Tversky A, eds. *Judgment under uncertainty: heuristics and biases.* New York: Cambridge University Press; 1982.
8. Baron J. *Thinking and deciding.* New York: Cambridge University Press; 1988.
9. Mellers BA, Schwartz A, Cooke ADJ. Judgment and decision making. *Annu Rev Psychol.* 1998;**49**:447–77.
10. Hunink M, Glasziou P, Siegel JE, et al. *Decision making in health and medicine: integrating evidence and values.* Cambridge: Cambridge University Press; 2001.
11. Sox HC, Jr, Blatt MA, Higgins MC, et al. *Medical decision making.* Stoneham (MA): Butterworths; 1988.
12. Stanovich KE, West RF. Individual differences in reasoning: Implications for the rationality debate? *Behav and Brain Sci.* 2000;**23**(5):645–26.
13. Kahneman D. Maps of bounded rationality: a perspective on intuitive judgment and choice. In: Frangsmyr T, ed. *Les Prix Nobel. The Nobel Prizes 2002.* Stockholm: Almqvist & Wiksell International; 2003.
14. Hogarth RM. Deciding analytically or trusting your intuition? The advantages and disadvantages of analytic and intuitive thought. In: Betsch T, Haberstroh S, eds. *The routines of decision making.* Mahwah (NJ): Lawrence Erlbaum Associates; 2005. pp. 67–82.
15. Lee TH. Interpretation of data for clinical decisions. In: Goldman L, Ausiello D, eds. *Cecil textbook of medicine.* 22nd ed. Philadelphia: Saunders; 2004. p 25.
16. Panzer RJ, Black ER, Griner PF. *Diagnostic strategies for common medical problems.* Philadelphia: American College of Physicians; 1991.
17. Strauss SE, Richardson WS, Glasziou P, et al. *Evidence-based medicine: how to practice and teach EBM.* 3rd ed. New York: Churchill Livingstone; 2005.
18. Chapman GB, Bergus GR, Elstein AS. Order of information affects clinical judgment. *J Behav Decis Making.* 1996;**9**:201–11.
19. Moskowitz AJ, Kuipers BJ, Kassirer JP. Dealing with uncertainty, risks, and tradeoffs in clinical decisions: a cognitive science approach. *Ann Intern Med.* 1988;**108**:435–49.
20. Kassirer JP, Kopelman RI. *Learning clinical reasoning.* Baltimore: Williams & Wilkins; 1991.
21. Joseph GM, Patel VL. Domain knowledge and hypothesis generation in diagnostic reasoning. *Med Decis Making.* 1990;**10**:31–46.

22. Patel VL, Groen G. Knowledge-based solution strategies in medical reasoning. *Cogn Sci.* 1986;**10**:91–116.
23. Wigton RS, Hoellerich VL, Patil KD. How physicians use clinical information in diagnosing pulmonary embolism: an application of conjoint analysis. *Med Dec Making.* 1986;**6**:2–11.
24. Groen GJ, Patel VL. Medical problem-solving: some questionable assumptions. *Med Educ.* 1985;**19**:95–100.
25. Brooks LR, Norman GR, Allen SW. Role of specific similarity in a medical diagnostic task. *J Exp Psych: Gen.* 1991;**120**:278–87.
26. Eva KW, Neville AJ, Norman GR. Exploring the etiology of content specificity: factors influencing analogic transfer and problem solving. *Acad Med.* 1998;**73**(10 Suppl):S1–S5.
27. Elstein AS, Kleinmuntz B, Rabinowitz M, et al. Diagnostic reasoning of high- and low-domain knowledge clinicians: a re-analysis. *Med Decis Making.* 1993;**13**:21–9.
28. Davidoff F. *Who has seen a blood sugar? Reflections on medical education.* Philadelphia: American College of Physicians, 1998.
29. Medin DL, Schaffer MM. A context theory of classification learning. *Psychol Rev.* 1978;**85**:207–38.
30. Norman GR, Coblentz CL, Brooks LR, et al. Expertise in visual diagnosis: a review of the literature. *Acad Med.* 1992;**66**:S78–S83.
31. Rosch E, Mervis CB. Family resemblances: studies in the internal structure of categories. *Cogn Psychol.* 1975;**7**:573–605.
32. Lemieux M, Bordage G. Propositional versus structural semantic analyses of medical diagnostic thinking. *Cogn Sci.* 1992;**16**:185–204.
33. Reyna VF, Lloyd FJ, Brainerd CJ. Memory, development, and rationality: an integrative theory of judgment and decision-making. In: Schneider S, Shanteau J, eds. *Emerging perspectives on judgment and decision research.* Cambridge: Cambridge University Press; 2003. pp. 201–45.
34. Reyna VF. How people make decisions that involve risk. a dual-processes approach. *Curr Dir Psychol Sci.* 2004;**13**(2):60–66.
35. Elstein AS. What goes around comes around: the return of the hypothetico-deductive strategy. *Teach Learn Med.* 1994;**6**:121–23.
36. Bordage G. Why did I miss the diagnosis? some cognitive explanations and educational implications. *Acad Med.* 1999;**74**:S138–S42.
37. Janis IL, Mann L. *Decision-making.* New York: Free Press; 1977.
38. Anderson RC, Pichert JW. Recall of previously unrecallable information following a shift in perspective. *J Verb Learning Verb Behav.* 1978;**17**:1–12.
39. Bartlett FC. *Remembering: a study in experimental and social psychology.* New York: Macmillan; 1932.
40. Hurwitz B, Greenhalgh T, eds. *Narrative based medicine: dialogue and discourse in clinical practice.* London: BMJ Books; 1998.
41. Charon R. Narrative medicine: a model for empathy, reflection, profession, and trust. *JAMA.* 2001;**286**(15):1897–902.
42. Sackett DL, Haynes RB, Guyatt GH, et al. *Clinical epidemiology: a basic science for clinical medicine.* 2nd ed. Boston: Little, Brown; 1991.
43. Knottnerus JA. Application of logistic regression to the analysis of diagnostic data. *Med Decis Making.* 1992;**12**:93–108.
44. Ebell MH. Using decision rules in primary care practice. *Prim Care.* 1995;**22**:319–40.

45. Meehl PE. *Clinical versus statistical prediction: A theoretical analysis and review of the evidence.* Minneapolis: University of Minnesota Press; 1954.

46. James PA, Cowan TM, Graham RP, et al. Family physicians' attitudes about and use of clinical practice guidelines. *J Fam Pract.* 1997;**45**:341–47.

47. Cabana MD, Rand CS, Powe NR, et al. Why don't physicians follow clinical practice guidelines? a framework for improvement. *JAMA.* 1999;**282**(15):1458–65.

48. Hayward R, Wilson MC, Tunis SR, et al. Users' guides to the medical literature. VIII: how to use clinical practice guidelines, A: are the recommendations valid? *JAMA.* 1995;**274**:70–74.

49. Wilson MC, Hayward R, Tunis SR, et al. Users' guides to the medical literature. VIII: how to use clinical practice guidelines, B: what are the recommendations and will they help me in caring for my patient? *JAMA.* 1995;**274**:1630–32.

50. Col NF, Eckman MH, Karas RH, et al. Patient-specific decisions about hormone replacement therapy in postmenopausal women. *JAMA.* 1997;**277**:1140–47.

51. Kempainen RR, Migeon MB, Wolf FM. Understanding our mistakes: a primer on errors in clinical reasoning. *Med Teach.* 2003;**25**(2):177–81.

52. Tversky A, Kahneman D. Judgment under uncertainty: heuristics and biases. *Science.* 1974;**185**:1124–31.

53. Elstein AS. Heuristics and biases: selected errors in clinical reasoning. *Acad Med.* 1999;**74**:791–94.

54. Eddy DM. Probabilistic reasoning in clinical medicine: problems and opportunities. In: Kahneman D, Slovic P, Tversky A, eds. *Judgment under uncertainty: heuristics and biases.* New York: Cambridge University Press; 1982. pp. 249–67.

55. Dawes, RM. *Rational choice in an uncertain world.* New York: Harcourt Brace Jovanovich; 1988.

56. Tversky A, Kahneman D. The framing of decisions and the psychology of choice. *Science.* 1982;**211**:453–58.

57. Tversky A, Kahneman D. Advances in prospect theory: cumulative representation of uncertainty. *J Risk Uncertain.* 1992;**5**:297–323.

58. Fischhoff B, Bostrom A, Quadrell MJ. Risk perception and communication. *Annu Rev Pub Health.* 1993;**14**:183–203.

59. Einhorn HJ, Hogarth RM. Decision making under ambiguity. *J Bus.* 1986;**59**(Suppl):S225–S50.

60. Dolan JG, Bordley DR, Mushlin AI. An evaluation of clinicians' subjective prior probability estimates. *Med Decis Making.* 1983;**6**:216–23.

61. Tversky A, Koehler DJ. Support theory: a nonextensional representation of subjective probability. *Psychol Rev.* 1994;**101**:547–67.

62. Rottenstreich Y, Tversky A. Unpacking, repacking, and anchoring: advances in support theory. *Psychol Rev.* 1997;**104**:406–15.

63. Redelmeier DA, Koehler DJ, Liberman V, Tversky A. Probability judgment in medicine: discounting unspecified probabilities. *Med Decis Making.* 1995;**15**:227–30.

64. Wolf FM, Gruppen LD, Billi JE. Differential diagnosis and the competing hypotheses heuristic: A practical approach to judgment under uncertainty and Bayesian probability. *JAMA.* 1985;**253**:2858–62.

65. Gruppen LD, Wolf FM, Billi JE. Information gathering and integration as sources of error in diagnostic decision making. *Med Decis Making.* 1991;**11**:233–39.

66. Edwards W. Conservatism in human information processing. In: Kleinmuntz B, ed. *Formal representation of human judgment.* New York, Wiley; 1969. pp. 17–52.

67. Kern L, Doherty ME. "Pseudodiagnosticity" in an idealized medical problem-solving environment. *J Med Educ.* 1982;**57**:100–104.
68. Hatala R, Norman GR, Brooks LR. Influence of a single example on subsequent electrocardiogram interpretation. *Teach Learn Med.* 1999;**11**:110–17.
69. Wason PC, Johnson-Laird PN. *Psychology of reasoning: structure and content.* Cambridge (MA): Harvard University Press; 1972.
70. Wallsten TS. Physician and medical student bias in evaluating information. *Med Decis Making.* 1981;**1**:145–64.
71. Poses RM, Cebul RD, Collins M, et al. The accuracy of experienced physicians' probability estimates for patients with sore throats. *JAMA.* 1985;**254**:925–29.
72. Bergus GR, Chapman GB, Gjerde C, et al. Clinical reasoning about new symptoms in the face of pre-existing disease: sources of error and order effects. *Fam Med.* 1995;**27**:314–20.
73. Gigerenzer G, Todd PM, ABC Research Group. *Simple heuristics that make us smart.* Oxford: Oxford University Press; 1999.
74. Barrows HS. Problem-based, self-directed learning. *JAMA.* 1983;**250**:3077–80.
75. Barrows HS. A taxonomy of problem-based learning methods. *Med Educ.* 1986;**20**:481–86.
76. Schmidt HG. Problem-based learning: rationale and description. *Med Educ.* 1983;**17**:11–16.
77. Norman GR. Problem-solving skills, solving problems and problem-based learning. *Med Educ.* 1988;**22**:279–86.
78. Gruppen LD. Implications of cognitive research for ambulatory care education. *Acad Med.* 1997;**72**:117–20.
79. Gruppen L, Frohna A. Clinical reasoning. In: Norman G, Van Der Vleuten C, Newble D, eds. *International handbook of research in medical education.* The Netherlands: Kluwer Academic Publishers; 2002. pp. 205–30.
80. Ludmerer KM. *Time to heal: American medical education from the turn of the century to the era of managed care.* New York: Oxford University Press; 1999.
81. Heneghan C, Badenoch D. *Evidence-based medicine toolkit.* 2nd ed. London: BMJ Books; 2006.
82. Fagan TJ. Nomogram for Bayes's theorem [letter]. *N Engl J Med.* 1975;**293**:257.
83. Schwartz A. Nomogram for Bayes's theorem. Available at: http://araw.mede.uic.edu/cgi-bin/testcalc.pl.
84. Lloyd FJ, Reyna VF. A web exercise in evidence-based medicine using cognitive theory. *J Gen Int Med.* 2001;**16**(2):94–99.
85. Eva KW. What every teacher needs to know about clinical reasoning. *Med Educ* 2005;**39**(1):98–106.
86. Norman G. Research in clinical reasoning: past history and current trends. *Med Educ.*2005;**39**(4):418–27.

CHAPTER 13

Improving test ordering and its diagnostic cost-effectiveness in clinical practice—bridging the gap between clinical research and routine health care

Ron Winkens, Trudy van der Weijden, Hans Severens, and Geert-Jan Dinant

Summary box

- In recent decades, the number of diagnostic tests ordered by doctors has increased enormously, despite the often absent or disappointing results from studies into their accuracy.
- Evidence-based clinical guidelines are needed to formalize optimal diagnostic performance. Both disease-specific and complaint-specific guidelines will be needed, but guidelines will not affect practice unless implemented properly.
- In applying a guideline recommendation to a unique individual, doctors will frequently have strong patient- or context-related arguments to deviate from the guideline. It is not known what optimal mean guideline adherence scores are for a group of professionals and for different diagnostic guideline recommendations.
- Interventions ideally provide both knowledge on what to do and insight into one's own performance. Such interventions are dissemination of guidelines and (computerized) reminders combined with audit, individual feedback, and peer review.

The Evidence Base of Clinical Diagnosis: Theory and Methods of Diagnostic Research. 2nd edition. Edited by J. André Knottnerus and Frank Buntinx. © 2009 Blackwell Publishing, ISBN: 978-1-4051-5787-2.

- There is no "one and only ideal implementation strategy." Although the evidence is somewhat conflicting, educational strategies, comparative feedback followed by peer group review, and (computerized) reminders seem to be promising strategies for optimizing test-ordering behavior. There is no evidence that multifaceted strategies are more effective than single strategies.
- In the selection of the implementation strategy, insight in modifiable barriers to change should play a role.
- Although the randomized controlled trial remains the "gold standard" for evaluation studies, inherent methodological challenges, such as the required randomization of doctors, need special attention.
- More attention must be paid to the perpetuation of interventions once they have been started and to the measurement and scientific evaluation of their effects over time.
- More research into the ways to improve test ordering is urgently needed, in particular for patients suffering from recurrent non-specific or unexplained complaints.

Introduction

An important part of making a proper diagnosis is using diagnostic tests, such as blood and radiographic investigations. In recent decades, the number of diagnostic tests ordered by doctors has increased substantially, despite the (often disappointing) results from studies into their diagnostic accuracy. Apparently, arguments other than scientific ones for test ordering are relevant. Furthermore, it might be questioned to what extent current knowledge, insights into a correct use of diagnostic tests, and results from research have been properly and adequately implemented in daily practice. This chapter discusses how to bridge the gap between evidence from research and routine health care.

The need to change

For several reasons, there is a need to improve test-ordering behavior. The use of medical resources in western countries is growing annually and consistently. In the Netherlands, for example, there is a relatively stable growth in the nationwide use of health care resources of approximately 7% per year. An annual growth in expenditure for diagnostic tests is also visible.

The following factors may be responsible for the increasing use of diagnostic tests:

1 The mere availability and technological imperative of more test facilities is an important determinant. In view of the interaction between supply and demand in health care, the simple fact that tests can be ordered will lead to their actual ordering. This applies especially to new tests, which are sometimes used primarily out of curiosity.

2 Another factor is the increasing demand for care, caused partly by the ageing of the population and an increasing number of chronically ill people.

3 Also, new insights from scientific evidence and guidelines often provide recommendations for additional diagnostic testing.

4 Doctors might wish to perform additional testing once an abnormal test result is found, even in the absence of clinical suspicion, while ignoring that a test result outside reference ranges may generally be found in 5% of a healthy population. A cascade of testing may then be the result.

5 Furthermore, over the years, higher standards of care (adopted by the public, patients, and health care professionals) and defensive behaviors from doctors have contributed to the increased use of health care services, one of them being diagnostic testing.

6 Because of recent changes in tasks of primary care, more patients with chronic disorders are monitored in primary care, causing a further increase in the numbers of tests.

Factors influencing test ordering

Despite the introduction of guidelines focusing on rational use of diagnostic tests, there are many factors that influence test-ordering behavior. All these factors make it difficult for doctors to adhere to guidelines. Such determinants of test-ordering behavior include doctor-related, patient-related, and context-related factors.

Doctor-related factors

In daily practice, reasons for doctors to ignore evidence-based recommendations are numerous and hard to grasp. The interdoctor variation in test-ordering behavior is higher than can be explained by differences in case mix between doctors.[1] Differences are not only seen between individual doctors but also between groups of doctors. For example, high users of imaging tests ordered more than four times more tests than low users, even after adjusting for practice size and working time factor.[2] On a group level, in one region the median number of tests ordered proved to be more than twice compared with a region with low numbers of tests ordered.[1]

According to diagnostic decision-making theories, the decision to order a test should at least be based on the pretest probability for a disorder and the seriousness of the suspected disorder. Other important considerations include the diagnostic value of the test, the consequences of the test result for further decision making and the risk or financial costs for the society and the patient.

Applying a guideline recommendation to an individual patient is complex and far from easy. Doctors will frequently have strong patient-related arguments to deviate from a guideline. This translation from a guideline recommendation to the individual patient may also be hampered because many guidelines are disease specific instead of symptom specific. In daily practice, diagnostic decision making may also be influenced or biased by professional-related determinants of test-ordering behavior, such as (in)tolerance of diagnostic uncertainty, bias toward action, the desire to end the consultation during high workload, personal routines, and working in a group practice.[1,3,4].

Patient-related factors

Barriers for adherence to guidelines may also be found in the interaction of the professional with the direct environment such as pressure by patients, leading to tactical motives for test ordering. The general practitioner (GP) may experience pressure from the patient or may assume that the patient needs reassurance by testing. In several studies, patient expectations on test ordering were assessed; percentages of patients desiring laboratory tests ranged from 14 to 22%.[5–8] In a cohort of patients presenting with medically unexplained symptoms, tests were ordered more often for patients who, before the consultation, expected that the GP would order one or more tests compared with patients without these expectations.[8] Complying with needs of the patient for reassurance through testing is seen as an easy, cost- and time-effective strategy.[3] While doing so, doctors should, however, keep in mind that patients tend to overestimate the qualities of diagnostic tests and appear to have high hopes for testing as a diagnostic tool. They expect diagnostic certainty without errors and consider a normal test result as a proof of good health.[9]

Context-related factors

Apart from doctor- and patient-related determinants of test-ordering behavior, also context-related factors play a role, such as the organization of how to order tests (problem-based order form, making thresholds or barriers for restricted tests), the remuneration system and its impact on supplier-induced demand, and, finally, financial incentives or regulatory sanctions. All these factors may explain differences in the volume of tests ordered between regions or countries, or even between university and nonuniversity hospitals.[1,2]

Can we make the change?

In terms of quality, improvement, and cost containment, there are sufficient arguments for attempting to change test-ordering behavior. Overall, the decision to order laboratory tests is the result of a complex interaction of often-conflicting considerations. Better knowledge of the professional's motives for ordering laboratory tests in the case of diagnostic uncertainty may steer interventions directed at improving compliance with guidelines or reducing unnecessary testing. Designers of interventions meant to improve test ordering should be aware of the numerous determinants and take contextual variables into account. It is recommended that certain steps be taken, from orientation to perpetuation. The individual steps are described in the implementation cycle.[10] Following this implementation cycle, we first need insight into the problem under study. Also, an assessment of actual performance (the level of

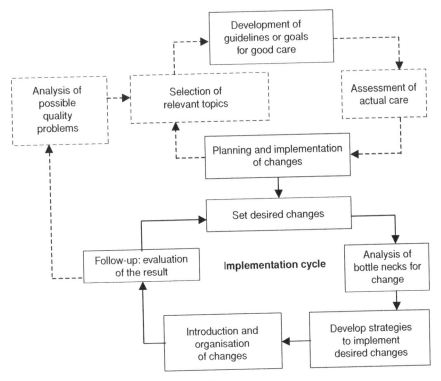

Figure 13.1 The implementation cycle.[10]

actual care) is needed. The problem needs to be well defined and must be made clear to those whose performance we wish to change. Next, the optimal—"gold standard"—situation should be determined and communicated as such. Usually this means the development and dissemination of guidelines. Then, the desired changes need to be determined and a guideline implementation strategy must be set up to achieve the actual change. After this, the results should be monitored. The outcome of this monitoring can be used as new input for further improvement and for defining new goals for quality assurance, thereby reentering the implementation cycle. These general rules apply not only to test-ordering behavior but also to other actions (such as prescribing drugs and referring to hospital care). Figure 13.1 highlights a number of steps in the implementation cycle.

Guideline development and implementation

Guidelines, protocols, and standards are needed to formalize the optimal practice situation. In the past, there have been various moves toward guideline development. Mostly, these guidelines are problem oriented and address clinical problems as a whole, such as taking care of diabetes patients, or diagnosing and managing dyspepsia. The diagnostic workup of a clinical problem and the resulting recommendations for specific tests—if necessary—are then important aspects to be dealt with. A good example of a comprehensive set of guidelines is the development of standards for Dutch GPs by the Dutch College of General Practitioners.[11] Starting in 1989, the college has set up more than 80 guidelines on a variety of common clinical problems. In the meantime, many of these standards have been revised in line with new evidence from scientific research. One of the guidelines specifically addresses the principles of rational ordering of blood tests.[12]

The development of guidelines does not automatically lead to the desired behavioral change, especially when their dissemination is limited to the distribution of written material. In other words, simply publishing and mailing the guidelines does not make clinicians act accordingly. Implementation strategies are needed to bring about change. Implementation includes a range of activities to stimulate the compliance with guidelines as shown in the implementation cycle.

Systematic development seems necessary to improve the effectiveness of interventions on implementation. Interventions should be targeted at barriers and stimulating conditions for working according to professional guidelines. The reasons that professionals have for noncompliance, be it professional or context related, should be thoroughly known. Possible methods for collecting these barriers can be both qualitative and quantitative. Unfortunately, in literature, little has been published so far on how to systematically translate knowledge on barriers and stimulating conditions into the contents of such quality improvement strategies.[13] The next section gives an overview of the experience so far with most of the guideline implementation strategies.

For obvious reasons we should seek and apply methods that both improve the rationality of test ordering and can stop the increase in the use of tests. Ideally, such instruments combine a more rational test-ordering behavior with a reduction in requests. To determine these, a closer look at the performance of the specific implementation strategies is needed.

However, not all of these instruments have been used on a regular basis. Some have been regularly applied on a variety of topics (such as changing test ordering), whereas others have been used only incidentally. Most implementation strategies try to change doctors' behavior. Although evidence showing relevant effects is required to justify their implementation in practice, because of the nature of the intervention it is not always possible to perform a proper effect evaluation. Especially in large-scale interventions, such as changes in the law or health care regulations (nationwide), it is virtually impossible to obtain a concurrent control group. Nevertheless, a number of (randomized) trials have been performed, albeit predominantly on relatively small-scale implementation strategies.

Is a change feasible?

Implementation strategies

A variety of implementation strategies is available. However, not all of them are successful: some strategies were effective, but others have been disappointing. There have been a number of published reviews focusing on the effectiveness of implementation strategies. Although their conclusions vary, some consensus can be observed: there are some implementation strategies that seem to fail and some that are at least promising.

Many different approaches have been adopted to improve doctors' performance. In 2004, a large systematic literature review was on effectiveness of guideline implementation strategies among medically qualified health care professionals with objective measures of doctor behavior or patient outcome.[14] Two hundred and thirty-five studies published before 1999 were included. The majority of the included studies (87%) observed improvements in care. The median absolute improvement in performance from the highest levels of evidence (cluster randomized controlled trials [RCTs]) is 8% for dissemination of educational materials, 7% for audit and feedback, 14% for reminders, and 6% for multifaceted strategies. The improvements are generally modest to moderate and there was no clear relationship between number of interventions and effect size.

Another systematic review focused on the effectiveness of strategies aiming at influencing test ordering.[15] In total, 98 studies published until 2001 were included; these included RCTs, quasi-experiments, controlled before–after studies, and interrupted time-series analyses of any intervention to influence the test-ordering behavior of any type of health care professional. Overall, results were heterogeneous due to differences in the type or intensity of the intervention, in the setting, or due to methodological differences between studies (such as differences in measurement periods). It was concluded that there is no overall rule for choosing the best intervention to influence test-ordering behavior, apart from the generally accepted rule to tailor the intervention to the barriers for change. In addition to professional-oriented interventions, it seems important to consider the use of interventions focusing on organizational factors. Moreover, it is not clear if multifaceted strategies have more impact than single strategies, but it seems important to focus the intervention at both the professional and the context.

There is a range of interventions that combine the provision of knowledge with giving more specific insight into one's own performance. Such interventions include audit, individual feedback, peer review, and computer reminders. Some examples follow.

Among the most frequently used basic interventions are the distribution of written material (such as protocol manuals) and educational meetings (such as training sessions or postgraduate education). Distribution of educational materials and educational meetings should be looked on as (necessary) parts of a multifaceted intervention.

Implementation strategies that have been used and studied regularly in the past are audit, peer review, and feedback. To that end, tests ordered are reviewed and discussed by (expert) peers or audit panels. Audit represents a monitoring system on specific aspects of care. It is often rather formal, set up and organized by colleges and regional or national committees.[16] The subject and the intensity of the related interventions of an audit system may vary strongly. The results of the audit are to be fed back to the professionals. In peer review, expert colleagues review actual performance.

Within this group of interventions, there is a huge variation in what is reviewed and discussed, in how often and to whom it is directed, and in the way the review is presented. Audit and feedback, both with and without information transfer, show consistent and sometimes even strong effects on both changing the absolute rate of test use ("modifying overuse") as well as on improving appropriateness of test use ("improving quality"). There is no clear trend toward a specific content of the feedback given, but feedback seems more effective when the information provided can be used directly in daily practice, when the doctor is individually addressed, and when the expert peer is generally respected and accepted.[15] An intervention with substantial effects, also proven in a randomized trial, was feedback given to individual general practitioners, focusing on the rationality of tests ordered.[17] After 9 years, there was a clear and constant reduction in test use, mainly due to a decrease in nonrational requests.[18]

Small-group quality improvement, including peer review, seems reasonably effective (median absolute improvement in performance about 10%).[19] Outreach visits and patient-mediated interventions seem promising but deserve more research.

An increasingly popular implementation strategy is through computer reminders. The use of computer reminders is stimulated by the explosive growth in the use of computers in health care. Having the same background and intentions as audit and feedback, reminders do not generally involve the monitoring of the performance of specific groups or individual doctors. Here the computer may take over, but the intention is still to make doctors comply with guidelines and to give insight into one's own performance. From the viewpoint of the observed clinician, "anonymous" computer reminder systems may appear less threatening: there are no peers directly involved who must review the actions of those whose behavior is monitored.

The results of computer reminders are promising. It appears to be a potentially effective method requiring relatively little effort. Reminders have significant but variable effects in reducing unnecessary tests, and seem to improve compliance with guidelines.[8,20] To date, there are relatively few studies on computer reminders. It may be expected, however, that in the near future more interventions on the basis of computer reminders will be performed as a direct spin-off of the growing use of computer-supported communication facilities in health care.

One reason for the increasing use of tests is that tests are both available and accessible. Organizational interventions are focused on facilitating desired behavior or reducing undesired or restricted (diagnostic) behavior. Consequently, a simple strategy would be to reduce the availability of tests on forms or to request an explicit justification for the test(s) ordered. Such interventions have by and large proved to be effective, with a low input of additional costs and effort: Zaat and Smithuis found reductions of 20–50%.[21,22] A drawback of these interventions, however, is that they risk a possible underuse of tests when the test order form is reduced too extensively and unselectively. Therefore, the changes to the form should be selected and designed carefully. Regulations include interventions where financial incentives or penalties can be easily introduced. Reimbursement systems by health insurance companies or the government may act as a stimulus to urge clinicians to move in the desired direction. Combinations of regulatory steps and financial changes are also conceivable. In several western countries, the health care system includes payment for tests ordered by doctors, even if the tests are performed by another professional or institution. Adaptation of the health care regulations could change this payment system, which might reduce the ordering of too many tests, thereby directly increasing clinicians' income. Even negative incentives for nonrational test ordering can be built in, acting more or less as a financial penalty. Little is known about the effect of financial interventions, but the three studies were not promising in their results.

Perpetuation and continuation
One aspect that needs more attention in the future is the perpetuation of interventions once they have been started. There is no assurance that effects, when achieved, will continue when the intervention has stopped. In most studies, the effects after stopping the intervention are not monitored. As one of the exceptions, Tierney performed a follow-up after ending his intervention through computer reminders on test ordering.[23] The effects of the intervention disappeared 6 months after stopping. On the other hand, Winkens found that feedback was still effective after being continued over a 9-year period.[17] This argues in favor of a continuation of an implementation strategy once it is started.

Evaluating the effects
There is a growing awareness that the effects of interventions are by no means guaranteed. Consequently, to discriminate between interventions that are successful and those that are not, we need evidence from scientific evaluations. However, after a series of decades where many scientific evaluations of implementation strategies have been performed and a number of reviews have been published, many questions remain and conclusions cannot yet be drawn. In a dynamic environment such as the (para)medical profession, it is almost inevitable that the effects of interventions are dynamic and variable over time too. Hence, there will always be a need for scientific evaluation.

As in all scientific evaluations, there are quality criteria that studies should meet.[24] Regarding these criteria, evaluation studies on implementation strategies do not essentially differ from other evaluations. The randomized controlled trial still remains the gold standard. However, there are some circumstances that need special attention, such as the risk of a Hawthorne effect due to a certain awareness. Especially in the field of implementation strategies, the nature of the intervention can cause some awareness among professionals, and therefore cause some effects, merely by the knowledge that one's behavior is monitored. Informed consent may cause such an awareness and situations where informed consent is not required can be beneficial.[25] Although it is impossible to blind doctors for participating in a RCT, alternative designs such as the balanced incomplete block design may assist in optimizing the experimental conditions and control for the Hawthorne effect.[26] Another striking issue is the following. In most studies on improving test-ordering behavior, the doctor is the one whose decisions are to be influenced. This automatically means that the unit of randomization, and hence the unit of analysis, is the individual doctor. As the number of doctors participating in a study is often limited, this may have a considerably negative effect on the power of the study. A potential solution to this problem may be found in multilevel analyses.[27]

Cost-effectiveness of implementation

As far as the cost-effectiveness of intervention strategies is concerned, those that combine good effects with the least effort and lowest costs are to be preferred. On the other hand, we may question whether strategies that so far have not proved to be effective should be continued. Should we continue to put much effort into CME, especially in single training courses or lectures? Whom should we try to reach through scientific and educational papers: the clinicians in daily practice or only the scientist and policy maker with special interest? Should we have to choose the most effective intervention method, regardless of the effort that is needed? If we start an intervention to change test ordering, does this mean it has to be continued for years? There is no general answer to these questions, although the various reviews that have been published argue in favor of tailor-made interventions and combinations of strategies focusing on the professional and the process and organization of care. How such a combination is composed depends on the specific situation (such as local needs and healthcare routines, and the availability of experts and facilities). General recommendations for specific combinations are therefore not possible or useful. However, if we look at costs in the long term, computer interventions look quite promising.

Studying costs of implementation strategies is only one side of the picture. For a full economic evaluation, two criteria are relevant: (1) Is an explicit comparison made between two strategies or between a strategy and usual care? (2) Are both costs and consequences of these strategies evaluated (Figure 13.2)?[28,29]

Outcomes and costs taken into consideration?

		Outcomes only	Costs only	Both outcomes and costs
Alternatives	No	Description of outcomes	Description of costs	Description of cost effects
compared?	Yes	Evaluation of outcomes	Evaluation of costs	Economic evaluation

Figure 13.2 Criteria for a complete economic evaluation (based on Drummond *et al.* 2005).[29]

It can only be determined whether an implementation strategy, such as educating doctors on test ordering, is value for money when this implementation strategy is compared with another strategy or when it is compared to usual care. In most cases of implementation of strategies to improve test-ordering behavior of doctors, a comparison will be made with usual care (no implementation strategy). This can either be done in a prospective study or by using a retrospective historical control. Apart from a comparison with care as usual, different implementation strategies for improving test-ordering behavior can be compared to determine which one offers best value for money (Figure 13.3). Obviously, a prospective study is the only option then.

The second prerequisite stated that both investment and result should be part of a full economic evaluation. This seems logical because it is impossible to define the efficiency of any activity in health care if investment expressed as costs is not explicitly related to the effects realized. Five types of economic evaluations can be identified.

1 *The cost-minimization analysis:* Only studying costs will offer a rather limited scope although this might be considered as one of the methods of a full economic evaluation. This is the so-called cost-minimization analysis. A cost-minimization analysis requires the knowledge or the evidence-based assumption that patient outcome will be equal in the compared strategies, irrespective of the fact that the implementation strategy is compared to another strategy or to care as usual. However, this situation is hardly ever the case. When an implementation strategy is effective, these effects are likely

Consequences of A compared to B

		A is worse than B	A is better than B
Costs of A	Higher	A inferior compared to B	Better outcome worth the higher costs?
Compared to B	Lower	Worse outcome acceptable, considering the lower costs?	A is dominant compared to B

Figure 13.3 Classification of the outcomes of economic evaluations comparing two alternatives.[28]

to lead to improvement of patient care as well. Therefore, most situations require an economic evaluation that includes measurement of the consequences or effectiveness. The consequences of implementation strategies to improve test-ordering behavior can be expressed in several ways. Process parameters and patient outcome can be distinguished. Process parameters can described as any parameter that values the process of the doctors' actions, for instance, the number of adequately ordered test per 1,000 patients, or the number of doctors who order tests properly. In fact, the ways to define a relevant process parameter are numerous and in a full economic evaluation this will lead to the so-called cost-effectiveness ratio that expresses efficiency of a strategy to improve test ordering: the extra costs per extra adequately ordered test, per doctor who ordered tests properly, per patient tested according to the recommendations in the guideline, and so. Because of the fact that any economic evaluation is an explicit comparison between several strategies, the cost-effectiveness ratio between strategies expresses the investment that is needed to achieve a higher effectiveness. Of course, in case one strategy is both cheaper and better than any other, this strategy is considered dominant and should be stimulated without any doubt.

2 *Cost-effectiveness analysis:* Using process parameters in an economic evaluation is based on one important, major assumption: the process parameter is positively correlated to patient outcome. Thus, for example, the higher the number of adequately ordered tests, the higher the patient outcome; more specifically, the patients that do not need to be tested are not bothered with the burden of testing or the consequences of false positive test results and the patients that need to be tested are indeed tested and benefit from the correct consequence of the test result, namely to treat or to refrain from treatment. Sometimes, however, the relationship between a process parameter and actual patient outcome is not known or uncertain. In that case, it is useful to determine patient outcome in evaluating strategies to improve test-ordering behavior. Patient outcome is, as can be expected, usually not influenced by a diagnostic test as such, but more clearly by the consequences of the test result. In this situation, the health status of a patient should be defined. In case this health status is defined in so-called disease specific values (e.g., blood pressure or diabetic regulation), these in fact reflect intermediate patient outcome. The efficiency of an implementation strategy in this situation is expressed as cost per blood pressure reduction or cost per adequately treated diabetic patient. An evaluation relating cost to a process parameter or to an intermediate patient outcome is called a "cost-effectiveness analysis."

3 *Cost–utility analysis:* Here, patient outcome is measured in quality of life, more specifically, in the utility or value that society gives to a patient's health status. For this measurement, several standardized instruments exist such as the EuroQol-5D or the Short Form 36. In this way the cost per QALY (quality adjusted life year) can be determined, an evaluation outcome that is hardly seen in implementation research.[30] A more convenient method to

determine the cost–utility of improving test-ordering behavior of doctors is to use the Mason model.[31] In this model, the previously mentioned process parameters are mathematically combined with cost per QALY data that might reflect proper test-ordering behavior and subsequent correct treatment of patients. This model shows that multiple factors of influence determine whether effort to achieve behavioral change is worthwhile. Of course, using the Mason model is only possible when the full economic consequences and patient outcome of proper test use or the compliance with the clinical guideline for test use are known from previous research.

Relevant behavioral change, at least from the viewpoint of policy makers, demands an implementation strategy that does not load test-treatment cost-effectiveness to such an extent that normal bounds of cost-effectiveness are exceeded.[31] An estimation of overall policy costs and benefits can be expressed in the following equation on policy cost effectiveness:

$$\Delta CE_p = \frac{1}{d.n_p.p_d.\Delta b_t}\Delta CE_i + \Delta CE_t = L_{CE} + \Delta CE_t$$

Here (slightly adapted from Mason) $\Delta b_t, \Delta c_t$, and ΔCE_t are the net health gain, cost of diagnostic and therapeutic care and test-treatment cost-effectiveness per patient ($\Delta c_t/\Delta b_t$); Δc_i, Δb_i, and ΔCE_i are the net cost, the proportion of patient care changed, and the implementation cost-effectiveness per practice ($\Delta c_i/\Delta b_i$); d is the duration of effect of the implementation method; n_p and p_d are the average practice size and population prevalence of the targeted condition; L_{CE} is the loading factor on treatment cost effectiveness.[31]

This formula shows the case when a change in health care is valued as a cost-effectiveness ratio and the performance indicator is the simple proportion of patients getting appropriate care. Where the loading is small, treatment and policy cost-effectiveness are very similar. If the loading is large, advanced use of a cost effective treatment may not be worth encouraging as a policy goal using the available implementation strategies.

4 *Cost-benefit analysis:* This is hardly used in evaluating activities in health care. In essence, patient outcome is expressed here in monetary units, something that is considered both difficult and unethical.

5 *Cost-consequence analysis:* The cost-consequence analysis has recently been introduced as an alternative economic evaluation. In the cost-consequence analysis, costs are not explicitly related to any process or patient outcome parameter using a cost-effectiveness ratio, but costs and consequences are simple listed, leaving the decision maker to make the balance between positive and negative consequences.[32]

In the economic assessment of treatment of patients, cost analysis is rather simple: just estimate or, when possible, determine the costs of treatment, costs of possible side effects, longer-term costs, possibly cost outside the health care sector such as expenses by patients (depending of the perspective used in an evaluation) or productivity costs due to a patients (in)ability to work.

In evaluating test-ordering behavior, things become more complicated. Of course, the costs of testing are relevant, but the costs of false negative and false positive test results are also relevant. When evaluating implementation strategies to improve test-ordering behavior, the complexity of the costing study increases. Consequently, the costs of implementation strategies can be split for different phases of the implementation process.[33] First, there are costs related to the *development of an implementation strategy*. For example, when implementing a computer system to improve test-ordering behavior, the computer software must be developed. Such costs are usually nonrecurrent and can therefore be considered fixed costs. Next, the costs of the actual *execution of the implementation strategy* are not relevant until the moment the strategy is executed. Such costs can be considered fixed (e.g., installing the computer system) or variable (the time of the doctor being trained or using the computer system). Finally, costs are sometimes associated with a *change in health care delivery* because of using an implementation strategy. These are the aforementioned costs of testing and treating patients.

In short, analyzing the full cost and consequences of strategies to improve test-ordering behavior of doctors requires an extensive analysis of a full range of costs and actual patient outcome. In case rational test ordering is—without any doubt—also efficient in terms of both subsequent treatment costs and patient outcome, such extensive analysis is not necessary. Otherwise, economic evaluation, from mathematical modeling of cost-effectiveness of process outcome to cost-effectiveness of patient care can be of help.

From scientific evidence to daily practice

An important objective in influencing test-ordering behavior is the change in the rationality and volume of tests ordered, thereby reducing costs or achieving a better relation of costs and effects. However, the ultimate goal is to improve the quality of care for the individual patient. To what extent are patients willing to pay for expensive diagnostic activities, weighing the possibility of achieving better health through doing (and paying) the diagnostics, versus the risk of not diagnosing the disease and staying ill (or getting worse) because of not doing so? In other words, how is the cost–utility ratio of diagnostic testing assessed by the patient? In this context the specific positive or negative (side) effects of (not) testing on the health status of the individual patient are difficult to assess independently of other influences. On the other hand, a reduced use in unnecessary, nonrational tests is not likely to cause adverse effects for the individual. An upcoming trend, predominantly in western societies, is the actual use of self-tests by consumers. It is not known yet what consequences this phenomenon will have on availability of facilities, cost-effectiveness of diagnostics in health care, and diagnostic performance by health care professionals.

Despite the increasing research evidence showing the need for changes in test-ordering behavior, doctors will always decide on more than merely scientific evidence when the question whether to order a test for a certain patient is at stake.[34] Low diagnostic accuracy or high costs of testing may conflict with a patient's explicit wish to have tests ordered or with the doctor's wish to gain time, the fear of missing an important diagnosis, his or her feeling insecure, and the wish of both patient and doctor to be reassured. These dilemmas are influenced by a variety of doctor and patient related aspects. Regarding the doctor, one could think of the way in which they were trained, how long they have been active in patient care, the number of patients on their list, their relationship with their patients, and their personal experience with "missing" relevant diseases in the past. The patient might suffer from a chronic disease, or from recurrent vague or unexplained complaints, making them question the skills of the doctor. For this latter category of patients in particular, doctors might order more tests than are strictly necessary. Research into the ways of improving test ordering in these situations is urgently needed.

References

1. Verstappen WHJM, ter Riet G, Dubois WI, et al. Variation in test ordering behaviour of general practitioners: professional or context-related factors? *Fam Pract.* 2004;**21**:387–95.
2. Verstappen WHJM, ter Riet G, Weijden T van der, et al. Variation in requests for imaging investigations by general practitioners: a multilevel analysis. *J Health Serv Res Policy.* 2005;**10**:25–30.
3. Van der Weijden T, Bokhoven MA, Dinant GJ, et al. Understanding laboratory testing in diagnostic uncertainty: a qualitative study in general practice. *Br J Gen Pract.* 2002;**52**:974–80.
4. Bugter-Maessen AMA, Winkens RAG, Grol RPTM, et al. Factors predicting differences among general practitioners in test ordering behaviour and in the response to feedback on test requests. *Fam Pract.* 1996;**13**:254–58.
5. Marple RL, Kroenke K, Lucey CR, et al. Concerns and expectations in patients presenting with physical complaints: frequency, physician perceptions and actions, and 2-week outcome. *Arch Intern Med.* 1997;**157**:1482–88.
6. Cohen O, Kahan E, Zalewski S, et al. Medical investigations requested by patients: how do primary care physicians react? *Fam Med.* 1999;**31**:426–31.
7. Froehlich GW, Welch HG. Meeting walk-in patients' expectations for testing: effects on satisfaction. *J Gen Intern Med.* 1996;**11**:470–74.
8. van der Weijden T, van Velsen M, Dinant GJ, et al. Unexplained complaints in general practice: prevalence, patients' expectations, and professionals' test-ordering behavior. *Med Decis Making.* 2003;**23**:226–31.
9. van Bokhoven MA, Pleunis-van Empel M, Koch H, et al. Why do patients want to have their blood tested? a qualitative study of patient expectations in general practice. *BMC Fam Pract.* 2006;**7**;75.
10. Grol RPTM, van Everdingen JJE, Casparie AF. *Invoering van richtlijnen en veranderingen.* Utrecht: De Tijdstroom; 1994.
11. Wiersma TJ, Goudzwaard AN. *NHG Standaarden voor de huisarts.* Houten: Bohn, Stafleu, van Loghem; 2006.

12. Dinant GJ, van Wijk MAM, Janssens HJEM, et al. NHG-Standaard Bloedonderzoek. *Huisarts Wet*. 1994;**37**:202–11.

13. van Bokhoven MA, Kok G, van der Weijden T. Designing a quality improvement intervention: a systematic approach. *Qual Safety Health Care*. 2003;**12**:215–20.

14. Grimshaw JM, Thomas RE, MacLennan G, et al. Effectiveness and efficiency of guideline dissemination and implementation strategies. *Health Technol Assess*. 2004;**8**(6).

15. Verstappen WHJM. Towards optimal test ordering in primary care. Thesis Maastricht University; 2004. pp. 33–56.

16. Smith R. Audit in action. London: BMJ Publishers;1992.

17. Winkens RAG, Pop P, Bugter AMA, et al. Randomised controlled trial of routine individual feedback to improve rationality and reduce numbers of test requests. *Lancet*. 1995;**345**:498–502.

18. Winkens RAG, Pop P, Grol RPTM, et al. Effects of routine individual feedback over nine years on general practitioners' requests for tests. *BMJ*. 1996;**312**: 490.

19. Verstappen W, van der Weijden T, Sijbrandij J, et al. Effect of a practice-based strategy on test ordering performance of primary care physicians: a randomized trial. *JAMA*. 2003;**289**:2407–12.

20. Buntinx F, Winkens RAG, Grol RPTM, et al. Influencing diagnostic and preventive performance in ambulatory care by feedback and reminders: a review. *Fam Pract*. 1993;**10**:219–28.

21. Zaat JO, van Eijk JT, Bonte HA. Laboratory test form design influences test ordering by general practitioners in the Netherlands. *Med Care*. 1992;**30**:189–98.

22. Smithuis LOMJ, van Geldrop WJ, Lucassen PLBJ. Beperking van het laboratoriumonderzoek door een probleemgeorienteerd aanvraagformulier [abstract in English]. *Huisarts Wet*. 1994;**37**:464–66.

23. Tierney WM, Miller ME, McDonald CJ. The effect on test ordering of informing physicians of the charges for outpatient diagnostic tests. *N Engl J Med*. 1990;**322**:1499–504.

24. Pocock SJ. Clinical trials: a practical approach. Chichester: John Wiley & Sons; 1991.

25. Winkens RAG, Knottnerus JA, Kester ADM, et al. Fitting a routine health-care activity into a randomized trial: an experiment possible without informed consent? *J Clin Epidemiol*. 1997;**50**:435–39.

26. Verstappen WHJM, van der Weijden T, ter Riet G, et al. Block designs in quality improvement research enable control for the Hawthorne effect. *J Clin Epidemiol*. 2004;**57**:1119–23.

27. Campbell MK, Mollison J, Steen N, et al. Analysis of cluster randomized trials in primary care: a practical approach. *Fam Pract*. 2000;**17**: 192–96.

28. Sculpher MJ. Evaluating the cost-effectiveness of interventions designed to increase the utilization of evidence-based guidelines. *Fam Pract*. 2000;S26–S31.

29. Drummond MF, Sculpher MJ, Torrance GW, et al. Methods for the economic evaluation of health care programmes. 3rd ed. Oxford: Oxford Medical Publications; 2005.

30. Schermer TR, Thoonen BP, Boom Gvd, et al. Randomized controlled economic evaluation of asthma self-management in primary health care. *Am J Resp Crit Care Med*. 2002;**166**:1062–72.

31. Mason J, Freemantle N, Nazareth I, et al. When is it cost-effective to change the behaviour of health professionals? *JAMA*. 2001;**286**:2988–92.
32. Mauskopf JA, Paul JE, Grant DM, et al. The role of cost-consequence analysis in health care decision making. Pharmacoeconomics 1998;**13**:277–88.
33. Severens JL. Value for money of changing healthcare services? economic evaluation of quality improvement. *Qual Saf Health Care*. 2003;**12**:366–71.
34. Knottnerus JA, Dinant GJ. Medicine-based evidence, a prerequisite for evidence-based medicine. *BMJ*. 1997;**315**:1109–10.

CHAPTER 14

Epilogue: overview of evaluation strategy and challenges

J. André Knottnerus, Ann van den Bruel, and Frank Buntinx

Summary box

- The first phase in the evaluation of diagnostic procedures consists of (1) specifying the clinical problem, the diagnostic procedures(s), and the research question, and (2) a systematic search and review of the literature, to decide whether the question can already be answered or whether a new clinical study is necessary.
- In preparing a new clinical study, the investigator must decide about the need for evaluation of (1) test accuracy in circumstances of maximum contrast or, as a further step, in the "indicated" clinical population; (2) the impact of the test on clinical decision making (3) prognosis; or (4) cost-effectiveness. The answers to these questions are decisive for the study design.
- Systematic reviews and meta-analysis, clinical decision analysis, cost-effectiveness analysis, and expert panels can help to construct and update clinical guidelines.
- Implementation of guidelines should be professionally supported and evaluated, in view of what is known about how clinicians approach diagnostic problems.
- Further developments in four fields are especially important: progress and innovation of (bio)medical knowledge relevant for diagnostic testing and its impact; the development of information and communication technology in relation to clinical research and practice; the changing role of the patient; and further exploration of methodological challenges in research on diagnostic problems.

The Evidence Base of Clinical Diagnosis: Theory and Methods of Diagnostic Research. 2nd edition. Edited by J. André Knottnerus and Frank Buntinx. © 2009 Blackwell Publishing. ISBN: 978-1-4051-5787-2.

Introduction

The chapters in this book speak for themselves and there is no need to repeat them or summarize their contents. However, a compact overview of important steps in the evaluation of diagnostic procedures may be useful. In addition, challenges for future work are outlined.

Important steps

Test development

As indicated in Chapter 3, any new test must first go through a phase of technical development and assessment.[1] This will often encompass basic biological and pathophysiological research. In this phase, candidate tests are being evaluated on whether and to what extent they can produce usable information under laboratory conditions. That is, the ability to detect a specified quantity of a certain component present in a sample (analytical sensitivity), to indicate its absence where appropriate (analytical specificity), and to obtain the same test result on repeated testing or observations (reproducibility). The phase of early development and assessment may also consist of behavioral research if psychological phenomena are to be diagnosed.

This book was focused on tests that are assumed to have successfully passed this early development and assessment phase, and then have to be evaluated as to their clinical and health care impact. In this context, the most important steps are represented in a flow diagram of the evaluation strategy (Figure 14.1), with reference to chapters in the book.

Clinical problem and research question

The first step is to specify the clinical problem and the diagnostic procedure(s) to be evaluated and the aim and research question of the study. Are we looking for the (added) diagnostic value of the procedure, or the impact of the procedure on clinical management, on prognosis and patient's health, or on cost-effectiveness?

As to diagnostic value, in Chapter 2 and 3, the importance of defining the research question and the contrast to be evaluated was emphasized, which is also crucial for the choice of the study design.[2] The following situations were distinguished: (1) single test: assessing the value of inserting a new test compared with not testing; (2) comparing tests: the (performance of a) new test with the best ones already available for the same diagnostic problem; (3) additional testing: estimating the value of further (e.g., more invasive) testing, given the tests already performed; and (4) comparing diagnostic strategies: to evaluate the most accurate or efficient diagnostic test set or test sequence for a certain diagnostic problem. A new test can also be less invasive, and therefore interesting to be inserted earlier in the process to preselect for more invasive tests. In line with this approach, three roles of new tests have been defined: (1) replacement, (2) triage, and (3) add-on.[3] A new test may replace

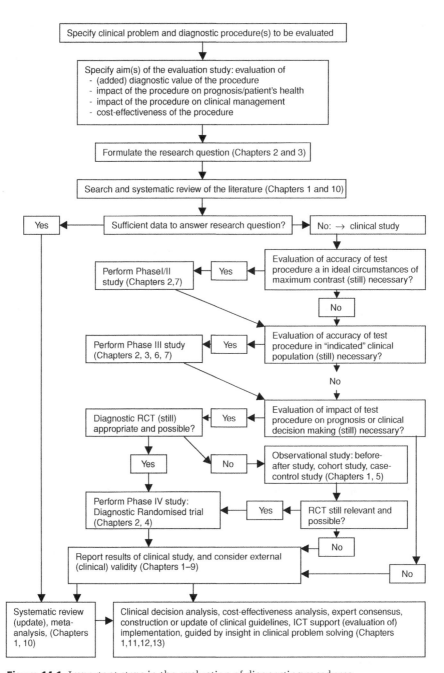

Figure 14.1 Important steps in the evaluation of diagnostic procedures.

an existing test if it is more accurate, less invasive for the patient, cheaper, easier to interpret, or yields quicker results. To be able to decide on this, the new test will need to be compared on these aspects with the existing test. Triage tests typically exclude the disease in a proportion of patients who no longer enter the further clinical pathway. However, triage tests may also be used to increase the proportion of patients entering the clinical pathway, by picking up cases that otherwise would have been missed. Triage tests are especially attractive if they are noninvasive for patients, simple to perform and cheap. Finally, a new test may be placed as add-on after an existing clinical pathway, if it is not only more accurate but also more invasive or expensive. It may then be only applied in a subgroup of patients.

The ultimate goal of health care is to improve patient outcome: expected harm of testing, such as burden, pain, and risk, should be weighed against expected benefit, such as improved life expectancy, quality of life, and avoidance of other test procedures. In addition, for policy decisions, weighing effects and benefits against costs, is important. As properly and directly evaluating these aspects (in the context of a randomized trial or otherwise in an appropriate observational study) is not always possible, studying the test's influence on the physician's thinking and management decisions may serve as a proxy. After all, in general, a patient's outcome cannot be influenced by diagnostic testing unless the physician is led to do something different than he would have done without the test result. The focus is then on change in diagnosis or treatment decision by the physician, by comparing the intended management before and after the test result is known. We have to consider, however, that change in management does not necessarily lead to an improved patient outcome: patients may not benefit from the change in therapy or even experience harm.

Cost-effectiveness goes beyond the individual risks and benefits. It addresses whether the cost of using a given test is acceptable to society and allows to make comparisons across a broader range of health interventions. Cost-effectiveness studies estimate a cost per unit of the effect measure, for example, cost per surgery avoided, cost per appropriately treated patient, cost per life year gained, or cost per quality adjusted life year (QALY) gained. Final outcomes, such as life years or QALYs gained, are preferred over intermediate outcomes. As data on outcomes and costs of diagnostic and subsequent therapeutic pathways are not always available from empirical observations, cost-effectiveness is often assessed on the basis of (additional) assumptions. The correctness of such assumptions of course determines the validity of the conclusions.

Systematic review
After having formulated the research question, we must search and systematically review the literature and decide whether sufficient research data—meeting appropriate quality requirements—are already available to answer the question. If this is the case, additional clinical research efforts are not

needed nor justified. If sufficient data are not yet available, a new clinical study should be considered if this is to be expected to add to the evidence base for giving a better answer.

Study design

To evaluate the diagnostic and clinical value of diagnostic procedures in relation to the defined contrast and test role, a variety of study designs, including observational and experimental approaches, are available. As emphasized before, choosing the most appropriate approach depends primarily on the research question. In preparing a clinical study, in summary, to choose the appropriate approach the following questions need to be answered: (1) is evaluation of accuracy of the test procedure in ideal circumstances of maximum contrast (still) necessary or (2) has this already been successfully achieved and should accuracy still be established in the "indicated" clinical population? (3) Is the impact of the diagnostic procedure on clinical decision making or prognosis yet unknown? (4) Should cost-effectiveness be evaluated? The answers to these questions lead to the appropriate study type, as shown in Figure 14.1. It is sometimes possible to include more than one type of design in one study. For example, test accuracy may be determined in the context of a randomized trial or a before–after study.

From results to practice

In preparing and reporting the results of a clinical study, the generalizability or external (clinical) validity should be carefully considered. In connection to this, additional evaluations in other populations representative of the target group to be tested are often important.[4] Especially in those cases where multivariable prediction rules or tests are derived, validation in an independent similar population of patients is necessary. If the study is unique with regard to clinical applicability, the results represent an important evidence base themselves. More often they contribute to a broader knowledge base and can be included in (an update of) a systematic review or meta-analysis. Clinical decision analysis, cost-effectiveness analysis, and expert panels are helpful in constructing or updating clinical predition rules[5] and clinical guidelines. The implementation of guidelines in clinical practice should be professionally supported and evaluated, in view of the acquired insights into the way clinicians approach diagnostic problems.

Challenges

Throughout this book, a comprehensive range ("architecture") of methodological options has been described. At the same time, it has become clear that there are important challenges for future work.

Developments in four fields are especially important. First, (bio)medical knowledge will continue to be expanded, cumulated, and refined. Second, information and communication technology (ICT) will further develop and its use in daily practice will be more and more facilitated. Third, the patient's role is an increasingly active one, with important implications for patient–doctor communication and the decision-making process. Finally, in research on diagnostic problems and procedures, methodological requirements, and innovations are to be further explored.

Biomedical progress and clinical epidemiological quality

Innovation of biomedical knowledge and understanding of pathophysiological processes are the principal requirements for the development and evaluation of better diagnostic tests. A clear example is the current work to develop DNA tests in various clinical fields. Increasingly, these will not only support genetic counseling and perinatal screening but also clinical diagnosis, prognostic assessment, targeting and dosing of therapeutics ("pharmacogenetics"), and targeting of interventions in the field of prevention, public health, and nutrition.[6,7,8]

A small number of people have specific genetic characteristics that make the chances to be or become diseased very high (e.g., trisomy 21 for Down's syndrome or BCRA polymorphisms for breast cancer). In such cases, individual genetic tests can provide substantial diagnostic information or even be the gold standard. Of many frequent diseases such as diabetes, cardiovascular disorders, and most malignancies, however, the risk increases or decreases according to the presence of genetic polymorphisms interacting with other polymorphisms and with environmental factors.[9] Much work in this field is being done, for example, in cardiovascular medicine,[10] oncology,[11,12] and psychiatry.[13]

Genetic characteristics can relate to the person (i.e., all his or her cells), the pathological cells only (e.g., tumor tissue), or a causing organism (e.g., a virus). Both in genetic patient testing and in DNA (or RNA) testing of causal agents, considerable efforts are still needed, not only in the laboratory but also in clinical research. Regarding the latter, the clinical epidemiological quality of many molecular genetic studies is generally poor and needs substantial improvement and development.[14,15,16] Furthermore, long-term follow-up to clinically validate diagnostic and prognostic predictions needs much more attention. At the same time, the methodology of using shorter-term intermediate outcomes must be better developed in a time of increasingly fast progress of knowledge and technology.[17] In addition, in view of the ambition to develop more targeted, perhaps even individualized, diagnostic and intervention processes, studies in large study populations will be increasingly unsatisfactory.[18] Research methodology will therefore be challenged to strengthen its tools for small group and even n = 1 studies. Also, ethical issues regarding the privacy of genetic information and the right to (not) know have to be dealt with.[19] In this context, doctors and patients, traditionally battling to reduce diagnostic and prognostic uncertainty, must also learn to cope with approaching certainty.[20]

ICT and the methodological agenda

Although until now computer decision support systems seem to have had more impact on the quality of drug prescriptions—avoidance of drug interactions, and high-risk group-targeted preventive care—than on diagnosis, the growing body and complexity of knowledge enhances the need for (online) diagnostic decision support systems. The development and evaluation of such systems will therefore remain an important challenge, as was outlined in Chapter 11. The same applies to the provision and maintenance of appropriate input, that is, valid and up to date diagnostic and prognostic knowledge.

Performing especially designed and organized diagnostic studies in large study populations is expensive and will necessarily always cover only a limited part of diagnostic management. Moreover, such studies may produce results with rather limited generalizability in place and time. Consequently, ways are sought to more efficiently and permanently harvest clinical knowledge and experience. It is worth considering whether and under what conditions accuracy studies, randomized controlled trials, quasi-experimental studies, and before–after studies can be more embedded in routine health care.[21] In view of continuity, up-to-date results, and (external) clinical validity, much can be expected from standardized clinical databases, with even international connections, also to be used as sampling frames for research. As these databases are closely related to or even integrated into routine health care, additional efforts are required to meet basic quality and methodological standards and to avoid biases.[22] In the context of such an integrated approach, also the implementation of new findings can be studied and monitored in real practice.

ICT progress has opened new ways of health care provision such as telemedicine and e-health. These innovations bring also new opportunities and challenges for dia-prognostic research. For instance, in addition to evaluating the quality and validity of diagnostic and prognostic triage by phone,[23,24] also the validity of telemedicine and e-mail assessments are now research topics. New methodological challenges in this context are related to the expectation that patients will increasingly have e-health consultations with physicians independent of distance, in principle without geographical limitations. This will, for example, have important implications for how to define the epidemiological numerators and denominators for such contacts, and, accordingly, for how to deal with spectrum and selection phenomena. Obviously, these developments are creating a new generation of research questions with a related methodological agenda.

Role of the patient, and self-testing

The role of the patient in diagnostic management is becoming more active. People want to be optimally informed and involved in the decision about what diagnostics are performed for what reason and want to know what the outcome means to them. Patient decision support facilities, at the doctor's office and at home, using e-health (e-mail or other Internet) services, are receiving increasing attention. Clinicians have to think about their possible role—interactively with the patient—in sifting, explaining, and integrating information via these facilities. Which level of certainty is worth which diagnostic procedures is not always similarly answered by patients and doctors. Patients' perceptions, preferences, and responsibilities should be respected and supported, not excluded, in clinical research and guidelines.[25] However, these features are not easily measurable and may show substantial inter- and intra-subject variability. A good patient–doctor dialogue therefore remains the core instrument of individual decision making.[26] Integrating patient preferences in diagnostic research and guidelines implies specific methodological challenges which only have begun to be appropriately addressed.

A phenomenon that increasingly comes forward is self-testing, as the market for so-called self-tests is growing fast, thereby responding to the wish of many people to be able to test themselves before or even without visiting a doctor. A substantial number of products and services have been introduced and are offered to the public via, e.g., pharmacies, drugstores, supermarkets, check-up centers, and the Internet, supported by television and newspaper commercials. Manufacturers claim not only that such tests enable users to detect disease in an early phase but also that this will benefit health. However, a recent analysis by the Health Council of the Netherlands[27] showed that only 3 out of 20 available self-tests represented a potentially useful addition. The other 17 did not meet general criteria of diagnostic validity, clinical utility, a favorable risk–benefit ratio, and cost-effectiveness. Given the developments in biomedical research, commercial interests, and market developments, it is to be expected that the increase in offered self-tests will continue. Accordingly, in the interest of the public and patients and their well-informed decision making, it is necessary formally to require an appropriately documented and convincing evidence base from manufacturers to justify their claims, to optimally inform the public, to monitor test follow-up, and to explore how useful self-tests can best be connected with state-of-the-art health care when needed. Also in this domain, there are various methodological challenges, such as evaluating test validity when applied by nonexperts in the context of daily life.

Other methodological challenges to keep us busy

In addition to the new issues mentioned in the two previous sections, also diagnostic research methodology in general must be further refined with respect to strategy, spectrum and selection effects, prognostic reference standards,[28] and the assessment of the clinical impact of testing. Data analysis needs progress in many aspects,[29] for example, with regard to "diagnostic and dia-prognostic effect modification" (which implies the study of factors influencing the diagnostic value of tests and interactions between tests), multiple test and disease outcome categories,[30] and estimation of sample size for multivariable problems. In addition, more flexible modeling is needed to identify alternative, clinically and pathophysiologically equivalent, but more comprehensive models, to optimally classify subgroups with varying sets of clinical characteristics.[31,32] For example, when using conventional statistical techniques, an infrequent symptom may not survive the selection process for the overall prediction model, while for the small subgroup where it is present it could be highly predictive. And, as another example, in the case that hemoglobin level would not be statistically selected for a prediction model because the strongly correlated hematocrit pushed it out, the model might not be applicable to patients with a missing value for hematocrit although the hemoglobin value may be available. More flexibility, for instance, by analyzing both pathways and integrating them in a more flexible model presentation, can help.

Better methods to improve and to evaluate external clinical validity, for example, in the context of daily practice, are also required. Furthermore, one must neither forget nor underestimate the diagnostic power of "real-life doctors' assessment": at least, the performance of proposed diagnostic innovations should be compared with the achievements of experienced clinicians, before such innovations are recommended as bringing new possibilities. We also need more understanding of the "doctor's black box" of diagnostic decision making, using cognitive psychological methods (Chapter 12). This can help in more efficient diagnostic reasoning and in the development of custom-made support systems.[33,34]

Efficiency and speed in the evaluation of the impact of diagnostic procedures can be gained if new data on a specific aspect (e.g., a diagnostic test) can be inserted into the mosaic of available evidence on a clinical problem (e.g., on the most effective treatment in case of a positive test), rather than studying the whole problem chain again whenever one element has changed. For this purpose, flexible scenario models of current clinical knowledge are needed.[35]

Systematic review and meta-analysis of diagnostic studies must not only be further improved[36,37,38] but also become a permanent routine activity of professional organizations producing and updating clinical guidelines. To increase comparability and quality, and to overcome publication bias, meta-analysis should not only be performed on already reported data but increasingly on original and even prospectively developing databases allowing individual patient data analysis. Such databases can originate from specific (collaborative) research projects, but sometimes also from health care (e.g., from clinics where systematic workups for patients with similar clinical presentations are routine, and where the population denominator is well defined). Accordingly, meta-analysis, evaluation research, and health care can become more integrated.

Although the methodology of diagnostic research is still lagging behind (and is even more complex) as compared to that of treatment research, in the past decades a lot of fundamental work has been done. Accordingly, important steps can now be made in the development of standards for the evaluation of the validity, safety, and impact of diagnostics, which is also necessary to control acceptance, maintenance, and substitution in the health care market. An important basic requirement is high quality and transparency of diagnostic research reports. The international agreement on Standards for the Reporting of Diagnostic Accuracy studies (STARD), described in Chapter 9, therefore deserves full support from the scientific and health care community[39] and, together with the tool for the quality assessment of studies of diagnostic accuracy included in systematic reviews (QUADAS),[38] also provides important input for standards for performing diagnostic research and for the evaluation of diagnostics for the health care market.

References

1. Van den Bruel A, Cleemput I, Aertgeerts B, et al. The evaluation of diagnostic tests: evidence on technical and diagnostic accuracy, impact on patient outcome and cost-effectiveness is needed. *J Clin Epidemiol.* 2007;**60**(11):1116–22.
2. Knottnerus, Muris JW. Assessment of the accuracy of diagnostic tests: the cross-sectional study. *J Clin Epidemiol.* 2003;**56**(11):1118–28.
3. Bossuyt PM, Irwig L, Craig J, et al. Comparative accuracy: assessing new tests against existing diagnostic pathways. *BMJ.* 2006;**332**(7549):1089–92.
4. Van den Bruel A, Aertgeerts B, Buntinx F. Results of diagnostic accuracy studies are not always validated, as shown in an empirical study. *J Clin Epidemiol.* 2006;**59**:559–66.
5. McGinn T, Guyatt G, Wyer P, et al. Diagnosis: Clinical prediction rules. In: Guyatt G and Rennie D (eds.): Users' guides to the medical literature, pp. 471–83. Chicago: AMA Press, 2004.
6. Ilkilic I, Wolf M, Paul NW. The brave new world of prevention? On the prerequisites and scope of public health genetics. *Gesundheitswesen.* 2007;**69**:53–62.
7. Afman L, Müller M. Nutrigenomics: from molecular nutrition to prevention of disease. *J Am Diet Assoc.* 2006;**106**:569–76.
8. Stover PJ. Influence of human genetic variation on nutritional requirements. *Am J Clin Nutr.* 2006;**83**:436S–42S.
9. Tucker G. Pharmacogenetics—expectations and reality: drug response and toxicity depend on genes, environment, and behaviour. *BMJ.* 2004;**329**:4–6.
10. Ginsburg GS, Donahue MP, Newby LK. Prospects for personalized cardiovascular medicine: the impact of genomics. *J Am Coll Cardiol.* 2005;**46**:1615–27.
11. Stoehlmacher J. Prediction of efficacy and side effects of chemotherapy in colorectal cancer. *Recent Results Cancer Res.* 2007;**176**:81–88.
12. Midley R, Kerr D. Towards post-genomic investigation of colorectal cancer. *Lancet.* 2000;**355**:669–70.
13. Perlis RH, Ganz DA, Avorn J, et al. Pharmacogenetic testing in the clinical management of schizophrenia: a decision-analytic model. *J Clin Psychopharmacol.* 2005;**25**:427–34.
14. Bogardus ST, Jr, Concato J, Feinstein AR. Clinical epidemiological quality in molecular genetic research. The need for methodological standards. *JAMA.* 1999;**281**:1919–26.
15. Ransohoff DF. How to improve reliability and efficiency of research about molecular markers: roles of phases, guidelines, and study design. *J Clin Epidemiol.* 2007;**60**(12):1205–19.
16. Porta M, Hernández-Aguado I, Lumbreras B, et al. "Omics" research, monetization of intellectual property and fragmentation of knowledge: can clinical epidemiology strengthen integrative research? *J Clin Epidemiol.* 2007;**60**(12):1220–25.

17. Kummar S, Gutierrez M, Doroshow JH, et al. Drug development in oncology: classical cytotoxics and molecularly targeted agents. *Br J Clin Pharmacol.* 2006;**62**:15–26.

18. Knottnerus JA. Challenges in dia-prognostic research. *J Epidemiol Community Health.* 2002;**56**: 340–41.

19. Health Council of the Netherlands: Pharmacogenetics. The Hague: Health Council of the Netherlands; 2000; publication no.2000/19.

20. Knottnerus JA. Community genetics and community medicine. *Fam Pract.* 2003;**20**:601–6.

21. van Wijk MA, van Der Lei J, Mosseveld M, et al. Assessment of decision support for blood test ordering in primary care: a randomized trial. *Ann Intern Med.* 2001;**134**:274–81.

22. Knottnerus JA. The role of electronic patient records in the development of general practice in the Netherlands. *Meth Info Med.* 1999;**38**:350–55.

23. Giesen P, Ferwerda R, Tijssen R, et al. Safety of telephone triage in general practitioner cooperatives: do triage nurses correctly estimate urgency? *Qual Saf Health Care.* 2007;**16**:181–84.

24. Derkx HP, Rethans JJ, Knottnerus JA, et al. Assessing communication skills of clinical call handlers working at an out-of-hours centre: development of the RICE rating scale. *Br J Gen Pract.* 2007;**57**:383–87.

25. Nease RF, Owens DK. A method for estimating the cost-effectiveness of incorporating patient preferences into practice guidelines. *Med Decision Making.* 1994;**14**:382–92.

26. Sackett DL. Evidence-based medicine. *Semin Perinatol.* 1997;**21**:3–5.

27. Health Council of the Netherlands. Annual report on screening for disease 2007—the self testing of body samples. The Hague: Health Council of the Netherlands; 2007; publication no. 2007/26.

28. Lijmer JG, Mol BW, Heisterkamp S, et al. Empirical evidence of design-related bias in studies of diagnostic tests. *JAMA.* 1999;**282**:1061–66.

29. Chan SF, Deeks JJ, Macaskill P, et al. Three methods to construct predictive models using logistic regression and likelihood ratios to facilitate adjustment for pretest probability give similar results. *J Clin Epidemiol.* 2008;**61**(1):52–63.

30. Biesheuvel CJ, Vergouwe Y, Steyerberg EW, et al. Polytomous logistic regression analysis could be applied more often in diagnostic research. *J Clin Epidemiol.* 2008;**61**(2):125–34.

31. Heckerling PS, Conant RC, Tape TG, et al. Reproducibility of predictor variables from a validated clinical rule. *Med Decision Making.* 1992;**12**:280–85.

32. Knottnerus JA. Diagnostic prediction rules: principles, requirements and pitfalls. *Prim Care.* 1995;**22**:341–63.

33. Friedman CP, Elstein AS, Wolf FM, et al. Enhancement of clinicians' diagnostic reasoning by computer-based consultation: a multisite study of 2 systems. *JAMA.* 1999;**282**:1851–56.

34. Elstein AS, Schwartz A. Clinical problem solving and diagnostic decision making: selective review of the cognitive literature. *BMJ.* 2002;**324**:729–32.

35. Knottnerus JA, van Weel C, Muris JW. Evaluation of diagnostic procedures. *BMJ.* 2002;**324**:477–80.

36. Irwig L, Tosteson AN, Gatsonis C, et al. Guidelines for meta-analyses evaluating diagnostic tests. *Ann Intern Med.* 1994;**120**:667–76.

37. Devillé WL, Buntinx F, Bouter LM, et al. Conducting systematic reviews of diagnostic studies: didactic guidelines. *BMC Med Res Methodol.* 2002;**2**:9.

38. Whiting P, Rutjes AW, Reitsma JB, et al. The development of QUADAS: a tool for the quality assessment of studies of diagnostic accuracy included in systematic reviews. *BMC Med Res Methodol*. 2003;**3**:25.
39. Bossuyt PM, Reitsma JB, Bruns DE, et al. Towards complete and accurate reporting of studies of diagnostic accuracy; the STARD initiative. *Clin Chem*. 2003;**49**:1–6.

Index

Page numbers in *italics* refer to figures; those in **bold** to tables.

Printed and bound by CPI Group (UK) Ltd, Croydon, CR0 4YY

Printed and bound by CPI Group (UK) Ltd, Croydon, CR0 4YY

27/10/2024

14580191-0004